GPs, Politics and Medical Professional Protest in Britain, 1880–1948

This book charts the journey of British General Practitioners (GPs) towards professional self-realisation through the development of a political consciousness manifested in a series of bruising encounters with government.

GPs are an essential part of the social fabric of modern Britain but as a group have always felt undervalued, clashing with successive governments over the terms on which they offered their services to the public. Explaining the background to these disputes and the motives of GPs from a sociological perspective, this research casts new light on some defining moments in the creation of the modern British state, from National Health Insurance to the National Health Service, and the history of the British medical profession. It examines these events from the point of view of the professionals intimately involved in and affected by them, using both established sources, like Ministry of Health records, an in-depth analysis of rarely studied records of professional bodies, and previously unresearched archive material. The result is a fascinating account of conflict and cooperation, and of heroic, and less-than-heroic, defiance of political authority, involving interactions between complex personalities and competing ideologies.

Scholarly yet readable, this book will be of interest to the general reader as much as to medical practitioners and historians.

Chris Locke is currently an honorary research fellow in the Department of History at the University of Sheffield. With postgraduate degrees in History and Law, he developed his interest in medical politics during a thirty-year career advising medical practitioners on contractual and policy matters.

Routledge Studies in Modern British History

The Beveridge Report
Blueprint for the Welfare State
Derek Fraser

The Modern British Data State, 1945–2000
Kevin Manton

Labour's Ballistic Missile Defence Policy 1997–2010
A Strategic-Relational Analysis
James Simpkin

Legacies of an Imperial City
The Museum of London 1976–2007
Samuel Aylett

Politics, Propaganda and the Press
International Reactions to the Falklands/Malvinas Conflict
Louise A. Clare

Oil for Britain
The United Kingdom and the Remaking of the International
Oil Industry, 1957–1988
Jonathan R. Kuiken

GPs, Politics and Medical Professional Protest in Britain, 1880–1948
Chris Locke

For more information about this series, please visit: https://www.routledge.com/history/series/
RSMBH

GPs, Politics and Medical Professional Protest in Britain, 1880–1948

Chris Locke

Routledge
Taylor & Francis Group

NEW YORK AND LONDON

First published 2024
by Routledge
605 Third Avenue, New York, NY 10158

and by Routledge
4 Park Square, Milton Park, Abingdon, Oxon, OX14 4RN

Routledge is an imprint of the Taylor & Francis Group, an informa business

© 2024 Chris Locke

ISBN: 978-1-032-57200-0 (hbk)
ISBN: 978-1-032-57201-7 (pbk)
ISBN: 978-1-003-43827-4 (ebk)

DOI: 10.4324/9781003438274

Typeset in Times New Roman
by codeMantra

Contents

Acknowledgements

This book is very much a solo project, if not the product of a personal obsession. It would not have been possible, however, without the encouragement of supportive colleagues, most notably my PhD supervisors in the History Department at the University of Sheffield, Dr Julia Moses and Professor Adrian Bingham. I am indebted to their continued generosity. During my research, I also benefitted from stimulating conversations with other academics and students at Sheffield, most notably Professor Julie Gottlieb and Dr Chris Millard, and constructive questioning from, among others, Professor Martin Gorsky of the London School of Hygiene and Tropical Medicine, and Dr Torsten Riotte and his colleagues in the History Department at Goethe University in Frankfurt. I wish to thank my friend Dr Adele Cresswell of Nottingham University's Business School for suggested reading on the sociology of the professions. I also wish to record my gratitude to my former tutor at St John's College, Oxford, Dr Ross McKibbin, for assuring me that I was not misguided in attempting to take up historical research into this subject after such a long career outside academia. My thanks are owed to the staff at the numerous libraries housing archival material I studied while preparing this book, particularly those at the British Library reading room at Boston Spa, Yorkshire, during the challenging conditions imposed by the COVID pandemic. I am especially grateful to the British Medical Association for giving me, over a period of many years, unfettered access to relevant records in their archival collections and extend particular thanks to their archivists Lee Sands and Dan Heather. I also wish to record my thanks to the Local Medical Committees (LMCs) who kindly permitted me to study their private archives and the staff who proved so hospitable and accommodating during my visits to their offices. These were Kelly Brown at Kent LMC, Peter Higgins and Stephen Toulmin at Lancashire and Cumbria LMCs, Miriam Adams at North Staffordshire LMC, and Belinda Smith at YOR LMC. Finally, I wish to thank my wife for her unfailing support and forbearance during the enforced absences which my research necessitated, and for helping me overcome my occasional frustrations with information technology. This book is dedicated to her and the rest of my family, living and deceased. It may also be viewed as a tribute to the many anonymous GPs whose labours form the subject matter of this book, in the hope that it may lead to a better understanding, if not appreciation, of their professional struggles.

Chris Locke
University of Sheffield

Abbreviations

APC	Association of Panel Committees
ARP	Air Raid Precautions
BMA	British Medical Association
BMJ	British Medical Journal
CEC	Central Emergency Committee
CMWC	Central Medical War Committee
EMS	Emergency Medical Services
GMC	General Medical Council
GP	General Practitioner
IAC	Insurance Acts Committee
LCC	London County Council
LGB	Local Government Board
LMC	Local Medical Committee
LMPC	Local Medical and Panel Committee
MOH	Medical Officer of Health
MPA	Medical Policy Association
MPC	Medical Planning Commission
MPU	Medico-Political Union, subsequently Medical Practitioners Union
MWF	Medical Women's Federation
NHI	National Health Insurance
NHS	National Health Service
NMU	National Medical Union
NUT	National Union of Teachers
PEP	Political and Economic Planning
PHC	Primary Health Centre
PLMO	Poor Law Medical Officer
PLMOA	Poor Law Medical Officers Association
PMPU	Panel Medico-Political Union
PMS	Public Medical Service

RAMC	Royal Army Medical Corps
RMO	Regional Medical Officer
SMA	Socialist Medical Association
SMSA	State Medical Services Association
TUC	Trades Union Congress

1   Introduction

General Practitioners (GPs) are an essential part of the social fabric of modern Britain. Regarded as the cornerstone of the National Health Service (NHS), they provide a personalised general medical service available to every citizen and mediate between individual patients and the state in matters of health, lifestyle, and access to welfare benefits and social services. Yet unlike other NHS doctors, GP principals are not state employees. Their independent contractor status guarantees them a limited freedom of action in professional matters of which they are fiercely protective, and, as this book shows, they have always been wary of attempts by politicians and administrators to manipulate or control them for political ends. GPs have, rightly or wrongly, earned a reputation among NHS managers and politicians for being 'bolshie'. Individually, they pose no threat to the political establishment, but their collective refusal to accept the received wisdom of policy makers, and willingness to highlight deficiencies in health service funding and administration, have alarmed and infuriated NHS officials and made them a target for ministerial opprobrium. While most GPs are too preoccupied with patient care to become actively involved in political activities, a substantial minority have felt less inhibited, some even daring to suggest that, due to their intimate daily interactions with patients, they know more about the health needs of the public than those in authority. Where did these attitudes and beliefs originate? Why do GPs put such a high value on their professional freedom, and why do they maintain such a distrust of, and disregard for politicians and representatives of the state? A desire to answer these questions provided the stimulus for the research on which this book is based. The story it affords is one which is, hopefully, of interest to the general reader as much as to medical practitioners and historians. It is an account of conflict and cooperation, heated debates, and heroic, and sometimes less-than-heroic, defiance of political authority; of interactions between complex personalities and competing ideologies; of altruistic self-sacrifice and hardship contrasted with materialistic self-interest and paternalistic complacency. Throughout their history, GPs as a group have felt perpetually undervalued and misunderstood. They despaired of the often-distorted views of them presented by politicians and the press which have, to

DOI: 10.4324/9781003438274-1

some extent, been accepted uncritically by historians. In the course of the present study, conflicting views of GPs and their activities in the political sphere are scrutinised and evaluated and, where appropriate, challenged or corrected.

The contemporary relevance of this study may not be immediately obvious without some context. At a special meeting in January 2016, called in response to a widely held belief that British General Practice was in crisis, the Conference of Representatives of Local Medical Committees (LMCs), the NHS GPs' representative bodies, passed a significant resolution. This was that 'should negotiations with government for a rescue package for General Practice not be concluded successfully within six months…the General Practitioners Committee should canvass GPs on their willingness to submit undated resignations'.[1] Spokesmen for the British Medical Association (BMA) acknowledged that resignation from NHS contracts was a measure of last resort for GPs, designed to provide publicity for their concerns and to 'up the ante' in negotiations with NHS England and the devolved administrations. In explaining his motives for proposing the motion in an article for an on-line journal, a representative of Buckinghamshire LMC referred to previous occasions on which GPs had successfully used the threat of mass resignation to persuade government to accede to their demands.[2] The most notable example was the settlement of the 'Family Doctors Charter' negotiations in 1965.[3] However, GPs' attempts to challenge government policy over terms offered for their services have a much longer pedigree. The origins of the action proposed on this occasion can be traced to the political crisis which began in 1911, when the Liberal Chancellor of the Exchequer, David Lloyd George, announced the health insurance provisions of his National Insurance Bill, and culminated the following year in the submission of 'pledges' by 27,000 doctors declining to participate in the Government's scheme.[4] As this book explains, the political ideology which lay behind this collective action was itself the product of a long gestation. The book begins by investigating the events, attitudes, and beliefs which helped to create that ideology and explains the profession's often difficult relationship with the Government in Britain immediately prior to and following the advent of National Health Insurance (NHI). This task involves an explanation of the even more problematic relationships existing between GPs and institutions offering health insurance for the working classes or facilitating delivery of medical care to them over a longer time period and extends to consideration of alternative forms of primary healthcare engaged in by GPs and their professional rivals. The book then charts attempts made by professional leaders to establish a constructive relationship with state representatives at local and national levels, the GPs' sacrifices during the First World War, and their frustrated expectations of post-war recompense. It documents the successes and failures of the BMA's attempts at collective bargaining and continued attempts by their professional opponents to establish rival organisations amid the economic and political turmoil of the interwar years. Finally, it assesses the situation of the 'panel' GPs in the interwar period with their middle-class insecurities and grievances, and the extent to which their fears of increasing lay control conditioned their attitudes towards the much-needed reorganisation and reform of medical services before, during, and immediately following the Second World War.

This study is confined to mainland Britain.[5] However, the preponderance of extant research material relating to GPs in England has inevitably resulted in a more limited focus on their counterparts in Wales and Scotland. For the most part, the experience of GPs in those two countries in this period was not dissimilar to that of English GPs, but uniquely national events, such as the GPs' conflicts with the miners of South Wales, or the Scottish Health Board's divergent approach to tackling lax certification, are given appropriate emphasis in the narrative. The time period chosen for this study also requires some explanation. The opening chapter describes, from a largely sociological perspective, the origins of General Practice, and the growth of a distinct professional identity during the course of the nineteenth century. The second chapter, focusing on the emergence of a political ideology and representative organisations, takes 1880 as its starting point, even though it mentions events preceding that date. In truth, a number of earlier dates could be chosen as the start date for GPs' political activity. However, it was from the 1880s that GPs collectively began to express solidarity with colleagues involved in local conflicts with friendly societies and provident dispensaries, and the first national bodies aiming to address GPs' well-rehearsed grievances using trade union-type tactics began to emerge. The 'political doctor' was not yet fully formed, and it would take three decades of struggle, and the stimulus provided by the new and potentially threatening system of NHI, to bring this evolving archetype to maturity. The 1880s and 1890s were nonetheless a formative period in the development of the GPs' political mindset and are identified accordingly as the starting point for this analysis. The end of point of 1948, as the date at which the NHI system, extensively documented in this study, was replaced by the NHS, requires no further justification.

Culture and ideology: the GPs' 'articles of faith'

Understanding GPs' belief systems is essential to comprehending their collective political consciousness during the period studied. Historians are perhaps more reluctant than sociologists to generalise about belief systems and culture, particularly when talking about a group as heterogeneous as GPs. Moreover, sociologists tend to over-generalise when talking about 'the professions' and even more so when talking about the 'medical profession', ignoring the often-significant differences which exist between different classes of medical practitioners in different countries and their social milieux during different time periods. Nevertheless, this study has derived useful insights from those who have written about the sociology of the medical profession and about points of similarity with other professions.[6] In applying sociological constructs to GPs in this time period, it is important to recognise that there are always exceptions, and the terms used should be viewed as non-empiric labels intended to aid understanding. As such, they are always open to challenge or alternative interpretation. Not all GPs in Britain necessarily subscribed, on a continuous basis, to all of the beliefs identified in this study as motivating them collectively, but there were three attributes which effectively all GPs during this period considered essential to their well-being and necessary to enable them to give their best to their patients. These were gentility (or 'respectability'); economic security; and professional and occupational autonomy. According to sociologists, these aspirations have been, to a large extent, common to all branches of the medical profession internationally.[7] In the case of British GPs during this period, however, they crystallised into a subset of principles which became collective 'articles of faith' which their representative bodies were sworn to defend at all costs. These comprised independent contractor status; the patient's right to free choice of doctor; and professional control over standards of competence and behaviour. Explaining why these principles were so important to GPs and the lengths they went to in order to preserve them is a central objective of this book.

When seeking to uphold these articles of faith both before and after the advent of NHI, the profession's leaders demonstrated a commitment to democratic self-government. This manifested itself in a form of corporatism through which GPs sought to expand their status and influence using collective bargaining. It also led to impassioned debates about the merits and disadvantages of medical trade unionism. This was, as will be seen, no idle question for the medical profession as it went to the heart of how doctors saw themselves and their position in society. As will be demonstrated, the National Insurance Act, despite the profession's significant misgivings about it, accorded GPs considerable professional autonomy and a major share in the administration of government social policy.[8] GPs were able to secure considerable freedom of action by effective engagement with the apparatus of the state at local level, through the Local Medical and Panel Committees (LMPCs), and at national level through the activities of the BMA's Insurance Acts Committee (IAC). This, at times, uneasy partnership involved what Harold Perkin, *pace* Colin Crouch, calls 'bargained corporatism', an explanation of which, and the various attempts made to exercise it by the profession's leaders, is offered later in this book.[9] Underpinning this strategy was a belief shared by doctors of every political persuasion which Perkin calls the 'professional social ideal', that is an ability to justify professional self-interest 'in terms of the service performed for society…and the principle of social justice'.[10] As will be demonstrated throughout this study, the medical profession's ability to conflate their professional interests with those of public proved to be a defining feature of their relationship with government and their attempts to influence public opinion during this period.

Historiographical context and use of research

Political history is, of course, not currently much in vogue among professional historians. It is seen as the preserve of the great and powerful of whom, perhaps, a disproportionate amount has been written already. Since the 'cultural' and 'material' turns, much historical research has understandably been focused on the lives of those excluded from the exercise of power, and especially marginalised groups who make up a considerable part of the intricate mosaic of modern society. Medical history has likewise been reoriented towards the experiences of patients and disease processes rather than the history of the medical profession. This book therefore risks being seen as regressive in being, ostensibly, concerned with political history, and with the activities of a group of individuals who are usually regarded as privileged and powerful. As will become clear, however, the subject of this book is not political history in the traditional sense. Nor are those with whom the book is chiefly concerned necessarily part of the political elite. The book is concerned with the social aspirations, beliefs, and rituals of a numerically small professional group desperate for security and recognition, who engaged, with some reluctance, in political activities in collective self-defence. Reacting to events outside their control, they became accidental participants in the expansion of state authority and the creation of what is now only parenthetically referred to as the welfare state. However, the individuals on whom this study is focused were, for most of the time period in which it is set, largely invisible. Apart from the few occasions when their 'revolts' briefly occupied the centre stage of national consciousness, GPs performed the difficult and unglamorous work it fell to them to undertake, unheralded and almost unnoticed by society at large. Whenever they did become the focus of attention by politicians or the press, it was usually in a negative respect and the often-ill-informed comments and criticisms to which they were occasionally subjected only served to fuel their professional insecurities and grievances. While they were, unquestionably, an important part of the social fabric, this importance was rarely, and then only begrudgingly, acknowledged by those exercising political power. It was the GPs' fate to be taken for granted by politicians and the public and perpetually misunderstood. One of the objects of this book is to rescue GPs from this obscurity, to correct some common misapprehensions about them and their motives, and to restore some balance to the narrative of events in which they played a sometimes central but not always appreciated part.

This study may be viewed as timely, given that almost all the previous studies of GPs' involvement in the events described were written more than 40 years ago. The most recent substantive analysis of General Practice in the late nineteenth and early twentieth centuries, *The Evolution of British General Practice, 1848–1948* by Anne Digby, published in 1999, has been rightly praised for the quality of its research and the insights it offers, as the numerous citations of it in this book offer testimony. But, being socio-economic in approach, it largely eschews the political dimension. In a final chapter on the NHS, Digby identifies the need for further focus on the 'interests and ideologies' of GPs between the 'legislative watersheds' of NHI and the NHS.[11] This is a challenge the present work seeks to address. Digby's work was intended to complement Irvine Loudon's equally worthy study of the earlier history of General Practice, *Medical Care and the General Practitioner, 1750 to 1850*, written a decade before, and of which notable use is made in the first chapter of this study.[12] The foremost works on GPs' political activities in the era of NHI are Frank Honigsbaum's 1979 work, *The Division in British Medicine: A History of the Separation of General Practice from Hospital Care, 1911–1968*, and the less well-known *National Health Insurance and the Medical Profession in Britain, 1913–1939*, by Norman R. Eder published in 1982.[13] Honigsbaum's book is a fascinating but eclectic and discursive work which is visibly less coherent than his later work on the origins of the NHS.[14] Norman Eder's detailed and balanced examination of GPs' interactions with NHI is solid and meticulous but is somewhat narrow in focus and now very dated in terms of recent historiography. Other useful sources of information about GPs' political activities include the works of David B. Green, a severe critic of the medical profession who makes no secret of his admiration for their antagonists, the friendly societies.[15] An advocate of what was later described as 'the big society', Green's work is unashamedly polemical and his analysis of the friendly societies has been superseded by more authoritative studies.[16] The only recent political study of note is one by Andrew Morrice on the BMA's involvement in trade union-like activity in the decade preceding the National Insurance Act.[17] No list of historians describing GPs and their struggles during the interwar period would be complete, however, without mention of Charles Webster, official historian of the NHS. His numerous published works are of unquestionable value to everyone interested in this subject and are frequently called upon in the later chapters of this analysis.[18]

Sources and methodology

This book draws on a wide variety of original sources. These include a systematic analysis of the relevant entries in the professional journals written and read by GPs from the 1880s to the 1940s, principally the *British Medical Journal* (*BMJ*), *Lancet*, and *Medical World*, the findings from which are correlated with previously unresearched records of internal discussions within the BMA which are kept in the BMA's archive and in the Wellcome Collection in London. It also draws on relevant ministerial records in the National Archive, Kew, along with parliamentary discussions and newspaper articles, extracts from Royal Commission and other reports and surveys as well as critical commentary from other journals. Other sources include biographies and memoirs of prominent personalities and, in order to reflect a broader, societal view of the developments under consideration, the surprisingly rich source of material available in contemporary fiction offering vivid descriptions, based on first-hand knowledge, of GPs' lives and work in this period. Use is also made, unashamedly, in this book of a wide range of secondary source material covering, *inter alia*, the history of state formation, health services, social security, the medical profession, the class structure, and the broader history of the period in Britain, with reference, where appropriate, to international comparisons. The evolving trends in historical scholarship are demonstrated by highlighting what are often widely differing opinions among established historians of the events and developments with which this book is concerned.

There are in this study two areas offering substantial additions to the canon of research into GPs in this period. The first relates to the LMPCs which have previously been almost completely ignored by historians. Digby's *Evolution of British General Practice*, for example, makes no mention of them. Even more surprising perhaps is the absence of any mention of LMPCs prior to the Second World War in Peter Bartrip's otherwise creditable history of the BMA, *Themselves Writ Large*.[19] In *The Division of British Medicine*, Frank Honigsbaum's only substantive reference to what he chooses to call, generically, LMCs, is contained in a footnote.[20] Norman Eder is the one historian to accord the LMPCs anything like the attention they deserve, influenced no doubt by an unpublished MD thesis on the subject by former BMA Chairman John Marks.[21] Eder's efforts were hampered, he regretted, by the unavailability of extant records. He assumed that the records of LMPCs, apart from those of the London Panel Committee located in the BMA archive, had been lost.[22] However, a recent survey of LMCs in mainland Britain revealed the existence of a limited number of LMPC records located in LMC Offices in North Staffordshire, Lancashire, Kent, and North Yorkshire. Information from these newly discovered records has been supplemented in this study by that gathered from archive material located in the Medical Collections of Manchester University's Central Library and the Cheshire County Public Record Office. Unfortunately, no LMPC records from Scotland or Wales came to light in this exercise. Analysis of these data has revealed how the LMPCs interacted with local Insurance Committees, with other LMPCs, the BMA's Insurance Acts Committee (IAC), the Medical Practitioners Union (MPU), the NHI Commissioners, and later the Ministry of Health, and how they sought to ensure the representation of their constituents' views. As will be demonstrated later in the book, this analysis suggests that their role in the local administration of NHI has been underappreciated and that the LMPC/IAC axis is key to an understanding of all political activities affecting or involving GPs during the interwar period. The second area of new research relates to Public Medical Services (PMS) schemes, of which there are occasional but incidental references in the official BMA histories and other works. Again, the absence of any substantive analysis of them is surprising. David B. Green, who disparaged these schemes as a professional attempt to counteract the influence of the Medical Aid Societies, is the only authority to have accorded them any significance. As this study shows, the coverage

offered by these schemes even at their greatest extent was nowhere near sufficient to provide the profession with a serious alternative to NHI or the NHS, but
the fact that, at key moments in this story, they gave every appearance of being
able to do so means that they were of more than purely symbolic significance for
medico-politicians and are undoubtedly deserving of further study.

GPs and the state

A central theme running though this study is the evolving relationship between
British GPs and the state before, during, and immediately following the interwar
period. Historians, such as Mary Poovey and Patrick Joyce, among others, have
argued that the state in late nineteenth- and early twentieth-century Britain was a
pluralist assemblage of interests and institutions – private, public, charitable, and
voluntary – and not confined to the narrow definition of central government and
its appointed office holders.[23] Pat Thane describes this as 'bounded pluralism'.[24]
More recently, James Vernon has argued that during the early twentieth century,
the Liberal British state extended its reach to tackle social problems which it
considered unrelated to or outside the control of the market economy and that
thenceforward, 'those who wished to be left alone by it had to demonstrate…ap-
propriate forms of self-government'.[25] In mediating between GPs and the apparatus of the state, this book suggests that the LMPCs and their national executive
may be seen as examples of the diffuse networks of power through which both
Liberal and Conservative governments of this period sought to exercise authority. Thanks to the limited degree of self-government they were accorded, GPs
were therefore effectively among those privileged groups Vernon describes.[26]

   However, as local defenders of GPs' professional interests and guarantors of
their claimed right to self-determination, LMPCs were, paradoxically, the means
through which, during periods of conflict, the profession mobilised resistance
to government authority. Thus, the relationship between GPs and the state during the period studied was characterised by alternating periods of harmonious cooperation, in which GPs were willing to work with the Government for
the public good, and mutual distrust and antagonism, in which the profession
showed a determination to resist government authority using all legal means
possible. As this study makes clear, the actions of GPs in the political sphere
were invariably driven by a desire to protect hard-won professional privileges
and to obtain a just reward for their contribution to the nation's well-being. But
they were not blind to the deficiencies of the system in which they worked,
and their leaders were sincere in their desire for improvements, manifested in
campaigns to secure an expansion in the range of services offered and extension of NHI to cover the dependants of the insured. By 1939, most GPs favoured the inclusion of hospital care and additional services in a comprehensive
state-funded service, provided that the distinction between private practice and
publicly subsidised services remained intact. Only a minority wished to erase

that distinction. Critics of professional privilege are accustomed to question the extent of medical altruism.[27] A number of historians have consequently dismissed the BMA's blueprints for the reform of health services in this period, arguing that they were suffused with self-interest.[28] One of the later chapters of this book is dedicated to a re-examination of the proposals the BMA put forward for the reorganisation of national health services in 1930 and subsequently, and the reception they received at the time. These are considered in the context of ongoing discussions throughout the 1920s and 1930s between the BMA and government, and with influential political interest groups with whom the profession was sometimes at odds, such as the Approved Societies and the Labour movement.[29] The profession, it is suggested, was willing to support the establishment of more comprehensive medical services to all who could not afford to pay for healthcare directly at the point of delivery, provided the GPs' articles of faith were respected and their economic security guaranteed. The events of the 1940s, beginning with the Medical Planning Commission and ending with the defeat of the BMA over Labour's plans for the NHS, are the subject of detailed scrutiny in the final chapters of this book. The arguments employed by the profession's leaders clearly echoed those used in previous conflicts but there is no simple explanation for what transpired. The outcome might, but for a series of chance events and miscalculations, have been very different, this book asserts, confounding the seemingly 'path dependant' views of an earlier generation of historians.[30] What is not disputed is that the conflict between the medical profession and the Labour Government during 1946–1948 helped determine the shape of the NHS and how doctors worked within it for decades to come. The actions of professional leaders in that conflict were conditioned by the beliefs and articles of faith which evolved during the late nineteenth and early twentieth centuries and were expressed and tested in more than 35 years of GPs' experience of NHI. That experience represents the constituent material on which most of this book is based, and is described, in what follows, in all its fascinating complexity.

Notes

1 Matthew Limb, 'GPs Threaten Mass Resignation.' *BMJ,* 352 (6 February 2016). p. i646.

2 James Murphy, 'What GPs Need to Know about Submitting Undated Resignations.' *Pulse*, 18 February 2016. www.pulsetoday.co.uk/your-practice/what-gps-need-to-know-about-submitting-undated-resignations/20031151.article

3 See *BMJ*, 2 July 1966, 'Report of Special Representative Meeting', Supplement, pp. 6–8.

4 Paul Vaughan, *Doctors' Commons: A Short History of the British Medical Association* (London, 1959). pp. 200–203.

5 Implementation of NHI in Ireland was confounded by the nationalist struggle for independence. See R.W. (Robert William) Harris, *National Health Insurance in Great Britain, 1911–1948* (London, 1946). p. 192, 'Why Medical Benefit did not extend to Ireland'. NHI was eventually extended to Northern Ireland in the mid-1920s.

6   These include, *inter alia*, Elliot Friedson, *The Profession of Medicine: A Study of the Sociology of Applied Knowledge* (New York, 1970); Phillip Elliot, *The Sociology of the Professions* (Basingstoke, 1972); Daniel Duman, 'The Creation and Diffusion of a Professional Ideology in Nineteenth Century England.' *Sociological Review*, 27 (1979). pp. 113–138.

7   See Noel Parry and Jose Parry, *The Rise of the Medical Profession a Study of Collective Social Mobility* (London, 1976). p. 32, 79; Dietrich Rueschemeyer, 'Professional Autonomy and the Social Control of Expertise,' in Robert Dingwall and Phillip Lewis (eds) *The Sociology of the Professions: Doctors, Lawyers and Others* (London, 1983). ch.2, p. 41; Friedson, *The Profession of Medicine*, pp. 10 and 174.

8   See Harris, *National Health Insurance*, pp. 133 and 143.

9   Harold Perkin, *The Rise of Professional Society: England since 1880* (2nd edn, Abingdon, 2002). pp. 286–287. This is explored in Chapters 4–6.

10 *Ibid.*, p. 288.

11 Anne Digby, *The Evolution of British General Practice, 1850–1948* (Oxford, 1999). p. 325.

12 Irvine Loudon, *Medical Care and the General Practitioner to 1850* (Oxford, 1986).

13 Frank Honigsbaum, *The Division in British Medicine: A History of the Separation of General Practice from Hospital Care, 1911–1968* (London, 1979). Norman R. Eder, *National Health Insurance and the Medical Profession in Britain, 1913–1939* (New York, 1982).

14 Bentley Gilbert, the distinguished historian of British National Insurance regretted that in Honigsbaum's book 'inferences drawn from the myriad of facts' were often 'confused, half-baked and sometimes wrong.' Bentley B. Gilbert, 'Review.' *Journal of Social Policy*, 10 (1) (1981). pp. 119–122.

15 David B. Green, *Working-Class Patients and the Medical Establishment: Self-Help in Britain from the Mid-Nineteenth Century to 1948* (Aldershot, 1985).

16 Principally, Simon Cordery, *British Friendly Societies, 1750–1914* (Basingstoke, 2003); Martin Gorsky, 'Friendly Society Health Insurance in Nineteenth Century England,' in Martin Gorsky and Sally Sheard (eds) *Financing Medicine: The British Experience since 1750* (Abingdon, 2006) pp. 147–164, and Bernard Harris, 'Social Policy by Other Means? Mutual Aid and the Origins of the Welfare State in Britain during the Nineteenth and Twentieth Centuries.' *Journal of Social Policy*, 30 (2) (2018) pp. 202–235.

17 Andrew Morrice, "Strong Combination': The Edwardian BMA and Contract Practice,' in Martin Gorsky and Sally Sheard (eds) *Financing Medicine: The British Experience Since 1750* (Abingdon, 2006). pp. 165–181.

18 The works of Charles Webster most frequently cited in this study are *The Health Services Since the War, Volume 1, Problems of Healthcare: The National Health Service before 1957* (London, 1988) and *The National Health Service: A Political History* (2nd edn., Oxford, 2002).

19 Peter Bartrip, *Themselves Writ Large: The British Medical Association, 1832–1966* (London, 1996).

20 Honigsbaum, *The Division in British Medicine,* p. 60, footnote.

21 John H. Marks, *The History and Development of Local Medical Committees, Their Conference and Its Executive*, Edinburgh University MD Thesis, 1974.

22 Eder, *National Health Insurance*, p. 194, note 72.

23 Mary Poovey, *Making A Social Body: British Cultural Formation 1830–1864* (Chicago, IL, 1995) p. 14; Patrick Joyce, *The State of Freedom: A Social History of the British State since 1800* (Cambridge, 2013). pp. 31–34.

24 Pat Thane, *Foundations of the Welfare State* (2nd edn., London, 1996). p. 291.

25 James Vernon. *Cambridge History of Britain: 1750 to the Present* (Cambridge, 2017). ch. 4, p. 146.

26 See Nikolas Rose, 'Government, Authority and Expertise in Advanced Liberalism.' *Economy and Society*, 22 (3) (1993). p. 285.

27 See, for example, Friedson, *The Profession of Medicine*, p. 91, and F.B. (Francis Barrymore) Smith, *The People's Health, 1830–1910* (Canberra, 1979). pp. 362, 386 and 414–417.

28 For example, Brian Abel-Smith, *The Hospitals 1800–1948: A Study in Social Administration in England and Wales* (London, 1964). p. 350.

29 *BMA Archive*, B/177/2/1, British Medical Association, *A General Medical Service for the Nation* (London, 1930).

30 For a thorough analysis and explanation of the evolution of historiography of the NHS, see Martin Gorsky, 'The British National Health Service 1948–2018: A Review of the Historiography,' in *Social History of Medicine*, 21 (3) (2008). pp. 437–460.

2 An uncertain profession

GPs' struggle for identity and status in the nineteenth century

No understanding of the collective mindset of GPs during the twentieth century and their activities in the political sphere is possible without an account of their struggle for recognition and acceptance in the preceding century. Central to this was their attempt during that period to secure some form of occupational closure, that is, to control the numbers of those eligible to become medical practitioners and to differentiate themselves more clearly in the eyes of the public from unqualified quacks and other would-be professionals. They sought to achieve this by various means. Firstly, by obtaining a measure of state recognition through professional registration; secondly, by establishing recognised educational standards; and lastly, through social acceptance of their claims to expert status. This chapter describes that process. It also describes the simultaneous emergence of a distinct professional identity borne of social and economic insecurity and a long-drawn-out process of professionalisation. This process involved GPs in conflicts with rivals within and outside the medical profession and uneasy relationships with lay authorities contracting with them to provide medical services to the working classes and paupers. It was affected by fluctuations in the number of qualified medical practitioners seeking to practise, and by the rising prestige of medical science. It was also affected by changing public attitudes towards sickness and its causes and the role of the state in maintaining the public's health. It was a process by which GPs moved from being barely educated tradesmen on the margins of respectable society to an estimable group of medical professionals performing a valuable public service but who were never quite able to achieve the economic security and financial rewards they believed they deserved. These developments created the conditions in which political activity was deemed necessary to achieve, and then protect, hard-won professional privileges. They also established the 'articles of faith' by which, as will be shown in the chapters which follow, GPs' professional representative bodies subsequently considered themselves bound.

DOI: 10.4324/9781003438274-2

Social recognition, the rise of medical science, and the quest for gentility

During the eighteenth century, the medical profession in Britain was effectively divided into three classes: physicians, surgeons, and apothecaries. Each had its own corporation which sought to maintain the professional privileges accorded to each rank of practitioner.[1] The first GPs, who emerged in the early nineteenth century, were a hybrid of all three. Being not exclusively within one class or another left these individuals unsure as to their identity and insecure about their professional and social status. What bound these practitioners together was their sense of 'otherness'. They were lacking a 'local habitation', in terms of a clearly demarcated position in social space, and even 'a name', being variously described as 'surgeon-apothecaries' or physicians, or surgeons, 'in general practice' though they frequently adopted the gendered, non-specific cognomen, 'medical men'.[2] The Apothecaries Act of 1815 had helped differentiate the surgeon-apothecaries from unqualified purveyors of medicines by ensuring that only those licenced by it could legally dispense medicines.[3] It confirmed their status as respectable professional men entitled to put letters after their name.[4] The first recorded use of the term 'general practitioner' was in 1818.[5] By the 1830s, this term had effectively replaced the other designations mentioned which by 1847, according to Churchill's Medical Directory, had been rendered obsolete.[6] During the 1830s, the tripartite distinctions, although recognised at least partially by statute, were becoming increasingly porous. In 1834, some 41% of members of the College of Surgeons of England also held the licentiate of the Society of Apothecaries and according to the Surgeons' president, G.J. Guthrie, of 6,000 members practising in London at that time, all but a few hundred were GPs.[7] Many physicians at that time also practised surgery, prompting a group of eminent physicians from London hospitals to conclude in 1834 that: 'There is no exact line to be drawn between the practice of the physician and that of the surgeon'.[8] In 1839, the *Lancet* described the GP as 'a new class…different from any hitherto known, formed by a combination of the three already in existence but having no exact resemblance to any of them'.[9] The colleges were nevertheless determined to maintain the time-honoured distinctions and the privileges afforded their membership and resisted calls by representatives of the GPs during the 1820s and 1830s to reform the system of education to make it less exclusive and more suitable to practitioners' professional needs.[10]

By the middle of the nineteenth century, GPs constituted the largest part of the medical profession in Britain; yet as a group, they were not yet comfortable with their identity and felt aggrieved by a lack of public recognition. The stratification of social classes which was a defining feature of nineteenth-century British society was something which GPs as an emerging social group were acutely conscious of. They liked to think of themselves as educated gentlemen and situated firmly within the newly emergent middle class, but their claims to higher social status were continually undermined by a lack of recognised educational standards, and economic conditions which periodically depressed their income and forced many of them to maintain links with the apothecary's trade.[11] In the opinion of polite society, GPs could not consider themselves gentlemen, or even respectable professionals, when they continued to dispense and sell medicines and other items to the public like common tradesmen.[12] Education and social class lay at the heart of the distinction between the GPs and the elite of the medical profession in the nineteenth century. Admission to the Royal College of Physicians of London was initially denied to anyone not possessing a degree from the Universities of Oxford or Cambridge. Although the requirement was later widened to include Scottish, Irish, and some continental universities, it was only when the University of London established the first university hospital in 1834 that the division between the elite education of the physician and the practical education of the surgeon began to break down.[13] The pre-eminence of the elite gentleman physician was due as much to his culture and his classical education as to his medical knowledge.[14] The principal division between the status physician and the GP was the latter's continued association with the dispensing and selling of medicines. Physicians despised anything which smacked of 'trade', considering it beneath the noble calling of a gentlemanly vocation.[15] The Royal College of Physicians therefore officially disdained anything resembling manual work, including surgery, and they regarded midwifery as the province of the lower ranks of the profession.[16] In 1827, the College President stated that midwifery was 'an act foreign to the habits of a gentleman of enlarged academic education'.[17] By then, however, it had already become 'the central point' of general practice and was relied upon as an economic staple by almost every GP.[18]

Elite physicians aside, medicine in the 1830s was, according to F.B. Smith, 'the metier of the outsiders' and those who 'lacked connections that promised fair progress in the law, the church or the armed services'.[19] Ian Inkster described GPs, in light of his study of their activities in early nineteenth-century Sheffield, as 'marginal men' with 'one foot in trade and another in a profession'.[20] The concept of marginality, developed by the sociologist Robert E. Park, relates to 'one who moves in more than one social world and is not completely at home in any'.[21] Inkster found the medical cohort he studied to be a socially mobile group in need of 'social comfort'. Professionalisation was the key to achieving social status and within a provincial context, medical men sought 'to legitimise their social and intellectual positions through social action'.[22] Their efforts to secure acceptance and gentility led them to becoming actively involved in, and undertaking prominent roles in, local politics, religion, charitable activities, and social reform. By the 1830s, Ivan Waddington estimates that GPs provided 90% of qualified medical care in England.[23] However, their continued association with the apothecary's trade diminished their standing in the eyes of many of the public who viewed them more as sellers of drugs rather than diagnosticians and prescribers of treatment.[24] They were described by one American observer in 1834 as 'a mongrel kind of doctor, man-midwife, surgeon and druggist, a true jack of all trades and master of none...used by the public yet looked upon by them with a sort of good-natured contempt'.[25]

Nineteenth-century GPs were conditioned by the struggle to achieve financial security in a volatile and often congested medical market. From the mid-century, the majority of practitioners saw their economic prospects improve as medicine became, in the words of Irvine Loudon, 'one of the commodities in growing demand through the birth of the consumer society'.[26] Their social status improved with increased levels of prosperity. But the picture was not a uniform one. Provincial GPs often occupied a higher social status than their contemporaries in London, but GPs were generally much more socially insecure than their eighteenth-century predecessors.[27] Loudon notes that the eighteenth-century surgeon-apothecary was more prosperous than the nineteenth-century GP, citing the relative cost of education which was the equivalent of a year's income for the former but more like four to five years for the latter.[28] By the mid-century, many GPs possessed a recognised medical qualification, either a university degree in medicine and surgery, or the licentiate of the Society of Apothecaries. But many had obtained their medical education by attending lectures at one of the many private medical schools which sprang up in London and some provincial cities in the early nineteenth century, followed by an apprenticeship under an established practitioner.[29] The typical young man entering a career in medicine in the nineteenth century was a grammar school boy.[30] Many could not afford to pay for an education beyond the age of 14 to 16 and so opted for an apprenticeship with an established practitioner as a means of gaining the experience necessary to practise. Abuse of apprentices was commonplace, and Loudon describes them as 'living automatons' indentured for five to seven years' service.[31] Evidence of the lack of concern shown by established GPs for the welfare of their apprentices and assistants is not hard to find. In 1847, one country practitioner spent more on his horse (£35 per annum) than he did on his assistant's salary (£30 per annum).[32] The exploited assistants ate with the servants, opened the door to private patients, delivered their medicines, and undertook the less glamorous work like treating paupers.[33]

To address the new GPs' desire for economic security and improved social status, numerous new associations were formed to represent their interests. A body calling itself the Association of Apothecaries and Surgeon-Apothecaries had existed since the turn of the nineteenth century and its membership continued to grow until the 1830s, after which 'it disappears from sight'.[34] The first association specifically set up to represent the interests of GPs, The Metropolitan Association of General Practitioners and Surgeons in General Practice, was established in 1836. It subsequently formed an alliance with a group calling itself The British Medical Association, but unrelated to the organisation subsequently bearing that name, and another body calling itself the National Association of

General Practitioners, in lobbying parliament to authorise the setting up of a separate College of GPs.[35] The campaign for reform of the education system was supported if not initiated by the *Lancet*, the medical journal established in London in the 1790s and which soon identified itself with the interests of the GPs and was the most ardent critic of their opponents both within and outside the profession.[36] Its editor from the 1820s to the 1840s, the GP and sometime MP, Thomas Wakely, railed against the self-serving and restrictive practices of the medical corporations and highlighted their abuses.[37] While he was at times supportive of the idea of creating a separate corporation for GPs, he was for the most part concerned to improve GPs' access to membership of, and representation by, the College of Surgeons.[38] The campaign for a separate College of GPs ultimately failed to bear fruit and after the passing of the Medical Act 1858, the idea was abandoned until eventually resurrected nearly a hundred years later.[39]

The motives of GPs supporting the campaign for reform of medical registration from the 1820s onwards were largely economic. It was generally accepted that the profession in the 1820s and 1830s was 'overcrowded' and registration was intended both to control the number of qualified practitioners entering the profession and to reduce competition from the unqualified.[40] Noel and Jose Parry describe the profession's efforts as a form of occupational closure.[41] The Apothecaries Act of 1815 had not prevented the public using unlicenced practitioners, and the poor in particular continued to make considerable use of them throughout the nineteenth century. These 'irregulars', as Loudon calls them – bonesetters, midwives, herbalists, faith healers, homeopaths, and purveyors of quack remedies – offered a cheaper alternative than the GP but were frequently guilty of defrauding and injuring, and occasionally killing, the unsuspecting sick and vulnerable.[42] However, by the mid-century, the itinerant irregulars were being supplanted by a new breed of 'literate and educated empirics', including the dispensing druggist who was for the GPs a much more immediate threat. The rise of the druggist increased the clamour among GPs for more stringent medical registration to curtail the scope of their rivals' activities.[43]

In their efforts to enlist parliamentary support in their battle with unqualified practitioners, the medical profession sought to differentiate themselves more starkly from the quacks and providers of folk medicine and homely remedies who could make no claim to scientific authority.[44] The 1830s witnessed the beginnings of the movement which resulted in the significant advancements in medical science, particularly in surgery, and which continued throughout the nineteenth century. Understanding of the human body and disease processes had been greatly enhanced by experiments in anatomy and surgery carried out in hospitals in Paris and French provincial cities during and after the Napoleonic era and eventually found its way into the teaching of medicine and surgery in the universities and private medical schools of Britain, as in the rest of Europe.[45] The Parisian school pioneered a rational scientific approach to clinical medicine building on Morgagni's work on morbid anatomy. Rejecting disease classifications based on symptoms alone, French surgeons and physicians focused on the systematic and objective observation of the phenomena of disease.[46] Diagnosis was revolutionised by the use of percussion and mediate auscultation and by the invention of the stethoscope by Laennec.[47] The popularity of a rationalist mode of enquiry and of the new techniques and instruments of diagnosis and surgery spread rapidly throughout Europe. The new approach was readily taken up in the London teaching hospitals such as St Bartholomew's from the 1830s.[48] In *The Birth of the Clinic*, the philosopher and social scientist Michel Foucault describes the flourishing of the new medical science in Europe in the early nineteenth century as the triumph of an empirically based rationalism over outmoded ideas about disease and the human body, as morbid anatomy exposed pathological processes to the discipline of 'the medical gaze'. This created a doctor-centred form of medicine in which the patient was objectivised as a medical problem or puzzle to be investigated and resolved.[49] GPs who had studied at medical schools and later in the voluntary hospitals which began to offer teaching to medical students in the early nineteenth century certainly absorbed something of the new scientific rationalism, but the culture of the medical profession in Britain at this time was still dominated to a large extent by natural theology.[50] Many scientists and doctors, including the young Charles Darwin, adopted a 'bi-textual' philosophy, that is, one founded on according equal validity to scripture and of the 'book of nature', and in which religion and science were finely balanced.[51] The growth of epidemiology brought a new dimension to the practice of medicine at this time. Following the cholera epidemics of the 1830s, doctors like John Snow, William Farr, and William Budd attempted to create a new medical science and formulate investigative tools as a solution to the challenges posed not only by the spread of disease but what they saw as a generalised problem of 'disorder' in society.[52] Carrying out epidemiological enquiries and complimenting their studies with microscopic investigations and animal experiments, they contributed to a growing interest in public health interventions and a belief that disease, and the social problems to which it gave rise, could be both controlled and conquered. The growth of statistics which accompanied and indeed underpinned both the sanitarianism of Edwin Chadwick and the utilitarians, and the public health movement championed by Sir John Simon, often involved GPs active in local statistical societies.[53]

The last decades of the nineteenth century saw the development of a succession of potent therapeutic and prophylactic agents which helped to promote popular faith in technological intervention to prevent or cure disease. Christopher Lawrence argues that this flowed from the respect Victorians and Edwardians increasingly accorded to the sciences and that in an era preoccupied with evolution, 'scientific interventions were increasingly equated with the idea of social progress'.[54] International scientific advances encouraged the public and the profession to associate science with the advancement of medicine.[55] But improvements in medical science, while very real, did not immediately translate into significant therapeutic advances in medical practice.[56] W. F. Bynum notes that scientists like Pasteur or scientifically inclined clinicians like Lister 'became public figures and thereby mediated the profession to the public'.[57] Belief in progress and the efficacy of medical science was not universal, however, and further public health measures and expansion of the state's role in health were opposed by a powerful alliance of anti-vivisectionists, anti-vaccinationists, and civil libertarians, uniting, in the words of Dorothy and Roy Porter, 'opponents of the principle of compulsion and a terror of medical tyranny'.[58] Roy McLeod characterises the activities of this alliance as civil disobedience and part of a wider public distrust of scientific medicine and preference for 'natural' methods of treatment.[59] The alliance had some success in preventing the extension of legal powers of compulsion but the extent and character of their support remain unclear. Although it counted among its supporters some prominent medical men, for some of its members, a distrust of the new medical science resulted in a general questioning of the status ascribed to the medical profession. When Alfred Russell Wallace gave evidence to the Royal Commission on Vaccination in 1889, for instance, he denounced what he called 'the insidious growth of the medical profession'.[60] This view found a strong supporter in George Bernard Shaw, who opined that he had 'never been able to perceive any distinction between the science of the herbalist and that of the duly registered doctor'. However, for Shaw, it was the 'doctor's dilemma', that is their need to square the needs of their patients with the necessity to earn a living which made the medical profession unfit to enjoy the respectability and status which society was apt to accord them. 'Private medical practice is not governed by science', he maintained, 'but by supply and demand'.[61]

The development of an increasingly scientific basis for medical practice coincided with increased demand for medical care from the new industrial middle classes. For the emerging middle classes, employing the services of a qualified medical practitioner became an indication of respectability and wealth. It was a status symbol and a valued commodity. Many middle-class women preferred to be attended in childbirth by a qualified physician rather than by an unqualified midwife.[62] Midwifery was both a source of income for the GPs and a convenient way of introducing themselves to, and winning the confidence and continued custom of, local families. The economic considerations of practising in large towns necessitated charging clients according to their perceived ability to pay. This allowed some GPs to build up large practices catering for all sections of the community. Outside London especially, the GP began to fill the space that would otherwise be occupied by a physician, surgeon, obstetrician, and apothecary. The GPs' more varied functions placed them in a different social position than their predecessors as they were able to secure a wider social composition in their clientele and were therefore 'less reliant on the demands of an influential few'.[63] The relationship between the British GP and their middle-class patients was one of mutual dependence based on common social values. Many heads of families were professional men themselves and recognised the value of medical expertise when it came to caring for their dependants.[64] Middle-class demand for medical care also owed much to changing social attitudes towards health and disease. Disease was no longer seen as a punishment for sin by many of the professional classes who put their faith in science and who subscribed to the belief that the malignant forces of nature could be controlled by man.[65] S.W.F. Holloway hypothesises that the middle classes necessarily placed a high premium on the maintenance of good health 'both as a prerequisite for success and as a necessary condition for the enjoyment and exploitation of success'.[66] Belief in social progress was combined in popular middle-class thought with an increasing belief in the virtues of 'rugged individualism' encapsulated in Samuel Smiles' *Self-Help,* in which the author maintained that 'practical success in life depends more upon physical health is than is generally imagined'.[67]

The nineteenth-century GP was faced with an ethical dilemma – the need to attract patients in order to make a living conflicted with the codes of practice associated with the higher status of the physician and diminished the GPs' claim to moral authority and scientific objectivity. M. Jeanne Peterson says, 'their social origins gave them no claim to gentlemanly status. Their professional activities were inimical to such claims'.[68] The quest for gentility and social acceptance in the late nineteenth century made the GP in many ways the epitome of the aspirant middle classes whose overwhelming desire was to achieve what contemporaries referred to as 'respectability'.[69] In 1885, the GP-turned-specialist Morrell Mackenzie described this thus: 'In the breast of the ordinary middle-class John Bull, no emotion is stronger than to appear "respectable"; in the heart of the medical body corporate this feeling is intensified almost into a passion'. He went on to say that doctors, being uncertain as to their position in the social scale, were 'naturally somewhat ticklish about the matter.'[70] The organisations representing the interests of GPs, including the Provincial Medical and Surgical Association established in 1832 and reconstituted as the British Medical Association in 1856, sought to unify the medical profession and lobbied parliament to introduce a unitary registration system.[71] The idea of a common medical registration was revolutionary, contradicting the idea of qualification embodied in the three corporations and medical estates.[72] It was particularly repugnant to the numerically small but highly influential physicians. But the numerical superiority of GPs, who in 1847 constituted 68% of doctors in London and 85% in the provinces according to Churchill's Medical Directory, coupled with the efforts of several vocal GP MPs like Wakely, meant that parliament could not continue to ignore the call for reform.[73] At a time when more than half the population in England still lived in rural areas, the provincial GP had a virtual monopoly of qualified personal medical care and even their harshest critics had to admit that they dominated the practice of medicine.[74]

Servants of the state? GPs and the poor law

GPs also monopolised a role which made them an essential part of Britain's social administration. This was in providing medical care for the destitute subject to the poor law. Before 1834, 'parish work' was not despised by medical practitioners as its rewards were broadly equivalent to those of private practice.[75] However, the Poor Law Amendment Act of that year saw the replacement of some 10,000 parishes, each with their own GP parish surgeon, with around 2,500 Poor Law Unions under whose direction recipients of poor law relief were more systematically incarcerated in local workhouses. This reorganisation drastically reduced the number of poor law medical officers (PLMOs) but substantially increased the workload expected of those that remained without any commensurate increase in remuneration.[76] Standards of care inevitably suffered along with the status of the post. Throughout the rest of the century, the PLMO was not a position to which a great deal of prestige was attached. For most GPs, such posts were short-term appointments seen as a supplement to an emerging private practice and a necessary stepping stone to greater and more rewarding opportunities.[77] Many took such posts merely to keep our competitors who might take away their private practice.[78] The poor law doctors were accountable to Boards of Guardians who were laymen elected to ensure that local rate payers' money was used sparingly and to enforce what the architect of the new poor law, Edwin Chadwick, called the principle of 'less eligibility'. The Guardians overseeing the workhouses were rarely generous in what they paid their PLMOs who were, moreover, expected to pay for the inmates' drugs out of their remuneration.[79] The PLMOs resented the power wielded over them by the Guardians and wished to be free of lay interference. However, they were members of a social world in which the Guardians held an important position locally as a source of private practice custom and patronage. Consequently, as Margaret Crowther puts it, 'Professional independence was not safeguarded in the desperate search for private custom'.[80] Posts continued to be sought after competitively as they provided their holders with 'a publicly guaranteed introduction to the neighbourhood'.[81] A survey in 1848 found that 19% of doctors held poor law appointments at that time and nearly double that percentage of GPs had occupied one of these posts at some point in their careers.[82]

One doctor concerned to improve the standard of care offered to sick paupers began a campaign to highlight the failings of the poor law system. Dr Joseph Rogers, described by Jeanne Brand as 'the idealistic champion of the oppressed', thereby became a leading figure in the humanitarian movement.[83] His lengthy battles with Guardians and the Local Government Board (LGB), which assumed overall responsibility for poor law services after 1871, were dutifully documented in letters to medical journals and the press, and led to him being viewed as a heroic figure by many doctors. Rogers linked the appalling conditions endured by the pauper sick in the workhouses to the weakness of the PLMOs relative to their employers.[84] In an attempt to improve their bargaining power, he established the Poor Law Medical Officers Association (PLMOA). This group was instrumental in securing the passage of the Metropolitan Poor Act of 1867.[85] The Act brought about reform of facilities for the sick poor in London, providing for the establishment of district asylums or infirmaries, separate from the workhouses, and funded by a Metropolitan Common Poor Fund. From the 1860s, the PLMOA were supported by central government inspectors in urging the building of dispensaries to cope with the swelling numbers of pauper sick, including those receiving outdoor relief in their own homes.[86] By 1886, there were 44 of these servicing the needs of the poor in London and in 1888 a House of Lords select committee recommended that its example be followed in other major cities.[87] Conditions in many infirmaries in the late nineteenth century, as in the workhouses generally, were nevertheless considered 'uniformly grim'.[88] They gradually improved as the volume of healthcare provision in the infirmaries increased significantly towards the end of the century. In 1861, they provided 50,000 beds; by 1911, the number was 121,000.[89] In 1871, the PLMOA submitted a carefully argued nine-point programme for reform of poor law medical services to the LGB, couching its arguments in terms of public utility and efficiency as much as simple humanity. When this was peremptorily rejected, 'an extended lull' fell over the medical officers' efforts to change central policy.[90] Nevertheless, doctors sharing Rogers' aspirations actively sought to raise the standard of care in the infirmaries where they worked to the level of the voluntary hospitals in which they had been trained.[91] As societal attitudes towards poverty and its causes began to change, some PLMOs, particularly those in the larger infirmaries who began to enjoy the title and improved status of 'Medical Superintendent', used moral indignation to browbeat boards of Guardians to institute improvements in facilities and nursing care as well as the availability of drugs and equipment.[92] The humanitarian spirit eventually affected the LGB leading them to sanction the widespread use of anaesthetics in the infirmaries in the 1890s.[93]

From the 1870s, the PLMOA concentrated on efforts to improve the working conditions of its members but this attempt to combine was largely ineffectual and they failed to become an effective pressure group. The PLMOs were notoriously badly paid, as the LGB acknowledged in its annual report in 1878.[94] As late as 1899, 32% of English Authorities paid their Medical Officers between £20 and £30 a year.[95] The only success the PLMOA achieved was in securing the right to superannuation, courtesy of an Act passed in 1895.[96] Crowther asserts that the workhouse doctors were to some extent hampered by their own professional interests. The PLMOA was a GPs' union whose role was largely defensive, and it was not as effective as the larger, and not exclusively medical, National Poor Law Officers Association.[97] Although the BMA sometimes gave support for their efforts and the *BMJ* offered them an accommodating platform from which to air their grievances, the PLMOA was strongly committed to private practice and certainly hostile to the idea of a centralised state medical service. Consequently, when some PLMOs accepted offers of full-time salaried posts, they soon found themselves isolated from the rest of the profession. Young and poor doctors were always tempted by the lure of a regular salary and pension. Established doctors meanwhile disparaged full-time status as it implied greater subordination to the Guardians. They were therefore prepared to accept inadequate remuneration for part-time posts in order to keep others out of their district.[98]

Following the Medical Act of 1858, PLMO appointments were confined, at the prompting of Sir John Simon, to those possessing dual qualifications in medicine and surgery. This led to a marginal increase in their status within the profession and in the eyes of the public.[99] Nevertheless, while the PLMOs shared to some extent in the growing esteem which the medical profession was beginning to enjoy at the end of the nineteenth century, they remained 'at the bottom of the hierarchy'.[100] The PLMO was expected to be a 'sanitarian, surgeon, psychiatrist, midwife, disciplinarian, as well as a physician'.[101] The larger voluntary hospitals added to the PLMOs' burdens by excluding patients with chronic illnesses, and infectious and venereal diseases knowing that 'they could not be denied entry to the workhouse'.[102] The range of diseases with which they engaged increased accordingly after 1880 and, as Angela Negrine has shown in her study of the Leicester Workhouse, 'progressive' PLMOs responded by offering treatments and practising techniques (like skin grafts for leg ulcers) rarely attempted elsewhere at that time.[103] Her microstudy confounds the traditional image of workhouse medicine given expression in the reports of the Royal Commission into the poor law published in 1909.[104] By the end of the century, many GPs starting out in practice found the range of work they were required to do in the workhouse infirmaries as broad as anything they might experience in the larger voluntary hospitals.[105] The experience gained compensated for the miserable conditions, the niggardly remuneration and the numerous indignities they claimed to have to endure at the hands of often uneducated and unsympathetic lay Guardians.

Professional registration and the rise of the expert

Those seeking to reform the educational establishment of medical practice in the mid- to late nineteenth century argued that it was in the public interest to streamline the entry requirements and enforce standards of practice within the profession. In the early 1850s, there were no less than 17 licencing bodies in Britain and Ireland – one of which was the Archbishop of Canterbury![106] Successive medical reform Bills were discussed and rejected by parliament due to coordinated opposition from the vested interests of the medical corporations before a compromise version of earlier Bills was finally passed as the Medical Act of 1858.[107] The Act established the General Medical Council (GMC) as an independent regulatory body. It was made up entirely of medical men tasked with ensuring that only those meeting specified educational and occupational criteria were registered as licenced practitioners, while denying registration to

those failing to meet those criteria or who were deemed by the Council as unfit to practise.[108] However, it provided only partial protection from competition
with unlicenced practitioners. It did not preclude the irregulars from practice but
only from government employment. Loudon says that the profession's claim to
expertise was not sufficient in legislators' minds 'to justify a monopoly which
would conflict with patients' liberties and the principles of laissez-faire'.[109] The
Act may have created common entry requirements and equality of medical practitioners before the law, but it did not wrest power from the Royal Colleges
who continued to be responsible for validating the educational requirements of
those seeking registration. Nor did it increase the status of GPs in comparison
with the professional elite as the old distinctions were replaced by a new one
between GPs and the growing number of hospital Consultants. The Consultants
continued to offer their services as GPs to the wealthy members of the industrial
merchant class and nobility.[110] The high fees they were able to charge together
with the steady income earned from teaching medical students obviated the need
to seek tenured hospital appointments. Being 'honorary' reinforced the Consultants' claim to being medical gentlemen untainted by an association with trade
and allowed them to maintain a sense of moral and social superiority over the
GPs.[111] As one writer stated in 1868, 'For this is a point on which society is very
tenacious; a gentleman must not engage in retail trade'.[112] While this attitude
prevailed, it was clear that although GPs and Consultants belonged to the same
profession, they did not belong to the same social class.[113]

The higher standards required by the Medical Act of 1858 reduced the number of qualified practitioners so that the growth in the number of doctors which
took place during the 20 years following the Act was outstripped by the growth
in the general population.[114] The financial situation and status of most medical
men during this period therefore improved accordingly. The higher incomes
also attracted a higher calibre of candidate for registration and a greater commitment from them to medicine as a life-long career.[115] According to Holloway, education was increasingly becoming a determinant of class position as
'achieved status was replacing ascribed status'.[116] However, the content of
medical education itself was not subject to proper regulation or enforced standards until the 1890s.[117] In 1879, the *Lancet* complained that 'the GMC has been
sitting on the subject of education for 20 years'.[118] A. J. Youngson maintains
that one of the reasons for this inertia was that the Council and the profession could not agree what the prime purpose of medical education was. While
some advocated the paramount importance of a good grounding in science,
others, like Sir John Simon, saw the principal purpose as being to inculcate
the knowledge and manners of an educated gentleman.[119] Prominent members
of the GMC argued about whether a basic grounding in science was more or
less important than knowledge of Latin or ancient Greek. Simon's views were
no doubt influenced by his experiences in the political sphere. In Youngson's
words: 'The men who governed Britain were educated gentlemen and if the

doctors were to influence public policy -as they wished to do- they had to be educated gentlemen also'.[120] However, by the end of the century, 'the necessity for medical education to rest on a scientific basis was not only acknowledged in principle but recognised in fact'.[121]

Improvements in medical knowledge reinforced the power of the practitioner vis-a-vis the patient. The more scientific and specialised the doctor's knowledge became, the less it was questioned by the layman.[122] The patient had to take the practitioner's services on trust. The growth of public trust in medical expertise was not due entirely to advances in medical science. It coincided with a growing public respect for expertise in all its various forms which was preceded by a whiggish belief in progress, the spread of scientific rationalism, and a decline in the authority of established religion.[123] According to Peterson, 'Experts gained status not because they could always act effectively but because only they could name, describe and explain'.[124] The growth of public trust in abstract systems of knowledge like orthodox medicine was, according to the philosopher Anthony Giddens, one of 'the consequences of modernity', although this trust was not fully realised until the end of the nineteenth century when the inclusion of science in school curricula conveyed an aura of respect for technical knowledge of all kinds.[125] The professions were among those who sought to capitalise on the growing respect for expertise. Public endorsement of the GP's advisory role was a measure of the rising esteem of the professions generally. The efforts of medical men to gain recognition based on science proved ineffective until their own leadership discovered the social value of that knowledge.[126] The rise of the professional classes in Britain during the nineteenth century saw the establishment of numerous professional societies and institutions regulating the professions such as Law, Architecture, and Engineering, for example, all of which involved control of entry via examinations.[127] This process coincided with the growth of the new 'redbrick' universities, many of which, by the 1860s, had their own medical schools. By these means, expertise was gradually institutionalised and obtained public and state endorsement. But along with the public's growing acceptance of doctors' status as expert professionals came an expectation of competence and clinical success. Those who 'paid the piper' were not always content with the tune they received and, when dissatisfied, had recourse to legal means of obtaining redress. The last few decades of the nineteenth century saw an increasing number of claims brought against medical practitioners in the courts. These were principally breach of contract claims as the concept of medical negligence had yet to be fully established but it led to the establishment of medico-legal defence organisations funded by practitioners' subscriptions.[128]

In his book *The Rise of Professional Society*, Harold Perkin documents the increasing influence of the professions in nineteenth-century Britain coinciding with government reliance on expertise a part of a growing compact between the state and the new professional middle class.[129] This helps in some way to explain the prodigious rise in the number of medical appointments which, from the middle of the century especially, provided an economic mainstay for many GPs.[130] The second half of the nineteenth century was thus a 'golden age' for appointments according to Anne Digby and testified to the value which both state and private institutions put on scientific medical knowledge.[131] Against a background of increasing state regulation of the conditions under which working people were employed, or individuals were cared for in charitable or state-sponsored institutions, the state had the need of medical officers to assist in the process of inspection and certification. Every organisation engaging with, caring for, or employing large numbers of people wanted its own medical officers to advise on medical aspects of their activities. The putative expertise of the medical officer lent a degree of scientific validity to whatever activities they undertook, measured, mediated, or certified. Victorian GPs were involved in certifying births and deaths, notifying infectious diseases, and served as public vaccinators. By the end of the century, the state had begun to call on GPs for 'a myriad of other duties under Acts relating to factories, vaccination, children, public health, workmen's compensation and housing' and thus became 'increasingly involved in social organisation and in matters of social policy'.[132] According to Rosemary Stevens: 'For the GP there had been a revolution; he had become central to the administration of public health and sanitary services as was acknowledged as a responsible public servant'.[133] The GP had thus become an instrument of the state without any conscious recognition of this having happened.

The ideal of the family doctor

In the second half of the nineteenth century, the market for healthcare was increased by clients whose socioeconomic status was relatively modest. The GPs' clientele now ranged from domestic servants and labourers to the minor gentry and professional people. For these, the GP had become by the second third of the nineteenth century the family doctor in effect and in name.[134] As the patronage of the elite became less important and the demand for medical care ceased to be concentrated in the higher status groups, the shift in the balance of power in the relationship from patients to doctor was accentuated.[135] Patients were more apt to respect the doctor and follow his advice, however, if he had the inbuilt confidence of the gentleman, and the appearance of professional respectability and good moral character. As Youngson puts it, 'Who the doctor is, is often more important than what he prescribes'.[136] The success of the GP was less dependent on medical science than on an ability to understand and respond to the social as well as medical needs of a diverse range of patients on a personal level. The general public's appreciation of the value of qualified medical practice was according to Peterson, 'less than wholehearted' and patients were more influenced by his behaviour, style of speech, morals, cleanliness and character.[137] The patient's faith in the GP was often influenced by his demeanour. Solemn professionalism, honesty, and kindliness counted for a lot, as did the GP's reputation and personal habits.

According to Christopher Lawrence, the family doctor 'reinforced the Victorian valuation of the family'.[138] The concept of the family doctor began in the late eighteenth century, but it was during the early nineteenth century that it came into its own.[139] It was immortalised by fictional representations of GPs in this period, such as George Eliot's Dr Lydgate and Thackery's Dr Thorne. These 'informed and sympathetic portraits' are 'atypical' according to Loudon. However, he acknowledges that they represented a popular view of GPs and the respect in which they were generally held by patients, if not their social superiors.[140] It was the personal attention and the continuity of care which the GPs' patients seemed to value most about the service they offered.[141] In contrast to the cold world of scientific laboratory medicines based on the consulting room or hospital, Loudon says, the family doctor provided a 'sympathetic understanding and familiar friendly face in times of distress'. The GP was 'comfortably old fashioned and unscientific, much to be preferred for minor and everyday complaints'.[142] Nicholas Jewson and Roy Porter support Foucault's view that between the eighteenth and the nineteenth centuries, the balance of power between doctor and patient shifted from a client dominated to a doctor dominated relationship.[143] But there may have been an extended period of 'dialectical exchange' between doctor and patient in Britain.[144] What Gordon Horrobin describes as 'biographical medicine' became the raison d'être of the GPs' work as they relied far more on the patient's narrative than on the latest diagnostic aids.[145] The essence of the family doctor was the combination of a clinical and pastoral role.[146] According to Anne Digby, 'palliation rather than cure was often the outcome of doctor-patient encounters'.[147]

The caring family doctor soon became 'a fictional stereotype'.[148] This helped in no small measure to influence the GPs' view of themselves or at least portrayed a heroic ideal which many of them aspired to but which increasing numbers of them were unable to live up to due to economic vicissitude. The 'heroic' view of the family doctor was shared both by patients and by the doctors themselves. In 1843 in his 'Address to a Medical Student', the physician W.A. Greenhill extolled the GP as 'the noblest member of the medical profession'. He continued that 'with his long and weary rides at all hours and in all weathers…surely we may call him the missionary of the profession'.[149] Horrobin describes the 'moral superiority' which the 'horse and buggy doctor' enjoyed compared with his hospital colleagues, based on what he describes as 'the mystery' of the personal encounter, often in the patient's own home. Like the priest, he says, 'the doctor deals with sacred matters'.[150] M. Jeanne Peterson describes medicine at this time as a 'sacred' profession, its membership a 'priesthood', and its knowledge 'a mystery'.[151] The delivery of care to patients in the community involved what Roy Porter calls 'complex social rituals'.[152] The trusting relationship which GPs had with their patients is perfectly illustrated in Ian McLaren's novel, *A Doctor of the Old School*, published in 1895, in which the eponymous hero is, like the priest, privy to the innermost thoughts of his patients who know he will keep their confidences until and even after death.[153] This ideal was encapsulated in Sir Samuel Luke Fildes' celebrated and reverential portrait 'The Doctor' which proved to be a hit with the public when it appeared at the Royal Academy exhibition in 1891 and was subsequently reproduced thousands of lithographic copies.[154] The fact that it was intended to reflect the selfless ministrations of a family doctor on the artist's own sick child added to its popular appeal. As one medical man was quoted as saying to a group of medical students: 'A library of books written in your honour would not do what this picture has done and will do for the medical profession'. He went on to exhort his audience to 'hold before you the ideal figure of Luke Fildes' picture and be at once gentlemen and gentle doctors'.[155]

Horrobin, Jewson, and others have argued that the rise in dominance of hospital medicine in the nineteenth century placed the GP in a position of clientship to the hospital while remaining in an entrepreneurial, patronage-based relationship with his, or her, own clientele. As a medical expert, the GP adopted a paternalistic stance which the non-expert patient was obliged to accept, but the GP served as an 'intermediate expert' between the patient and the specialist.[156] The old antagonisms between the specialist and generalist branches of the profession were still strongly evident by the end of the nineteenth century; however, with Consultants in Loudon's words, 'accusing GPs of clinical ignorance, inefficiency and outdated knowledge while the GPs, firmly wedded to the concept of the family doctor, claimed the monopoly of sensitivity and compassion in the care of the sick'.[157] Rosemary Stevens says that by the turn of the twentieth century two 'medical archetypes' had developed: 'the hospital consultant, a brilliant, bluff empiricist, inspiring his group of students at the bedside with a barbed self-conscious wit; and the kindly, omnicompetent general practitioner who knew and was loved by all his patients'.[158] Although something of an exaggeration these images were, she says, 'perhaps true of many men who were in practice at the turn of the century'. In 1900, the first edition of a periodical called *The General Practitioner* summed up the differences, as the GPs themselves saw them, between the two branches of the profession. It contrasted family doctors as 'all-round men, who understand that the body is a unit, the parts of which are related and must work together harmoniously to produce health' with specialists, 'whose minds are narrowed, judgement-biased and unbalanced by disproportionate knowledge of one subject' knowing nothing of 'the constitutional idiosyncrasies of the individual... essential to correct diagnosis and treatment'.[159]

Individualism, collectivism, and professionalisation

When looking at Britain during the nineteenth century, it is possible to discern a tension between, on the one hand, a dynamic individualism, and on the other increasing acceptance of the concept of society and the state as an 'organism', ac-companied a collectivist approach to tackling social problems.[160] Individualism, manifested in entrepreneurialism, is sometimes seen as one of the ideological pil-lars of the political and economic doctrine of *laissez-faire*.[161] The mid-nineteenth century was an era of unprecedented social mobility, fuelled by enterprise and facilitated by the industrial revolution and the opportunities offered by an ex-panding overseas empire. In the absence of anything resembling an education 'system', those who rose through the ranks as businessmen, bankers, and fac-tory owners were often self-educated. Inspired by the exploits of those who had achieved success through their own diligence, hard work, and determination and in overcoming adversity and the setbacks and handicaps of humble beginnings, Samuel Smiles' *Self-Help* perfectly captured the zeitgeist of mid-nineteenth-century Britain.[162] This Bible of Victorian individualism succeeded in inspiring a new generation to believe that anyone could achieve great things through a combination of thrift, hard work, determination, and healthy habits. Many GPs, like the novelist Francis Brett Young's eponymous hero, Dr John Bradley, found solace and inspiration in it as they struggled to progress their hard-won careers.[163] It is perhaps no coincidence that Smiles himself was once a GP who, as it turned out, was more successful as an administrator, publisher, and writer than he ever was as a doctor.[164] Smiles extols the humble origins of many of the great men, and occasionally great women, he deems exemplars. He was not alone in this. Rationalists, protestant nonconformists, and followers of Darwin and Spencer were equally contemptuous of obstacles to advancement placed in individuals' paths by poverty or lack of education. All these groups recognised that life for the majority of human beings involved hardship and struggle. Overcoming these obstacles was for some of these groups an enlightening and character-building experience, while for others it was largely a case of 'survival of the fittest'. All of them recognised, however, that, for the resolute, such trials often proved the catalyst for creativity and ingenuity, leading to prosperity and self-realisation.

The self-directed and self-funded nature of medical education encouraged self-reliance. The difficulty of navigating one's way through qualification and registration in such a haphazard and incoherent system plagued with nepotism, preferment, and class prejudice, and into practice as a GP, required huge re-serves of determination and personal resilience. In that sense, the GP was the epitome of the self-made man (or woman). The obstacles faced by women en-tering the profession in the last decade of the nineteenth and early decades of the twentieth century, well described by Anne Digby, were so great that only the most determined and resilient succeeded and, as in many of the professions effectively closed to women, those that did so had to prove themselves to be su-perior to their male counterparts.[165] However, few GPs, even the most successful ones, could expect to become rich as a result of their medical labours. All they could hope for was a steady income sufficient to secure a comfortable middle-class existence and, if they were lucky, an entrée into the more select circles of upper-middle-class professional society.[166] There were some among them, however, who knew how to make the most of their situation and not infrequently exploited their professional colleagues in so doing.

By the turn of the twentieth century, the GPs' ontological attachment to self-employed contractor status, which gave them the (theoretical) freedom to accept or refuse work, was one of the ways in which they defined themselves collectively. For many GPs, life was one of drudgery and hard work. While GP principals were theoretically their own boss, they were a servant to many masters. They were, however, free to accept as much work as they felt able to undertake. Although their lot often involved overwork and financial worry, the GPs had valuable 'cultural capital' – that is, membership of an increasingly respected profession with a claim to a higher calling of public service, an education, and practical knowledge of the healing arts, and a tenuous claim to familiarity with some of the new medical scientific discoveries.[167] This cultural capital was, moreover, transferable. If the GP failed to make a good living in his or her chosen location, they could always pack up and try their luck elsewhere. Perkin refers to itinerant professionals with no loyalty or ties to a specific geographical location as 'spiralists'.[168] Once they had found a favourable professional niche, however, spiralist GPs usually set about cultivating their social position within the local community they found themselves in using their cultural capital for all it was worth. Echoing Inkster's findings, Digby finds that GPs often ended up as pillars of their local communities, serving as magistrates, school governors, churchwardens, freemasons, and officers in the St John's Ambulance Brigades.[169] Harry Eckstein states that medicine in Britain 'possessed an extraordinary immunity from the more obvious signs of social exclusiveness'. He characterises it as a career open to talent which was thus 'universalistic' as opposed to more 'particularistic' professions like the law, the church, and the armed forces.[170] It was therefore a profession particularly attractive to the self-educated and entrepreneurial sections of the lower middle classes. Many GPs came from modest backgrounds, particularly the graduates of Scottish and Irish universities.[171] One contemporary opined that most medical men were the sons of 'men of the secondary professional classes or tradesmen'.[172] One successful GP, the author of *The Story of a Toiler's Life,* began life as a labourer in county Cork.[173]

Peterson ascribes the failure of the medical profession to attract entrants from the higher echelons of society to a perception that medics were not truly independent, being at the beck and call of patients, as well as charitable hospital committees, poor law Guardians, and the like. The profession could not offer what the Victorian gentlemen most desired, she says, which was 'power'. [174] There is some truth in this, and Peterson is right to list these concerns among the principal reasons why, as will be seen, GPs fought so hard to free themselves from lay control and resisted any diminution of their clinical autonomy. But this is only half the story. Despite the restrictions, slights, and humiliations, GPs sometimes endured, and the vicissitudes of making a living in a competitive and sometimes hostile economic environment, general practice still offered a measure of free-dom and self-determination rarely found elsewhere. The clergy were still subject to ecclesiastical preferment; the military were part of a strict hierarchy governed by Queen's regulations. Even Barristers and solicitors had arguably less freedom to determine their own work than GPs. The sociologist Elliot Friedson argues that medicine is the only profession that has been truly autonomous.[175] The GP and BMA Secretary Alfred Cox appears to have agreed, stating that 'a doctor in practice is, or used to be, as much his own master as anyone can be'.[176] GPs may have been 'marginal men' but, as already acknowledged, they were 'self-made' men and, latterly, women. For these individuals, the life of the GP, for all its tribulations, was one of opportunity, with cultural capital of education and expertise offering at least geographical if not social mobility. Individuals from lower-middle-class families with a natural spirit of independence, a desire for self-improvement, and increased social status and economic reward, with an aptitude for learning and hard work, were predisposed to want to become GPs. There was no automatic right to a successful career in or a rewarding livelihood from general practice, so such individuals had to be risk takers. These individu-als were not team players. They wanted to be their own boss. The profession of general practice offered few perks, but the absence of rules and minimum of regulatory interference accorded them great freedom of action. The former GP Sir Arthur Conan Doyle, inventor of the fictional detective Sherlock Holmes, sums this up in his semi-autobiographical novel, *The Stark Munro Letters,* when his hero, musing on the opportunity of starting his own practice, says: 'If there was the promise of poverty and hardship, there was also that of freedom. I would be my own – my very own. I had youth and strength and energy, and the whole world of medicine packed in between my two ears.'[177]

However, the nature of general practice, whose practitioners operated in isola-tion without scrutiny or control, served to reinforce those attributes of individu-alism, entrepreneurialism, risk taking, etc., in a case of nature and experience being mutually reinforcing. The philosopher Pierre Bourdieu talks of an 'un-conscious sense of the possible' inclining individuals to seek the conditions and ergo the 'field' which will best suit them adding that 'actors gravitate towards those social fields (and positions within those fields) that best match their dis-positions'.[178] The British GP offers in many ways a perfect example of what Bourdieu describes. Given that GPs were individualists, however, whether natu-rally, by reason of temperament, or experientially, as a result of operating in a competitive market for their services, how can one explain in sociological terms the development of a collective ideology? The answer most frequently cited by historians and sociologists is professionalisation. For GPs in Britain, this pro-cess involved essentially four elements. The first was *differentiation*. As quali-fied medical practitioners, GPs made strenuous and largely successful efforts to distinguish themselves from competitors they believed themselves superior to, that is, unqualified quacks and other recognised but evolving healthcare professions such as midwives, nurses, health visitors, and pharmacists. Noel and Jose Parry describe this 'occupational closure' as a consequence of a desire for 'upward collective social mobility'.[179] This differentiation was reinforced by state recognition under the Medical Acts of 1858 and 1886. At the same time, GPs experienced a common sense of being looked down on as generalists by medical professionals who laid claim to higher status through specialism. This encouraged a defensive self-assertion through which GPs extolled the benefits and minimised the limitations of the family doctor's role.

The second factor involves *standards of education*. During the second half of the nineteenth century, GPs fought and eventually won a battle against the medical corporations to obtain conjoint examinations in medicine, surgery, and midwifery.[180] This combination of qualifications was essential to render them educationally fit to meet the medical needs of the broadest range of potential clients. The celebrated physician George Birkbeck had noted in 1834 that the GP was popular with middle-class families because their combined expertise in medicine, surgery, and midwifery made them a cheaper alternative to employing each of those professionals separately.[181] The streamlining and regulation of medical education establishments, the specification of a minimum numbers of years spent in training to become a doctor, and the eventual abolition of medical apprenticeships contributed to medicine's prestige. It also led to an increase in the price of medical education which made it less open to individuals from poorer backgrounds.

The third element of professionalisation was *public and state recognition of expertise*. The increasing importance of Public Health in British society, reinforced by advances in medical science linked to ideas of social progress, increased the value of medical knowledge.[182] This was testified by the growth in the number of Medical Officer appointments of which GPs enjoyed a virtual monopoly. Peterson says that 'the rise of the expert required social acceptance not of the fact of expertise...but of the equation of expertise with authority'.[183] The final element involves *self-regulation and common standards of behaviour*. Resisting lay control over their activities was a defining feature of the GPs' collective experience in the nineteenth and early twentieth centuries. Although subject to minimal external scrutiny, the threat posed to GPs' incomes and status by uncontrolled market forces led to the establishment of new intra-professional bodies designed to moderate and advise on professional etiquette and 'ethics'. As Parry and Parry explain, professionalisation represents 'a strategy for controlling an occupation in which colleagues who are in a formal sense equal, set up a system of self-government'.[184] These bodies, as will be seen in the next chapter, played an important part in the development of GPs' representative organisations in the early twentieth century. Those same organisations made it their business to resist any attempt by lay authorities to challenge GPs' clinical autonomy or dictate how they exercised their professional responsibilities.

But, given that GPs were largely 'solitary beasts' often working excessively long hours, competing vigorously with each other as well as with rival occupations, and therefore having limited time for social interaction, how were they able to communicate with one another, recognise collective professional needs, and establish common cause? GPs did sometimes meet one another professionally in, for example, medical societies and BMA branches and mix in similar social circles. But it was primarily the journals like the *Lancet* and *BMJ, The General Practitioner* and later *Medical World,* which, by articulating commonly held beliefs, reinforced a sense of professional identity. They provided a rallying point for the numerous campaigns which GPs fought and a means of advertising to other practitioners the times and locations of local and national meetings which of those GPs who were able to, could attend, to participate in the formation of collective policy or identify champions to form new representative organisations. Pierre Bourdieu says that groups often exist in a 'space of relationships' that is as real as geographical space.[185] GPs rarely interacted in social space before the momentous events of 1911 gave them cause to. Yet, they shared a virtual social space in that they imbibed and shared similar ideas based on a similar educational background and common professional experiences which they exchanged through letters to journals and occasional interactions in local medical societies. Digby talks about this in terms of a kind of cultural 'diffusion' or 'replication' 'working vertically, through medical education, and horizontally, through professional imitation'.[186] Their collective mentality was increased by endogamous marriage and shared lifestyles, all of which served to create a 'homogeneity of kind'.[187] This was reinforced by having common enemies of which the nineteenth-century GP had many. They were opposed within the profession by the elite physicians and surgeons anxious to keep them at arm's length and in a dependent position, something which only increased as the elite metamorphosed into the new class of hospital Consultants; they faced competition and criticism from other professions vying to assert themselves, principally midwives, nurses, and druggists; and there were the perennial alternative practitioners and commercial interests behind quack medicines.

GPs also shared with other members of the profession the opprobrium heaped on them by those critical of medicine and disbelieving of its benefits, including those from the anti-science movement and civil libertarians. Finally, there were powerful groups which sought to control that part of the medical market devoted to sickness insurance clubs, for the benefit of their members and subscribers, namely the friendly societies, trade unions, and the insurance 'combine' of which more will be said in subsequent chapters. Many of these groups accused the medical profession in general, and GPs in particular, of venality and self-interest. The GPs' defence was to point to what Perkin describes as 'the professional social ideal'. Doctors obviously made much of their professional vocation and the spirit of public service exemplified by the Hippocratic oath. According to Daniel Duman, 'the ideal of service allowed the profession to reconcile the concept of the gentleman with the necessity of working for a living and to formulate a definition of their relationship with clients and with society'.[188] Elliot Friedson disputes this, arguing that 'there is no reliable information to demonstrate that a service orientation is ever widespread among medical professionals'.[189] However, as early as 1823, the London Association of apothecaries and surgeon-apothecaries stated that 'public advantage' had a place in their deliberations and that 'the association was actuated by far more philosophical views than mere calls for private interest'.[190] As T.H. Marshall was later to observe, it was in every doctor's long-term interest to ensure that the public received an honest, conscientious, and effective service.[191] Echoing this, Loudon comments that while the Medical Act of 1858 had been described as a prime example of professional consolidation and monopolisation based on material self-interest, 'it was commonly agreed that the professional man's self- interest was the best guarantee of good public service'.[192]

Conclusion

The process of professionalisation was stimulated by GPs' search for identity and their overarching desire for status and security. For some sociologists and historians, GPs' attempts to create new educational standards affecting recruitment were an attempt to control the market. These authorities view the establishment of representative organisations in the form of medical practitioner associations and guilds at local and national levels, as a means to that end. Echoing Terence Johnson's views on client control, Parry and Parry are disparaging of what they see as a legally enforceable monopoly.[193] David B. Green likewise sees the efforts of GPs to resist control of their work and to take collective action in defence of higher fees as anti-consumer. He attacks the GMC ban on advertising on the same grounds.[194] His views contrast with those of the Fabians Sidney and Beatrice Webb, who in their 1910 treatise, *The State and the Doctor*, acknowledged that rates paid to doctors were 'scandalously inadequate'.[195] They agreed with many professional spokesmen that the best guarantee of a good service for the public was to ensure that the medical profession was adequately trained, remunerated, and respected.[196] The principal area of contention for them lay in the degree to which the profession was left free to self-regulate or was subject to the control of local or central government.

In the final decades of the nineteenth century, it became clear to many GPs that they were faced with an existential dilemma. They recognised that, to preserve their autonomy as individualist actors within their field, they would have to temporarily set aside their competitive instincts and bind themselves together as a professional group in corporate self-defence and even, should it prove necessary, collective bargaining. For GPs, improving their social status and autonomy was dependent on maintaining a decent standard of living and to achieve this, they were forced to adopt collectivist measures. The organisations which were created or evolved to help GPs fulfil that objective employed different tactics according to the personalities and political leanings of those leading them, but they were all focused on the achievement and maintenance of three things: gentility, economic security, and professional autonomy. The next chapter considers how they set out to achieve this.

Notes

1 The Royal College of Physicians of London (founded 1518), Edinburgh (1681), and Ireland (1667 and 1692); The Royal College of Surgeons of Edinburgh (1778), London (1800), and England (1843); and the Worshipful Society of Apothecaries, London, founded 1617 and given authority to licence medical practitioners under the Apothecaries Act 1815.
2 Irvine Loudon, *Medical Care and the General Practitioner, 1750–1850* (Oxford, 1986). pp. 160–161.
3 *Ibid.*
4 *Ibid.*, p. 175.
5 S.W.F. Holloway, 'Medical Education in England 1830–1858: A Sociological Analysis', *History*, 49 (167) (1964). p. 311.
6 Loudon, *Medical Care and The General Practitioner*, p. 225.
7 *Ibid.*, pp. 309–310.
8 *Ibid.*, p. 307.
9 M. Jeanne Peterson, *The Medical Profession in Mid-Victorian London* (London, 1978). p. 182.
10 *Ibid*, pp. 53–76; see also Rosemary Stevens, *Medical Practice in Modern England: The Impact of Specialization and State Medicine* (New Haven, CT, 1966). p. 23.
11 Loudon, *Medical Care and The General Practitioner*, p. 202.
12 See Jacqueline Jenkinson, 'A 'Crutch to Assist in Gaining an Honest Living': Dispensary Shopkeeping by Scottish General Practitioners and the Responses of the Medical Elite 1852 – 1911.' *The Bulletin of the Society for the Social History of Medicine*, 86 (1) (2012). pp. 1–36.
13 Peterson, *The Medical Profession in Mid-Victorian London*, p. 68.
14 *Ibid.*, p. 19. Ivan Waddington, *The Medical Profession in the Industrial Revolution* (Dublin, 1984). p. 19.
15 *Ibid.*, p. 21.
16 Loudon, *Medical Care and The General Practitioner*, p. 93.
17 Brian Abel-Smith, *The Hospitals 1800–1948: A Study in Social Administration in England and Wales* (London, 1964). p. 22.
18 Loudon, *Medical Care and The General Practitioner*, p. 93.
19 F. B. (Francis Barrymore) Smith, *The People's Health, 1830–1910* (Canberra, 1979). p. 346.
20 Ian Inkster, 'Marginal Men: Aspects of the Social Role of the Medical Community in Sheffield, 1790–1850,' in John Woodward and David Richards (eds), *Healthcare in Popular Medicine in Nineteenth Century England: Essays in the Social History of Medicine* (London, 1977). p. 129.
21 Robert E Park, 'Human Migration and the Marginal Man.' *American Journal of Sociology*, 33 (1927–1928). pp. 881–893.
22 Inkster, 'Marginal Men', p. 129.

23 Ivan Waddington, 'General Practitioners and Consultants in Early Nineteenth-Century England; The Sociology of an Intra-Professional Conflict,' in John Woodward and David Richards (eds), *Healthcare in Popular Medicine in Nineteenth Century England: Essays in the Social History of Medicine* (London, 1977). p. 178.

24 Peterson, *The Medical Profession in Mid-Victorian London*, p. 133.

25 Attributed to a Professor of Materia Medica at Pennsylvania University. Loudon, *Medical Care and The General Practitioner*, p. 203.

26 *Ibid.*, p. 129.

27 *Ibid.*, pp. 200–202.

28 *Ibid.*, p. 230.

29 Ernest Muirhead Little, *History of the British Medical Association, 1832–1932* (London, 1932). p. 7. See also Peterson, *The Medical Profession in Mid-Victorian London*, p. 86, and Loudon, *Medical Care and The General Practitioner*, pp. 177–179.

30 Loudon, *Medical Care and The General Practitioner*, p. 53.

31 *Ibid.*, p. 177.

32 Smith, *The People's Health*, p. 357.

33 *Ibid.*, p. 358.

34 *Ibid.*, p. 174.

35 Peterson, *The Medical Profession in Mid-Victorian London*, p. 23.

36 *Ibid.*, p. 54.

37 E.S. (Ernest Sackville)Turner, *Call the Doctor: A Social History of Medical Men* (London, 1958). pp. 155–160.

38 Loudon, *Medical Care and The General Practitioner*, pp. 160–161.

39 The College of General Practitioners was established in 1952 and received its Royal Charter in 1972. See www.rcgp.org.uk/about-us/the-college/who-we-are/history-heritage-and-archive.aspx

40 Peterson, *The Medical Profession in Mid-Victorian London*, p. 116.

41 Noel Parry and Jose Parry, *The Rise of the Medical* Profession: *A Study of Collective Social Mobility* (London, 1976). p. 79.

42 Loudon, *Medical Care and The General Practitioner*, p. 209.

43 *Ibid.*, pp. 130, 133 and 210.

44 Little, *History of the BMA*, pp. 274–275.

45 William F. Bynum, *Science and the Practice of Medicine in the Nineteenth Century* (Cambridge, 1994). p. 75.

46 Kenneth D. Keele, 'Clinical Medicine in the 1860s,' in F.N.L Poynter (ed.), *Medicine and Science in the 1860s* (London, 1968). p. 1.

47 *Ibid.*

48 *Ibid.*, p. 2.

49 Michel Foucault, *The Birth of the Clinic: An Archaeology of Medical Perception*, trans A.M Sheridan Smith (New York, 1975). p. 195.

50 Janis McLarren-Caldwell, *Literature and Medicine in Nineteenth Century Britain* (Cambridge, 2004). p. 6.

51 *Ibid.*, pp. 8–20.

52 Christopher Lawrence, *Medicine in the Making of Modern Britain 1700–1920* (London, 1993). p. 50.

53 *Ibid.*, p. 44.

54 *Ibid.*, p. 75.

55 Bynum, *Science and the Practice of Medicine*, p. 220.

56 Waddington, *The Medical Profession in the Industrial Revolution*, p. 197.

57 *Ibid.*

58 Dorothy and Roy Porter, 'The Politics of Prevention: Anti-vaccinationism and Public Health in Nineteenth Century England.' *Medical History*, 32 (1988). p. 231.
59 Roy M. MacLeod, 'Law, Medicine and Public Opinion: The Resistance to Compulsory Health Legislation, 1870–1907.' *Public Law* Summer (1967). p. 211.
60 Alfred Russel Wallace, *Vaccination a Delusion, Its Enforcement a Crime* (London, 1898) quoted in Porter and Porter, 'The Politics of Prevention', p. 238.
61 George Bernard Shaw, Preface to *The Doctor's Dilemma* (London, 1906). Penguin edn. 1946, p. 68.
62 Margaret Stacey, *The Sociology of Health and Healing* (London, 1988). p. 87.
63 Inkster, 'Marginal Men', p. 131.
64 Lawrence, *Medicine in the Making of Modern Britain*, p. 70.
65 Holloway, 'Medical Education in England', p. 319.
66 *Ibid.*
67 Samuel Smiles, *Self-Help* (London, 1859). Oxford World Classics edn. 2002, p. 263.
68 Peterson, *The Medical Profession in Mid-Victorian London*, p. 197.
69 Loudon, *Medical Care and The General Practitioner*, p. 274.
70 Quoted by Peterson, *The Medical Profession in Mid-Victorian London*, p. 251.
71 Little, *History of the BMA*, pp. 61–66.
72 Peterson, *The Medical Profession in Mid-Victorian London*, p. 33.
73 Loudon, *Medical Care and The General Practitioner*, pp. 225, 268.
74 *Ibid.*, p. 268.
75 *Ibid.*, p. 232.
76 *Ibid.*, pp. 238–239.
77 *Ibid.*, p. 239.
78 *Ibid.*, p. 246.
79 Margaret Anne Crowther, *The Workhouse System, 1934–1929: The History of an English Social Institution* (London, 1981). p. 163.
80 *Ibid.*, p. 172.
81 Jeanne C. Brand, *Doctors and the State* (Baltimore, MD, 1965). p. 88.
82 Loudon, *Medical Care and The General Practitioner*, p. 239.
83 Brand, *Doctors and the State*, p. 86.
84 Crowther, *The Workhouse System*, p. 162.
85 Brand, *Doctors and the State*, p. 100.
86 *Ibid.*, p. 98.
87 *Ibid.*, pp. 99 and 103.
88 Harry Eckstein, *The English Health Service: Its Origins, Structures and Achievements* (Cambridge, MA, 1964). p. 34.
89 Crowther, *The Workhouse System*, p. 167.
90 *Ibid.*, pp. 101–103.
91 Abel-Smith, *The Hospitals*, p. 71.
92 *Ibid.*, pp. 96–97.
93 Brand, *Doctors and the State*, p. 105.
94 Abel-Smith, *The Hospitals*, p. 92.
95 Joan Lane, *A Social History of Medicine: Health, Healing and Disease in England, 1750–1950* (London, 2001). p. 64.
96 Brand, *Doctors and the State*, p. 106.
97 *Ibid.*, p. 169.
98 *Ibid.*, pp. 167–170.
99 *Ibid.*, p. 88.
100 *Ibid.*, pp. 167–169.

101 *Ibid.*, p. 164.
102 *Ibid.*, p. 163.
103 Angela Negrine, 'Practitioners and Paupers: Medicine at the Leicester Union Workhouse, 1867–1905,' in Jonathan Reinarz, and Leonard Schwarz (eds), *Medicine and the Workhouse* (Rochester, NJ, 2013). pp. 196–197.
104 *Report of the Royal Commission into the Poor Laws and Relief of Distress 1905–1909.* Cmd. 4499, 1909, passim.
105 Crowther, *The Workhouse System*, pp. 164–167.
106 Loudon, *Medical Care and the General Practitioner*, pp. 194–195.
107 Stevens, *Medical Practice in Modern England*, p. 23.
108 See www.gmc-uk.org/about/who-we-are/our-history.
109 Loudon, *Medical Care and The General Practitioner*, p. 36.
110 Waddington, 'General Practitioners and Consultants in Early Nineteenth Century England', p. 171.
111 Loudon, *Medical Care and The General Practitioner*, p. 227.
112 Isaac Ashe, *Medical Education and Medical Interests* (Dublin, 1868). p. 14.
113 Peterson, *The Medical Profession in Mid-Victorian London*, p. 243.
114 Waddington, *The Medical Profession in the Industrial Revolution*, p. 148.
115 *Ibid.*, pp. 152 and 198.
116 Holloway, 'Medical Education in England', p. 315.
117 A. J. (Alexander John)Youngson, 'Medical Education in the Later Nineteenth Century: The Science Take-Over.' *Medical Education* (1989). p. 480.
118 *Ibid.*
119 *Ibid.*, p. 484.
120 *Ibid.*
121 *Ibid.*, p. 488.
122 Holloway, 'Medical Education in England', p. 317.
123 Peterson, *The Medical Profession in Mid-Victorian London*, p. 268. See also Jose Harris, *Private Lives, Public Spirit: Britain 1870–1914* (2nd edn, London, 1994). pp. 59–60 and 176–177.
124 Peterson, *The Medical Profession in Mid-Victorian London*, p. 286.
125 Anthony Giddens, *The Consequences of Modernity* (Cambridge, 1990). pp. 84 and 89.
126 Peterson, *The Medical Profession in Mid-Victorian London*, p. 286.
127 Harold Perkin, *The Rise of Professional Society: England since 1880* (2nd edn, Abingdon, 2002). p. 87.
128 The Medical Defence Union, the first organisation of its kind in the world, was established in 1885. See www.themdu.com/about-mdu/our-heritage
129 Perkin, *The Rise of Professional Society*, pp. 286–288.
130 Peterson, *The Medical Profession in Mid-Victorian London*, p. 110.
131 Anne Digby, *The Evolution of British General Practice, 1848–1948* (Oxford, 1999). p. 79.
132 Stevens, *Medical Practice in Modern England*, p. 35.
133 *Ibid.*
134 Loudon, *Medical Care and The General Practitioner*, p. 275.
135 *Ibid.*, p. 199.
136 Youngson, 'Medical Education in the later Nineteenth century', p. 485.
137 Peterson, *The Medical Profession in Mid-Victorian London*, pp. 90–91.
138 Lawrence, *Medicine in the Making of Modern Britain*, p. 70.
139 Irvine Loudon, 'The Concept of the Family Doctor.' *Bulletin of the History of Medicine*, 58 (3) (1984). pp. 347–352.

140 *Ibid.*
141 *Ibid.*, pp. 358–359.
142 *Ibid.*
143 Nicholas Jewson, 'Medical Knowledge and the Patronage System in Eighteenth-Century England', *Sociology*, 8 (1974). pp. 369–385. Roy Porter, 'Lay Medical Knowledge in the Eighteenth Century: The Evidence of the Gentleman's Magazine.' *Medical History*, 29 (1985). pp. 138–168.
144 McLarren-Caldwell, *Literature and Medicine in Nineteenth Century Britain*, p. 144.
145 Gordon Horrobin, 'Professional Mystery: The Maintenance of Charisma in General Medical Practice,' in Robert Dingwall and Phillip Lewis (eds) *The Sociology of the Professions: Doctors, Lawyers and Others* (London, 1983). p. 100.
146 Loudon, *Medical Care and the General Practitioner*, p. 277.
147 Digby, *The Evolution of British General Practice*, p. 13.
148 Loudon, *Medical Care and The General Practitioner,* p. 275.
149 *Ibid.*, p. 206.
150 Horrobin, 'Professional Mystery', pp. 100–101.
151 Peterson, *The Medical Profession in Mid-Victorian London*, p. 282.
152 Roy Porter, 'The Patient's View: Doing History from Below.' *Theory and Society*, 14 (2) (1985). p. 175.
153 Ian Maclaren, *A Doctor of the Old School* (London, 1895). pp. 75–85.
154 'The Doctor' by Sir Samuel Luke Fildes R.A. (1891) now part of the Tate Gallery Collection, London.
155 Peterson, *The Medical Profession in Mid-Victorian London,* p. 131.
156 Horrobin, 'Professional Mystery', p. 96.
157 Loudon, 'The Concept of the Family Doctor', p. 360.
158 Stevens, *Medical Practice in Modern England*, p. 33.
159 Peterson, *The Medical Profession in Mid-Victorian London*, p. 273.
160 See Harris, *Private Lives, Public Spirit*, pp. 220–232.
161 A view popularised by the Victorian jurist A.V. Dicey among others when describing the influence of Jeremy Bentham but now seen as an oversimplification. See Arthur J. Taylor, *Laissez-Faire and State Intervention in Nineteenth Century Britain* (5th edn, Basingstoke, 1985). pp. 32–38.
162 Smiles, *Self-Help*, passim.
163 Francis Brett Young, *Dr Bradley Remembers* (London, 1938). p. 222.
164 Peter W. Sinnema, Introduction to the Oxford World's Classics edition of Samuel Smiles' *Self-Help* (Oxford, 2002). pp. xiv–xvi.
165 See Digby, *The Evolution of British General Practice*, p. 162.
166 *Ibid.*, pp. 261–262.
167 Perkin, *The Rise of Professional Society,* pp. 7–8; Giddens, *The Consequences of Modernity,* pp. 88–89; Pierre Bourdieu, 'The Forms of Capital,' in H. Lauder, P. Brown, J-A. Dillabough and A. H. Halsey (eds) *Education, Globalisation and Social Change* (Oxford, 2006). p. 107.
168 Perkin, *The Rise of Professional Society*, p. 11.
169 Digby, *The Evolution of British General Practice*, pp. 263–271.
170 Eckstein, *The English Health Service*, p. 50.
171 See Jacqueline Jenkinson, 'More 'Marginal Men': A Prosopography of Scottish Shop-keeping Doctors in the Late Nineteenth and Early Twentieth Centuries.' *Social History of Medicine*, 29 (1). (2015) pp 89–11 and 102–103.
172 Peterson, *The Medical Profession in Mid-Victorian London,* p. 197.
173 James Mullin, *The Story of a Toiler's Life* (London, 1921). UCD ed., 2000, p. 23.

174 M. Jeanne Peterson, 'Gentlemen and Medical Men.' *Bulletin of the History of Medicine*, 58 (4) (1984). pp. 457–473.

175 Elliot Friedson, *The Profession of Medicine: A Study of the Sociology of Applied Knowledge* (New York, 1970). p. 143.

176 Alfred Cox, *Among the Doctors* (London, c.1949). p. 82.

177 Arthur Conan Doyle, *The Stark Munro Letters* (London, 1898). ch. X, 21 May 1882.

178 Pierre Bourdieu, *The Logic of Practice*, trans by R. Nice (Cambridge, 1990). p. 59.

179 Parry and Parry, *The Rise of the Medical Profession*, p. 79.

180 Waddington, *The Medical Profession in the Industrial Revolution*, p. 126.

181 *Ibid.*, p. 25.

182 Bynum, *Science and the Practice of Medicine in the Nineteenth Century*, p. 220.

183 Peterson, *The Medical Profession in Mid-Victorian London*, p. 286.

184 Parry and Parry, *The Rise of the Medical Profession*, p. 83.

185 Pierre Bourdieu, 'The Social Space and the Genesis of Groups.' *Theory and Society*, 14 (6) (1985). pp. 723–744.

186 Digby, *The Evolution of British General Practice*, p. 11.

187 Parry and Parry, *The Rise of the Medical Profession*, p. 77.

188 Daniel Duman, 'The Creation and Diffusion of a Professional Ideology in Nineteenth Century England.' *Sociological Review*, 27 (1979). p. 114.

189 Friedson, *Profession of Medicine*, p. 81.

190 Loudon, *Medical Care and The General Practitioner*, p. 154.

191 T.H. (Thomas Humphrey) Marshall, 'The Recent History of Professionalism and Social Policy', *Canadian Journal of Economics and Political Science*, 5 (3) (August, 1939), reprinted in T.H. Marshall, *Sociology at the Crossroads* (1963). pp. 150–170.

192 Loudon, *Medical Care and the General Practitioner*, p. 299.

193 Parry and Parry, *The Rise of the Medical Profession*, p. 78.

194 David B. Green, *Working-Class Patients and the Medical Establishment: Self-help in Britain from the Mid-Nineteenth Century to 1948* (Aldershot, 1985). p. 132.

195 Sidney and Beatrice Webb, *The State and the Doctor* (London, 1910). p. 253.

196 Samuel Squire Sprigge, *Medicine and the Public* (London, 1905). p. 233.

3   Political representation

The fight for autonomy and 'the battle of the clubs', 1880–1911

Throughout the nineteenth century, income was crucial to GPs' status. They saw themselves as deserving a central position in middle-class society, but their incomes sometimes failed to match their expectations of 'fair reward' and led to resentment of their wealthier physician colleagues. The poverty of the Scottish GP in particular was proverbial, and it was for that reason that they, like many doctors operating in urban areas occupied by the poor, were reluctant to abandon their association with retail trade.[1] GPs discovered that higher incomes and the respect of the public were often tied together. The marginal status of the profession made them feel acutely the need to 'keep up appearances' in their efforts to gain recognition as gentlemen. An adequate income allowed practitioners some freedom from the need to please every patient, while a marginal or substandard income accentuated and compounded feelings of inferiority and dependency.[2] Anne Digby describes the market for medical services in the late nineteenth century as 'a diffuse, fluid and heterogenous medical pluralism which enabled sufferers to choose from other alternatives according to their perceived effectiveness'.[3] In the final two decades of the century when, as will be shown, there were more doctors than ever competing for patients, GPs collectively faced a concerted threat of competition from several directions. In addition to continued and vigorous competition from the unqualified, GPs in urban areas now faced competition from voluntary hospital outpatient departments and dispensaries and from newly established specialist hospitals. The biggest threat to their collective well-being, however, came from attempts by lay institutions to control and restrict GPs' access to the increasingly significant part of the medical market which was funded through sickness benefit insurance. These institutions inhibited the patient's free choice of doctor, undermined GPs' professional autonomy, and ultimately represented a threat to their independent contractor status itself. Their efforts therefore offered the greatest stimulus to medical trade unionism and engendered a more widespread professional interest in political questions. As will be demonstrated, a minority of GPs were actively if intermittently involved in political activities of various sorts throughout the second half of the nineteenth century.[4] The dilemma for those seeking to organise GPs for political

DOI: 10.4324/9781003438274-3

ends in this period was how to persuade individuals plying their trade as independent tradesmen to set aside their competitive instincts and band together against external threats. Fear of these threats propelled British medical practitioners towards actions which would inevitably bring them into conflict with the state.

Contract practice and the first examples of medical combination

According to Irvine Loudon, to achieve prosperity, the nineteenth-century GP needed at least three things: an average of 15–20 visits a day, an efficient pharmacy run by their apprentice or assistant, and the minimum of bad debts.[5] In the absence of these things, many GPs relied on other forms of medical income. Work as a PLMO was, as has been seen, a good way of supplementing income from a limited private practice, but a great many more GPs took care to cultivate opportunities to obtain income from 'contract practice'. This was the generic term used to describe the various schemes by which GPs were contracted to provide medical care for individuals, usually working-class men and, less commonly, women and children, for whom regular contributions were paid into a collective sickness insurance scheme or 'club'. Many GPs ran their own sickness clubs for families to ensure that their poorer patients could spread the cost of medical treatment which would otherwise have been unaffordable. But, as the nineteenth century progressed, practice sickness clubs were gradually eclipsed by larger and less geographically specific schemes run by friendly societies, trade unions, and eventually commercial insurance companies. The most popular and common were those run by friendly societies. These fraternal membership organisations had emerged in the eighteenth century and grown in popularity, following legal recognition, state sanction, and a degree of state regulation at the turn of the nineteenth century.[6] Some of them were small, local societies comprising a few hundred members or less, while others, like the Hearts of Oak, the Oddfellows, or the Foresters, became large and influential national bodies comprising thousands of members organised through a federated network of local branches or 'lodges'. All espoused some occupational, religious, or philanthropic purpose.

Doctors had not commonly been employed by friendly societies before the 1840s.[7] The societies were at that time chiefly concerned to offer benefits during sickness rather than curative treatment.[8] The role of the GP medical attendant with whom the societies contracted was generally concerned with confirming if sickness and 'lying in' claims were genuine and, after 1858, providing death certificates as a necessary precondition for payment of burial costs.[9] Gradually, however, the friendly societies began to offer treatment from the GPs they had contracted with, recognising that, if successful, such ministrations would offset the cost of sickness benefits. Martin Gorsky states that medicalisation of friendly society sickness benefits arose for actuarial reasons, that is, to properly assess risk and 'moral hazard' (i.e., false claims) as the societies became larger and more impersonal.[10] The 'club' doctors were therefore contracted to attend on and provide medicine to members for an annual fee per member based on the number of subscribers. From the mid-nineteenth century to the first decade of the twentieth century, this was, usually, between 2s and 5s per patient annum, out of which the doctor was expected to provide and pay for medicines needed by the patient.[11] All but a small proportion of friendly society subscribers were adult males. For GPs competing with each other for patients in an overcrowded medical market, clubs offered both a guaranteed steady income and the opportunity which being the club doctor offered to introduce themselves to future custom from the wives and families of club members. In 1870, the *Lancet* opined that 'in towns the wives of club members are often fruitful vines'.[12] Many GPs ran their own sick clubs for women and children only.[13] In Gateshead, the Doctors' family clubs' subscription was 3d a week and according to local GP, Alfred Cox was 'the only way poor people could pay for medical attendance'.[14]

An appointment as a club or lodge doctor not only offered the prospect of a steady if modest income, it also spared the GP the inconvenience of collecting fees from patients and the risk of bad debts.[15] The principal benefit of club medicine, however, was that it extended working-class acceptance of qualified practitioners rather than quacks, and entrenched scientific medicine within the fields of life and sickness insurance.[16] For David B. Green, the friendly societies were the epitome of working-class thrift and self-reliance, and doctors' complaints about them were founded in self-interest and class prejudice.[17] He regards efforts by doctors to join together to demand higher fees from them as protectionist and anti-consumer.[18] However, more recent studies have shown that fees for doctors' services rose broadly in line with general wage levels.[19] The quality of medical care provided to members of friendly societies was often felt to be below the standard offered to fee-paying clients and was widely disparaged. Sidney and Beatrice Webb quoted a 'respectable medical witness' who asserted that 'club practice is most distasteful. No practitioner remains a club doctor any longer than he can possible help'.[20] The *BMJ* confirmed the view that club practice was no more than a stepping stone to something better when its editorial opined in 1895 that 'no one surely will suggest that the position of dispensing or club doctor is sufficiently attractive as an ultimate goal to make men study medicine as a science'.[21] To the friendly societies' complaints that their members sometimes received cursory treatment from club doctors, the GPs responded that the large number of patients and the niggardly remuneration offered prevented them from giving their best to the patient in each case.[22] The profession at that time was arguably less concerned about the level of fees paid for medical attendance, however, than about the societies' refusal to apply an income limit to membership. This meant that prosperous artisans and others whose income had increased to the level at which the doctors felt they could afford to pay privately for treatment obtained medical services 'on the cheap'. If unchecked, this kind of behaviour, the doctors felt, would undermine their ability to maintain a gentlemanly income from private practice.[23] Ernest Little, historian of the BMA, notes that the medical profession had always adjusted its fees to the financial status of its patients, but 'the societies professed themselves unable to see why the same advice and medicine given to a rich man should cost more than when given to a poor one'.[24]

Relationships between friendly societies and the doctors with whom they contracted did not seriously deteriorate until the last few decades of the nineteenth century.[25] But there had been concerted attempts by groups of doctors to obtain increased fees using trade union type tactics from a much earlier date. Professional objections to friendly society medical clubs began as early as 1837, in Cricklade and Wooton Bassett, and the first boycott by an 'organised medical profession' over what were perceived to be inadequate terms and conditions occurred in Sunderland in 1844.[26] The earliest evidence of doctors signing pledges not to work for a friendly society club occurred in the same year in Pickering in North Yorkshire.[27] The most concerted attempts at 'combination' however, took place in the late 1860s. In Birmingham, with the encouragement of the *BMJ* and support of the *Birmingham Daily Gazette*, doctors working for local friendly societies sought improvements in workload and fees, and enforcement of an income limit on subscribers. Their campaign culminated in 1868 in the signing of a pledge of solidarity by 168 doctors.[28] The same year saw a rash of medical trade union-like activity as friendly society sickness club medical officers sought, with mixed success, to secure a standardised rate of 5s per patient, in Oldbury and Wednesbury, and in Southampton. Doctors in these areas found themselves dismissed from their posts by the societies and responded by organising boycotts.[29] In Oldbury and Wednesbury, doctors sought to ostracise newcomers taking up boycotted posts, pledging 'neither to meet them professionally or socially (or)…meet in consultation any physician or surgeon who recognises them'.[30] The attention given to these disputes in the *BMJ* and the *Lancet* had the effect of normalising to some extent these kinds of actions among rank and file practitioners, even though they might offend the delicate sensibilities of elite doctors who were nevertheless enjoined to support their less wealthy colleagues. The continued failure of attempts by GPs to band together to resist unsatisfactory terms was invariably due to undercutting by fellow doctors. Boycotts failed because there was always some doctor desperate enough, or unprincipled enough, to ignore the local profession's call for solidarity.[31] This was an inevitable result of overcrowding of the medical market and its consequential lack of opportunities for advancement for many young doctors.[32] 'A Poor Club Doctor' writing to the *BMJ* in 1867 described the difficulties of persuading colleagues to boycott a club that had unjustly injured his reputation. Even when his colleagues supported him, outsiders were brought in and when eventually the club offered to meet his terms if he would resume the role, a local man still undercut him.[33] Ernest Little concluded that 'The strength of the position of the societies lay in the lack of union among medical men'.[34]

One means by which the profession sought to prevent undercutting was by establishing an agreed tariff of fees. The most widely quoted tariff was that created by the Manchester Medical Ethical Society in 1865. This enjoyed wide currency among GPs and was revised and re-circulated several times over the next 40 years. Established in 1847, the original objects of the Society were 'to maintain the honour, and interests of the profession and to promote good fellowship among its members'.[35] Its tariff became a point of reference in disputes with friendly societies and Poor Law Unions alike about the market rate for GP services.[36] The 1879 version reflected the commonly held practice of setting fees according to the client's ability to play and was 'fixed at such a rate that even the humblest member of the profession need not hesitate to make it the basis of his charges'.[37] The tariff used house rentals to determine ability to pay and based the fee on the value of the practitioner's time and skill.[38] It may seem strange that something calling itself an ethical committee should be concerned with setting a tariff of fees. In the twentieth century, medical ethics came to be understood as principally about doctors' behaviour towards patients and consideration of their best interests. In the eighteenth and nineteenth centuries, however, ethics had more to do with moderating doctors' relationships with each other. The first modern code of ethics in Britain was devised by Thomas Percival in 1794 in an attempt to prevent his 'quarrelsome colleagues' at the Manchester Royal Infirmary falling out with each other. Subsequent generations felt that his use of the word ethics was a misnomer because what he was describing was not ethics but etiquette.[39] In the absence of any agreed codes of behaviour, the fees tariff was simply one means by which to identify those inclined to depart from behavioural norms.[40]

Efforts to improve the status of GPs were undermined, however, by an explosion in the number of those seeking to join the medical profession occurring in the late nineteenth century, a phenomenon which occurred across Europe and the USA.[41] The number of those entering the medical profession in Britain increased by 62.7% between 1881 and 1911.[42] This resulted in the creation of what Anne Digby describes as an 'emerging professional proletariat' who were forced to appeal to the lower end of the market for medical services.[43] It thereby contributed to what many saw as a lowering of standards of practice as new arrivals resorted to offering only the simplest and most inexpensive remedies to their poorer patients and undercut established doctors. Digby states that these 'sixpenny doctors' adopted 'an economically rational strategy, maximising numbers through having a faster throughput at a low fee'.[44] The lowering of standards of medical care dented the reputation of the profession, however, and encouraged the belief that money was their prime consideration. In Francis Brett-Young's novel, *Dr Bradley Remembers,* 'Scottish invaders' threaten John Bradley's friendly society contract work by offering to undercut his fees.[45] Echoing the commonly held view of Scottish doctors as interloping 'sixpenny men', Dennison, the hero of Frank Layton's novel, *The Old Doctor*, explains to Dix, a naïve newcomer, that his best club pays him 3s 6d per member but 'McFadd has been at them. Says he'll take them on at three shillings. Naturally they want me to do the same'.[46] Dennison bemoans the insecurity of club work stating that:

> A lodge surgeon is liable to be kicked out of his job at the end of any year – because he is too strict in the matter of beer; because he refuses sick notes when he considers them uncalled for; because someone else…will do the work for less.[47]

Alfred Cox observed that club practice in those days was 'a sort of guerrilla warfare between the doctors and the promoters of the clubs. The latter very often played off one doctor against the others and appointed the man who accepted the lowest terms'.[48] Controversially perhaps, he states that 'It was no secret that many of these appointments were obtained by bribery and corruption'.[49] The friendly societies were not, however, the only threat faced by GPs in the final decades of the nineteenth century.

The rise of medical guilds and associations

Competition from the unqualified was not greatly affected by the passing of the Medical Acts of 1858 and 1886. Working-class patients continued to make significant use of unlicenced practitioners until well into the twentieth century. A government survey in 1910 found that in 82 out of 217 towns, surveyed unlicenced medical practice was either increasing or taking place to a large extent and in 75 to a limited extent. Unlicenced practitioners included prescribing chemists, herbalists, bonesetters, Christian scientists, faith healers, abortionists, and venereal disease specialists. Bonesetters, in particular, enjoyed a positive reputation, the miners' friendly societies accepting certification from them as equivalent to those of a qualified medical practitioner.[50] When seeking to distinguish themselves from the unqualified, GPs relied on their putative expertise and the growing prestige of medical science. But these were not so easily invoked when facing competition from specialists in hospital outpatient departments which increasing numbers of patients attended for treatment between the 1870s and the turn of the twentieth century. Taking the London Hospital in Whitechapel as an example, annual outpatient attendances had averaged 3,000–7,000 between 1750 and 1840 and then rose steeply. By 1870, there were 52,000 attendances and by 1900, 200,000 new cases were attending annually and a similar pattern appears to have occurred in most of voluntary hospitals in London and the provinces.[51] By providing care free of charge to the poorest sections of the community and at affordable rates to others of modest means, these departments denied income to GPs struggling to make a living in an overcrowded market. Contemporary commentator H.N. Hardy noted that in South London, discerning patients would send for the GP or go to them for medicine in bad weather but 'in fine weather they all flock to the hospitals'.[52] He added that London hospitals charged as little as 1s for small operations when the GP charged 1s or even 1s 6d for a visit and medicine.[53] Run by Consultants who extolled the merits of their specialist knowledge above that of the humble GP, outpatient departments gradually became extensions of specialist inpatient units rather than general clinics.[54] In 1872, the *BMJ* identified this factor as the main cause of the stagnation in GPs' income, commenting that: 'the indifference and traditions of successful and eminent practitioners at the head of consulting practice are among the chief causes which combine to stereotype, and therefore relatively to depreciate, the remuneration of practitioners in general'.[55] GPs were not alone in viewing these developments with alarm. The Charity Organisation Society voiced concern that free care encouraged pauperism and that voluntary hospitals wasted charitable resources by treating a mix of patients including those who could afford to pay for their care.[56] Competition from Consultants made GPs wary of the suggestion that the medical profession should adopt the kind of referral relationship that existed between barristers and solicitors.[57] However, by the 1880s, this was already becoming a reality. During the last three decades of the nineteenth century, the emergence of specialist hospitals, in London principally, increased GPs' insecurities about hospital-based competitors.[58] In an article in the *Fortnightly Review* in 1885, Morrell Mackenzie, a former GP who opened the country's first specialist Ear, Nose and Throat hospital, wrote that 'the family Doctor…comes to look upon the specialist as a receiver of stolen goods if not the actual thief'.[59] Writing a year later in the *BMJ*, one GP stated that 'the whole struggle between the general practitioner and consultant is one of bread'.[60]

GPs' income was further threatened by the rise of provident dispensaries attached to hospitals. Funded by regular patient subscriptions, the dispensaries were intended primarily for those of lower- and middle-range incomes, and were popularly seen, like friendly society schemes, as a form of self-help which 'maintained the dignity and independence of the subscriber, removing the stigma of charity and pauperism'.[61] One of the most egregious examples of provident dispensary 'abuse', from the GPs' point of view, involved the Coventry Dispensary, of which by 1900 approximately half of that city's population had become subscribers. The Doctors' objections to this featured in a long-running correspondence with the BMA aired in the *BMJ* and the local and national press. The establishment of a rival scheme run by the doctors themselves failed to diminish its appeal.[62] During the 1880s and 1890s, GPs regularly wrote complaining letters to the *BMJ* and the *Lancet* about this 'hospital abuse'.[63] Among the most ardent complainants was a Liverpool GP, Dr Robert Rentoul. In 1883, he wrote that 110 doctors had signed resolutions condemning abuse of hospital outpatients.[64] Three years later, he announced that an organisation calling itself 'The Association of General Practitioners' was to be formed 'with the aim of forcing consultants to confine themselves to consulting practice'.[65] Other Associations were formed with similar intentions. One calling itself 'The General Practitioners' Union' gave evidence to the Parliamentary Select Committee on Metropolitan Hospitals during 1890–1893.[66] Another, 'The Incorporated Medical Practitioners' Association', wrote to the *BMJ* in 1896 complaining 'that it is undesirable for those holding honorary appointments to see patients for a fee at such charitable institutions'.[67] Judging by the reports referring to hospital abuse after this date, it does not seem as if the efforts of any of these associations were particularly effective and as Keir Waddington says, 'they invariably proved stillborn'.[68] However, the voluntary hospitals' trustees acknowledged the accusation that their charitable status was occasionally misused and responded by making more systematic use of hospital almoners to interrogate patients about their financial circumstances. This policy helped slow, though it did not stop, the rise in hospital outpatient usage by large sections of the community in the period leading up to the passing of the National Insurance Act. After 1913, the Act 'achieved something hospital doctors and general practitioners had not been able to do', according to Waddington, by reducing admissions and making outpatient departments serve a more consultative role.[69] Despairing of being able to prevent poor patients from using the provident dispensaries, some GPs concluded that they needed to take matters into their own hands. In 1889, the previously mentioned Dr Rentoul drew up proposals for a 'public medical service' based on the model offered by the hospital dispensaries, which he envisaged being state sponsored but run by GPs themselves.[70] The announcement of his proposals in the *BMJ* aroused great interest and a lively correspondence ensued, leading to debates at meetings in a number of BMA branches. Most doctors commenting felt the proposals impractical and some feared that they would lead to a reduction in levels of fees charged by GPs for their services.[71] The BMA established a committee to investigate the idea which submitted its findings for BMA branches to vote on later the same year. A clear majority rejected Rentoul's ideas as impractical, unnecessary, and undesirable. This rejection did nothing to stop the hospitals' incursions into the GPs' business nor the GPs' efforts to resist them, but the 'Rentoul plan' did succeed in stirring medical thinking about organised medical services and about a potential role for the state in curative medicine. This was a subject which others with a less protectionist motivation were to return to in earnest a few decades later.

The growing might of the friendly societies

Rentoul also thought that his plan would provide an antidote to the increasing power of the friendly societies. GPs' problems with friendly societies were not purely about remuneration. The doctors complained that, while robbing them of a sizeable proportion of their potential income, the societies undermined professional autonomy by requiring their contracted GPs to follow the rigid dictates of lay managing committees. Many commentators highlighted the fact that GPs strongly disliked lay control of their activities. A *BMJ* article in 1875 stated that a committee 'being wholly composed of working men, is not a pleasant master for an educated man to serve under'.[72] In 1895, the Manchester Medical Guild opined that 'it is neither necessary or desirable…that members of our profession…be permitted to become paid servants of a lay committee…or used as a source of profit by lay speculators in medical attendance'.[73] Some doctors complained of 'degrading bondage' as when a doctor's assistant offended a member of a miners' institute he had treated by declining to have a drink with him and was told: 'You're nowt but a servant, my b….. servant!'[74] James Mullin was another doctor offended by the way members of the colliery clubs treated their medical attendants. He wrote: 'I could only shape my feelings into unutterable maledictions, not on the tyrannical colliers, but on that man or body of men who first put the collier's foot on the neck of the doctor by introducing contract practice'.[75] For many doctors, however, the tyranny of club practice was compounded by the behaviour of club members. 'A surgeon' writing in the *BMJ* in 1896 opined that 'no patient is as exacting as a club patient'.[76] Another correspondent wrote of club practice in 1900 that the doctor's duty 'to the patient was apt to be forgotten in his indignation at being sweated by a hundred boorish taskmasters'.[77] One GP wrote to the *Lancet* citing numerous examples of insolence, disrespect, and discourtesy by club members and their officers, and a total disregard or advice given. This resulted in excessive consumption of medicines provided, he complained, stating, 'If objection was raised to an insult, you were immediately reminded that you were paid to do the work'.[78]

An attitude which irked the GPs greatly, and which continued under NHI, was the idea that they had a 'right' to send for the doctor even for trivial matters because 'they had paid for his services already'.[79] Members of colliery clubs were notorious for expressing this feeling. The GP James Mullin illustrates this graphically in his memoirs. He states that, when experiencing discomfort of the most trivial nature, the attitude of the colliers was to call for the doctor stating: 'why shouldn't he come and cure at once? Are we not his master, do we not keep the roof over him, the clothes on his back, feed his family and provide him with a horse when he ought to tramp around like the rest of us?'[80] GPs continued to complain also about the granting of benefits of club membership to the well to do who could afford private fees. In 1894, the BMA's Oxford branch complained that the Banbury Medical Aid Association solicited membership 'from high and low, rich and poor' for the same subscription and that their membership included 'the Mayor of Banbury and many others of like standing'.[81] Disdain was often not one-sided in this relationship. An early commentary on NHI noted that the hoped-for custom of the club members' families could not be relied on 'owing to the prevalent idea that the club doctor is an inferior sort of practitioner, and if attendance on the family is required for which an ordinary fee is to be paid 'a proper doctor' as they say, is often called in'.[82] E.S. Turner states that 'as an exercise in snobbery', friendly society members often called an outside doctor to attend their families on the grounds that 'the club doctor was not good enough'.[83] The low estimation of club doctors' services is testified by the comment by 'a surgeon' in the *BMJ* in 1896 that 'Working people judge that things that are cheap are invariably nasty'.[84]

Another of the GPs' complaints about club practice concerned the issue of certification for sickness benefit purposes. Doctors complained that this often brought them into conflict with both members and club committees.[85] They were criticised if they were too willing to accept the members' word and issued too many certificates, as this served to diminish the society's funds, but were likely to incur the hostility of influential committee members if they failed to issue them with certificates when requested.[86] Alfred Cox, the future BMA medical secretary, experienced this dilemma. He had received no complaints about his service, he reported, but after offending the secretary's brother-in-law 'by refusing to certify him for a slight ailment', he was dismissed when a vote to change doctor was taken by a meeting attended by only 30 out of 300 members.[87] Questionable certificates were sometimes issued however, for quite different reasons. Doctors sometimes colluded in certifying as sick elderly claimants for whom the boundaries between 'sickness', 'unemployment', and 'old age' were increasingly blurred.[88] Another contemporary noted that many men awaiting the outcome of applications under the Workmen's Compensation Act were advised by their lawyers to remain off sick and claim money from clubs on legal and not medical grounds.[89] Many GPs resented being forced to become members of the societies they were contracted to and the requirements of membership, such as being obliged to march in their annual parades. In 1900, a Surrey Doctor informed the *Lancet* that he had been dismissed as a medical officer of a small friendly society for challenging the 'customary' deduction of a membership fee from his remuneration.[90] Not all GPs found this such an imposition, however. The Derbyshire GP, Harry Pooler, wryly notes in his memoirs that he was 'two or three sorts of Oddfellow, the same number of Foresters, a Druid, a Loyal Caledonian Cork, a Royal Antediluvian Buffalo and…a Rechabite'.[91] The East End GP Harry Roberts was likewise bemused rather than irritated by his induction into the ancient order of Buffaloes with its 'ceremonial knocks; passwords; grips; regalia; drawn swords' and by having to pay court to its chief officer, who was a local dustman![92]

In 1895, the newly formed Manchester Medical Guild published a report on 'Provident Medical Aid'. It stated that the provident principle was in itself 'commendable' but that the methods of carrying it out were such as 'to incur the just opprobrium of the medical profession' for whom they had become 'grinding tyrannies'.[93] The guild's report is instructive in cataloguing the often-overlapping professional grievances.[94] Sick club rates in Manchester at that time were usually 3s per patient per annum but were often as low as 2s 6d. Repeating the now familiar complaint, the report regrets that 'the club doctor does not usually become the family doctor as well', suggesting that many wives and children used the free dispensaries instead. Sick club medical officer posts were thus regarded as 'underpaid offices'. The report concludes that rates offered by friendly society clubs were generally too low and offered recommended fees for treatment, pre-admission medicals, and sick notes. Duties should be standardised, it suggested, and, repeating a familiar complaint, friendly societies 'should relieve the attendance upon those whose pecuniary status renders them improper recipients at the club rate'.[95] The report then details objections to the provident dispensaries established in Manchester and Salford in 1875 which, in addition to those already mentioned, included 'unethical touting' for members by advertising and canvassing which destabilised other clubs such as those run by GPs themselves. The report concludes with a list conditions essential to professional recognition of provident schemes and dispensaries. In other parts of the country, however, provident schemes were beginning to coalesce into something altogether more threatening from the doctors' point of view.

Medical Aid Institutes, the GMC, and medical trade unionism

The last few decades of the nineteenth century saw a steady increase in friendly society membership. Estimates vary as to the total membership of friendly societies at this time, but the most recent and authoritative calculation suggests that there were 3,318,000 members in 1889–1891 rising to 7,884,000 in 1905.[96] These included trade union-run friendly societies or industry-specific Medical Aid Societies established by trade unions or taken over by them from employers. The most successful of these were those catering for miners, steelworkers, and railwaymen and their families. A number of commercial insurance companies also established provident-based Medical Aid Societies which were condemned by the profession for their habit of touting for customers and sweating their contracted medical attendants. In the 1890s, GPs' misgivings about contract practice were accentuated by the prevalence of medical institutes. These were set up by federations of friendly societies, trade unions, or insurance companies in specific localities and often employed whole-time salaried medical officers and ancillary staff to provide medical services for subscribers and, not infrequently, their dependents, from a central facility. This facility, usually known as a medical institute but sometimes called a dispensary, typically comprised consulting rooms and a pharmacy and often rudimentary operating and diagnostic facilities. The institutes were managed by, usually joint, committees of society or union members.[97] The first medical institute, the Preston Associated Friendly Societies Provident Dispensary, opened in January 1870 and was, according to Green, a response to the demands for better pay and conditions by local doctors through what the local friendly societies called the 'Preston medical trades union'.[98] However, the institutes were not, he says, merely an attempt to frustrate the doctors but were a considered response to the failings of the lodge system. Firstly, they addressed the issue of doctors not giving their best to club members, because of the competing demands of other clubs and private patients, by employing GPs and ancillary staff on whole-time contracts. Secondly, they overcame the increasing tendency of club doctors to prescribe rather than supply medicines, on the grounds that they were too expensive to be met from the members' capitation fees, by purchasing their drugs at wholesale prices and supplying them direct through their own dispensaries. Thirdly, they overcame the problem of dependants falling outside benefits of society membership by providing for the whole family through a single subscription.[99] In the 1870s, most medical institutes typically charged 8s per year for the whole family compared with the usual 3s 6d or 4s for the single member charged elsewhere. By 1877, medical institutes had been founded in Bradford, Derby, Newport, Nottingham, Worcester, and York.[100]

For many GPs, the medical institutes compounded the problems of club practice by further restricting competition. As with the poor law medical officers, it was alleged that posts were often offered to those willing to accept the lowest remuneration and that they were mercilessly 'sweated'. Some doctors working in them complained of an intolerable workload, one example noted in the *Lancet* being a single GP responsible for over 3,000 patients, sometimes attending well over a hundred patients a day.[101] In Northampton, three doctors were required to care for 14,369 patients.[102] Posts in medical institutes were nevertheless said to appeal to 'the humbler sort' of doctor who could not afford to buy or set up their own practices and would otherwise be condemned to the equally exacting servitude of an assistantship to another GP. One institute medical officer wrote to the *Lancet* claiming that, contrary to what many colleagues were saying, 'I find it a very pleasant and comfortable berth. I am not at all overworked'. He added that the profession would never succeed in preventing doctors from working in institutes, while 'the scandal' of GP principals earning £1,000 per annum but offering their assistants as little as £60–£70 per annum continued.[103] In a letter to the *Lancet* in 1892, another GP also disputed the claims of 'sweating' by critics of the institutes stating, 'We, Sirs, have escaped from the slavery, the hard work and bad pay which were ours as assistants to medical men, to comparative freedom, comparative ease and comparative affluence'.[104] As with PLMO appointments, younger doctors had fewer qualms about accepting salaried posts in the institutes. There is ample evidence of the extent of competition for these. At Worcester in 1871, for example, there were 30 candidates for a post paying £170 a year (with a house) and in 1905 the Lincoln Oddfellows had 22 applications for an annual salary of £240.[105] In 1879, the Friendly Societies Medical Alliance (FSMA) was established to promote the development of medical institutes. By 1883, there were 32 institutes and by 1898 about 40, with a total of 213,000 members and employing 75 medical officers.[106] Green alleges that GPs objected to the inclusion of women and children within the institutes' coverage and the establishment of 'juvenile clubs', fearing that these developments would lead to the demise of private practice.[107] However, against this it should be remembered that the clubs for women and children which many GPs ran were often a 'charitable exercise', given the frequency with which patients proved unable to keep up their subscriptions.[108] The altruistic Harry Roberts came up with a solution to overcome his East End patients' fears of incurring excessive bills by allowing them to purchase a weekly card entitling them to unlimited attendances and medicines.[109] As the *BMJ* pointed out in 1895, contract practice had in it 'an element of charity. It does not pay; the doctor cannot live on it alone'.[110] In an obvious dig at the institutes, the Manchester Medical Guild's report on Provident Medical Aid said that sick clubs 'are more truly representative of honest providence than any other scheme of organized provident medical aid met with in practice'.[111]

GPs also objected to the fact that the institutes, like the friendly societies generally, did not normally offer the patient a choice of doctor. Institutes usually employed a single medical officer but by the 1900s, most were allowed to employ one or more assistants, thereby offering members a 'limited choice' of doctor.[112] Some of these found themselves doing the lion's share of the work and greatly resented the cut of their remuneration made by their principal. An illustration of this, albeit from one of the medical institutes still operating after the advent of National Insurance, is provided by A.J. Cronin in his celebrated novel, *The Citadel*.[113] Many doctors came to believe that those who accepted club or institute posts with intolerable working conditions were guilty of 'infamous conduct in a professional respect' which deserved to be investigated and punished by the GMC.[114] In 1892, at the prompting of the Medical Defence Union, the GMC investigated a GP from Stourport Worcestershire who was accused of 'covering', that is conniving at provision of medical services by unqualified persons, through the Stourport Amalgamated Friendly Societies and Medical Aid Association. The accused was, however, let off with a caution.[115] The following year, a committee set up by the GMC submitted a critical report into medical institutes. It recommended that a medical practitioner should be deemed guilty of 'infamous conduct' if (a) they held an appointment whose duties were so onerous that they could not do justice to the sick under their care, (b) they issued certificates not justified on medical grounds, or (c) accepted employment by an association which employed canvassing to attract members.[116] However, the committee's report was not adopted. GPs suspected that this was because the GMC was largely made up of Consultant physicians and surgeons who had little interest in contract practice. Dr W.H. Rowthorn wrote to the *BMJ* in 1900 complaining of the GMC's 'dog in the manger' attitude stating, 'So long as the GMC is composed of professors and consultants the general practitioner will have to wait in vain for anything of a really beneficial nature'.[117] The editor of the *Lancet* agreed, noting that 'it happens that those who have few or no grievances are exactly those who would have most influence in obtaining redress'.[118]

In 1895, Dr Leslie Phillips, the Secretary of the Medical Defence Union, sent a memorial to the GMC in which he condemned the 'sweating' of medical men by Medical Aid Societies as 'a serious danger to the welfare of the public and the profession'.[119] In 1897, a number of individuals and associations lobbied the

GMC to launch a further investigation into the way Medical Aid Societies and institutes operated, one of which was from 'the medical men of Norwich' requesting the GMC's views on its dispute with the Norwich Medical Institute.[120] The GPs argued that the conditions of service were 'detrimental to the public and derogatory to the profession' and therefore considered it unprofessional for any medical man to be associated with the institute which, the GPs also argued, constituted a 'trading body' making profits which were invested in real estate.[121] The GMC again declined to act but appointed a subcommittee which spent two years consulting with aggrieved GPs and the friendly societies about contract practice. It concluded that the principal point of contention was remuneration, subdivided into related grievances about the inclusion, as members, of women and children, and of individuals wealthy enough to pay directly for their own care.[122] The outcome was a proposal to establish a 'conciliation board consisting of representatives from both sides 'to discuss and, if possible, determine, the points at issue'.[123] This never met, however. According to Green, this was because 'the BMA kept dragging its feet'. But when the BMA did meet a delegation from the friendly societies in 1909, no agreement could be reached on the sticking point of a wage limit because, he admits, the societies 'disliked the idea intensely'.[124]

Discussion of means to tackle the abuses by which GPs considered themselves to be beset frequently turned to the tactics adopted by trade unions. Andrew Morrice notes that the success of British trade unions in improving their members wages and working conditions was not lost on the GPs who attended those workers.[125] Trade union tactics were plainly employed in the dispute in Cork in southern Ireland in 1894 where, in response to an organised boycott by a local medical association, the local friendly societies brought in 'scab' medical labour to break the 'strike'.[126] The setting up of a defence fund to support those who had been dismissed offered a precedent for later action by the BMA, and in the journals, doctors openly referred to those failing to heed the call to solidarity as 'blacklegs' and 'strike breakers'.[127] In a letter to the *BMJ* in 1896, Dr James Dalgleish praised the Lincoln GPs who had stood firm against the efforts of those seeking to subvert the boycott of friendly society posts ending that he hoped 'the men of Lincoln will show no white feather'.[128] Alfred Cox explained that when setting up a local GP association in Gateshead, 'I had become friendly with some of my patients who were keen trade unionists and I wondered why we should not adopt some of their methods'.[129] The association he founded in 1898 with 15 fellow GPs was active until 'the BMA came alive' in 1902. It managed to raise the minimum fee for midwifery and negotiate a fee of 3s 6d as the minimum friendly society per annum payment in place of the 'Dutch auction' which had previously taken place. Cox continued his crusade to improve the lot of local GPs when he became the Honorary Secretary of the BMA's Gateshead division, at which time he received 'some useful tips' for his organisational work from his 'trade union friends'.[130] Cox was not alone in his efforts to improve GPs' circumstances, but his success led him to be invited to assist in other areas. Edward Jepson, who helped found the Durham County Medical Union with the intention of improving the lot of the colliery doctors, made Cox an honorary organiser.[131] Together, they gradually 'wore down the opposition', forcing the miners, who at that time were enjoying an unprecedented level of prosperity, to increase the doctor's pay to 9d per patient per fortnight.[132] Writing in the *Manchester Guild Quarterly* in 1899, Dr Jepson criticised those 'low types' who 'do not think it wrong to take advantage of a dispute' and take away a fellow GP's post. The Northern Medical Unions had therefore established a new disciplinary system, he reported, whereby cases of 'blacklegging…will be tried and investigated' by a 'judicial committee' involving Consultants and anyone found guilty 'will be boycotted by the whole profession'.[133] Cox then helped form the Northumberland Medical Union of which he became the Honorary Secretary.[134] His association was hailed as an example to others by the *Lancet*'s deputy editor, Squire Sprigge.[135]

Although these tactics had been employed at various times and places in Britain and Ireland prior to 1900, militants within the GP community were also inspired by continental examples. In the first of his celebrated series of articles in the *Lancet* under the heading 'The battle of the clubs', Adolphe Smith reported on a strike by doctors in Brussels in 1895 organised by the *Syndicat Médicale* in which would-be strike breakers were deterred by ostracisation.[136] The actions of the strikers were, Smith notes, supported by socialists and local trade unionists. In 1900, H.N. Hardy wrote expectantly of the first International Congress of Medical Ethics taking place in Paris that year which would deal with questions of relations between medical men and the state 'or other collectivities such as clubs and dispensaries, *on the best trade-union lines*' (emphasis added).[137] It was Germany, however, that offered the best illustration of what doctors could achieve when they were prepared to stand together and adopt trade union tactics. The most powerful doctors' trade union, which had started in Leipzig and was therefore known colloquially as the *Leipziger Verband*, had by 1911 a membership of 95% of German medical practitioners and successfully coordinated strikes and boycotts of local sickness insurance societies (*Krankenkassen*) across the country. Between 1910 and 1911, there were said to have been 1,022 conflicts between doctors and the sickness insurance societies in Germany of which 921 were allegedly decided in the doctors' favour.[138] The union, also known as the *Hartmannbund*, after its founder, Dr Herman Hartmann, was by then confident of obtaining state approval of the principle of the patient's free choice of doctor.[139] The President of the BMA applauded their success in his address to the Association's annual meeting in 1911.[140]

By 1900, there were a plethora of ethical or political organisations representing GP interests in Britain, some national, some local. In addition to the two medical defence societies which had been formed in the 1880s, the Medical Defence Union and the London and Counties Medical Protection Society, there were two national bodies campaigning against hospital 'abuses', and nearly 30 local 'ethical and medical defence associations' and 'guilds'. There was also a national Colliery Surgeons Association, a Police Surgeons Association, and a Poor Law Medical Officers Association.[141] To these must be added the seven regional federations established to represent women doctors which subsequently coalesced into the Northern Association of Women Doctors and the Association of Registered Medical Women.[142] For Alfred Cox, 'The multiplicity of organisations was bad' and underlined the need for to concentrate the GPs efforts under one strong body.[143] Cox's preference was for the BMA but when he helped form associations in the northeast of England, the BMA seemed reluctant to involve itself in local disputes and completely eschewed any notion of becoming a trade union for doctors. The specialist physician Herbert Woodcock recognised that district associations like that formed by Cox and Jepson were meeting an urgent need not met by the unwieldy BMA branch structure, commenting: 'Somehow the BMA cannot get close hold of the districts and these local associations can'.[144] While expressing hopes for what the reform of the BMA's branch structure could achieve, the *Lancet's* deputy editor, Samuel Squire Sprigge, observed that 'much of the work of protecting the practitioner from the effect of unfair competition has fallen on local organisations'.[145] H.N. Hardy made the case for the BMA becoming a trade union but claims that the idea was, for the Tory-inclined majority of the BMA's Council, the proverbial 'red rag to a bull'.[146] He was at pains, however, to differentiate that form of trade unionism characterised by 'tyrannical oppression of workmen' by unscrupulous and self-serving officials 'which should be avoided by all honourable men', from the more beneficial kind of combination demonstrated successfully, he opined, in the dispute in Cork. Hardy felt inspired by European examples such as the formation of a medical ethical society in France, stating, 'The leaders of the BMA will, doubtless, learn some instructive lessons from countries in which the principles of trade unionism have been carried out by medical societies for years'.[147] Squire Sprigge reflected the conventional view, however, when stating that what was needed was 'medical combination in an intelligent form, a professional union based on the public needs and not a trade union directed towards the amelioration of a class against the community'.[148]

Among the evidence that many GPs were inclined towards trade unionism at this time are glowing references made by some GPs to the National Union of Teachers (NUT). In his presidential address to the Lancashire and Cheshire Branch of the BMA in 1897, Dr Samuel Woodcock described them as an 'admirable example of what may be accomplished by efficient local organisation'.[149] In the introduction to the report of the Manchester conference of medical organisations in 1900, the NUT is held up as an example of what GPs should aspire to. Formed only in 1870, the NUT had a membership comprising 90% of elementary school teachers paying an annual subscription which was one third that of the BMA. It was 'always consulted by the government on any question of importance bearing on education and had two representatives (sic) in parliament'. In 1900, it had 430 branches with an aggregate membership of 40,000.[150] 'The problem with the medical profession', the author of the introduction opines, is that 'it does not contain men as business-like and as devoted to the its interests as the teachers have shown themselves to be in theirs'.[151] The key to the NUT's success was said to lay in having 'active branches and a proper system of delegation and accountability with an annual conference as ultimate arbiters of policy'.[152] This was a message not lost on those seeking to reform the BMA.

The Manchester conference, the BMA, and the report on contract medical practice

While bemoaning the proliferation of medical bodies representing GPs, there was, Cox notes, 'a growing desire among these bodies for some kind of national action'.[153] The cry was taken up by the Manchester Medical Guild, when it convened a conference of like-minded organisations in 1900. The Guild had been established in 1895.[154] Its objectives were not purely to bring about improvements in its members' remuneration and working conditions but also to promote 'cooperation for the common good' and 'guide medical opinion on all matters affecting the profession'.[155] The Guild worked closely with the Manchester Medical Ethical society to produce a joint report containing a medical fees tariff.[156] From this and subsequent annual reports in the early 1900s, it appears that the Guild was determined to enforce adherence to its recommended minima by what they called the 'club pledge', the first mention of which occurs in their annual report in 1903.[157]Although the idea of practitioners signing written undertakings to support collective bargaining had by this time a long history, the prestige of the Manchester Guild and its ability to self-publicise through its own quarterly journal may have served to reinforce the idea of pledges in the minds of many within the profession, and thereby influence the thinking of those behind the pledges of non-cooperation with the National Insurance Act collected by the BMA in 1912.

The three-day conference took place during 1–3 May 1900 in the Memorial Hall, Albert Square, Manchester.[158] All medical societies and BMA branches in England and Wales were invited to send representatives and 35 organisations did so, including six BMA branches.[159] When it convened, the emergence of a rival body to the BMA 'appeared to be on the cards'.[160] Writing to the *BMJ* in the lead up to the conference, the Manchester Guild's secretary, Samuel Crawshaw, wrote that it would take too long to reform the BMA in the way the GPs wanted. Moreover, as currently constituted, the Association was unrepresentative of the profession as its meetings were dominated by Consultants, he said; it was undemocratic in its decision-making, and ineffective in influencing policy.[161] Crawshaw was careful to praise the BMA for its contribution to the development of medicine and to the charge that the BMA was yet capable of becoming an effective medical trade union he wrote that to do so 'would assuredly destroy it for scientific work, for it is evident that the majority of the men who have made it successful as a scientific body, that is the consultants, would at once be excluded'.[162] The conference began, however, with a report on the Medical Acts and their shortcomings by a Consultant member of BMA council who was sympathetic to the GPs' calls for reform, Mr Victor Horsley.[163] Later, Mr R.B. Anderson of the Corporate and Medical Reform Association read a paper on 'medical polity' in which he condemned the Royal Colleges, the BMA, and the GMC as 'medical oligarchies' which had failed to serve the interests of the profession. The 'new polity', he said, must 'render the profession self-governing and place the profession in a more proper rank in the state and in better relations with the government'.[164] On the third day of the conference, debate on medical organisation began in earnest when Dr Crawshaw proposed that 'no scheme of medical organisation can be considered satisfactory' unless it provided machinery comprising local district associations formed to discuss medical ethical or medico-political topics to which all practitioners in the locality had the right to belong; an annual conference of delegates of those associations; and a central executive nominated and elected annually by those local associations.[165] Crawshaw explained that the local associations should cover so small an area that 'every member would find no difficulty in getting to the meetings after his day's work was done'.[166] The present BMA branches, he said, were too large and unwieldy. For example, the Lancashire and Cheshire branch was 100 miles long and 50 miles wide, so attendance involved the loss of a day's work for some practitioners.

The debate reached its climax in the afternoon session when Dr Garrett Horder of Cardiff proposed that the conference appoint a 'provisional committee' to carry out its decisions and that it be instructed to request the BMA to organise a permanent 'ethical department', failing which it was to encourage the principal organisations committed to more effectively represent the GPs to amalgamate or form an entirely new representative organisation.[167] During the debate, however, some of the leading lights of the independent associations declared that their energies would be better directed towards 'capturing' the BMA.[168] Alfred Cox was one of these and his intervention proved decisive. Decrying the multiplication of associations, he argued that, although it urgently needed reformation, beginning with its branch structure, the BMA was the 'proper body to undertake the work'. He stated that, 'The Association had existed for 60 years and had obtained a position of importance which ought not to be thrown away'.[169] He therefore proposed a new resolution calling on all local medical organisations to convert the BMA Council into 'an energetic body really representative of the majority of members'.[170] The resolution was passed but many GPs were sceptical, Cox noted, including one who had made a name for himself at the conference, James Smith Whitaker, the founder of the Great Yarmouth Practitioners Association and who was not then a BMA member. However, he agreed to serve with Jepson and Cox on the provisional committee which was to negotiate with the BMA.[171]

Although the *BMJ* made no announcements regarding any of these events, it was clear that many in the BMA recognised how close they had come to facing a new and effective rival for their GP membership. An extraordinary general meeting of the Association was consequently held in London on 18 July to consider proposals for an amended constitution and more considered proposals presented for debate at the subsequent Representative Meeting in Ipswich.[172] An invitation was meanwhile extended to the provisional committee established at the Manchester conference to meet with BMA Council during that meeting. Cox notes that, 'We had an unexpectedly favourable reception…with the result that a constitutional committee was appointed with full power to make recommendations about the constitution of the Association'.[173] Half of the committee was nominated by the Council but included internal proponents of reform like Horsley, and the other half included external critics like Cox and Whitaker, who soon impressed with his skills as a 'draftsman and conciliator'.[174] Several of the provisions recommended by the committee and adopted at the BMA's annual meeting in Cheltenham in 1901 were 'lifted' from the Guild conference resolutions.[175] In particular, the primary unit of local organisation in the Association would henceforward be 'divisions' of similar size to parliamentary constituencies and whose meetings were likely to be better attended than those of branches, which were thereafter more like regional committees of divisions.[176] The divisions would send representatives to an annual meeting of the Association, thereafter renamed the Annual Representative Meeting (ARM) which would serve as the parliament of the Association, determine BMA policy, and hold the Council, as the BMA's executive, to account. Council members could attend and speak at the Representatives' meeting but were prevented from voting and the Council were duty bound to comply with any resolution passed by a two-thirds majority.[177] These proposals were passed with few objections by a meeting attended by over 800 members, the few dissenting voices expressing the familiar fear that the BMA was becoming more like a trade union.[178] The *Lancet* opined that 'disaster was averted', and 'the threat of the guilds' had been 'repulsed'.[179] But this was largely because the BMA had adopted many of their ideas.[180] Another factor was the BMA's decision to neutralise the influence of some of its more effective critics, that is Whitaker and Cox, by making them into 'BMA men'. Whitaker was appointed the BMA's first medical Secretary in 1902 and Cox became his deputy in 1908.[181]

One of Whitaker's main tasks was to take charge of all committees dealing with medical political and organisational affairs.[182] He immediately set about establishing a Central Ethical Committee.[183] This committee made it a priority to establish 'ethical rules' which the new divisions, acting as what Squire Sprigge later described as 'courts of honour', could attempt to regulate professional behaviour and punish 'infamous conduct'.[184] 'Courts of honour' were an established feature of medical practice in Prussia in the late nineteenth century and were given state sanction by the 'Honour Court law' of 1899.[185] Many British doctors hoped for something similar to be established, including H.N. Hardy who stated in 1900 that 'A court of medical ethics of some sort is badly needed in the profession'.[186] In practice, the divisions' response to the 'unethical' behaviour on which they passed judgement involved boycotting of designated friendly society and medical institute posts and ostracising those who ignored the boycott and applied for them. In 1900, the *BMJ* had begun to publish 'warning notices' against taking such appointments. These were successfully applied in Durham, Gateshead, Walsall, and Rotherham.[187] They became more regular after 1905, when the Central Ethical Committee's model rules were approved at the ARM in Bradford and were thereafter referred to as the 'Bradford Rules'.[188] The list of posts deemed worthy of such condemnation was determined by the newly established Contract Practice Subcommittee and referred to colloquially as the 'blacklist'. Blacklisted advertisements were accompanied by the injunction 'Consult the secretary of the local BMA Division before applying' or similar wording.[189] The *BMJ* and the *Lancet* continued to print letters from irate GPs, however, about the abuses of club practice and the insidious growth of medical institutes and a *BMJ* editorial in 1903 noted continuing difficulties with clubs and Institutes in Sheerness and Birmingham.[190] Shortly after therefore the Representative Meeting asked the Association's Medico Political Committee to investigate club abuses and in 1904, it issued 12,000 questionnaires as part of an inquiry into contract practice.[191] The report of the inquiry was published in the *BMJ* in July 1905.[192]

The value of the report's conclusions must be qualified by the limited number of responses on which it is based. Only 13% responded and only 856 of the 1,548 respondents were actually engaged in contract practice at that time.[193] The report nevertheless captures the feelings of many GPs and is consistent with the correspondence which had appeared in both professional journals over several years. It reflected both the minority who had positive things to say about club practice and the majority who did not. The report cited many examples of 'sweating' by friendly societies and their Institutes and abuse by patients. For example, a man who made £30,000 on the sale of public house paid his doctor 1d a week. Another doctor wrote, 'I pay the railway porter one shilling for bringing up a parcel to the house; he pays his doctor a shilling a month for his family and himself'. A London doctor complained of being driven out of his home by tipsy members of one of his clubs. His neighbour helped 'somewhat roughly' to clear them out but in consequence the doctor was forced to resign from his post. However, a South London doctor noted, 'I never had anything but the most cordial relations with any of my clubs'.[194] The report showed that 24% of clubs paid less than 4s per annum, 52% between 4 and 5s, and 24% over 5s per patient per annum. It revealed that 82% of GPs' own clubs included all family members and 90% included juveniles from birth, whereas only 5% of friendly societies admitted families and 69% juveniles between the ages of one and six years old. Interestingly, however, only 53.5% of respondents considered their remuneration from club practice inadequate.[195]

Meanwhile, an opportunity arose for the BMA to flex its newly developed muscles in defence of its GP members in the case of a dispute in South Wales with the Miners' Medical Aid Association in Ebbw Vale. Like many of the miners works clubs originally run by mine owners and managers, responsibility for this scheme had recently been devolved to a workmen's committee which in 1905 unilaterally changed their medical officers' contracts from a capitation to a salaried basis. When the doctors subsequently refused an instruction to relinquish their rights to private practice, the doctors were dismissed and replaced by 'blacklegs'.[196] The case quickly became an ideological battleground for the BMA over the extent of lay control of medical practice in which the Association sought to mobilise the whole profession.[197] Attempts to resolve the dispute through mediation by the local MP failed. A temporary truce was agreed by which the dismissed doctors were able to resume their posts but the dispute rumbled on, heightened to some extent by the advent of National Health Insurance, until 1915.[198] Some doctors had become convinced that the best way to counter the spread of medical institutes was to set up similar services run by the doctors themselves but, crucially, offering the patients a genuine free choice of doctor. The first of these, adopting the title 'Public Medical Service' (PMS) popularised by the 'Rentoul plan' in the 1880s, opened in Coventry in 1893 in response to the threat posed by the Coventry provident dispensary. It became a model for several others which were to follow.[199] Concern at the threat posed by both medical institutes and provident dispensaries prompted the BMA's Medico Political Committee to instruct its Contract Practice Subcommittee to draw up a model PMS scheme. This followed recommendations included in its Contract Practice report in 1905.[200] The model was developed, taking account of examples of district-wide schemes run by GPs themselves such as those operating at that time in Coventry and Hampstead.[201] The objective was to provide for workers and their families below a defined income limit a comprehensive family medical service offering a range of benefits similar to those being offered by the Institutes and Dispensaries. Significantly, however, the professional schemes would be open to all qualified local doctors and would therefore offer the subscriber free choice of doctor.[202] The PMS would be administered by committees of local doctors and made no provision for lay involvement in their management. It was thus an example of medical paternalism in its purest and most unapologetic form. The BMA spent several years refining the model scheme. It hoped that it would eventually be taken up by doctors across the country, thereby replacing, without the need for compulsion, all existing club contractual arrangements, which would inevitably look inadequate by comparison.

The BMA was given a new impetus to develop such a model by the Royal Commission of inquiry into the poor law when it delivered its report in 1909.[203] The BMA was equally alarmed by both the majority and the dissenting minority reports.[204] The majority report recommended *inter alia* an extension of existing friendly society club practice. The minority report's proposal for 'straightening out the tangle' of overlapping and uncoordinated medical services, however, was a state-controlled, non-contributory scheme administered through local government agencies. It was to be available to all citizens below an accepted income limit and delivered by salaried doctors.[205] While the majority report's recommendation was unwelcome to the GPs, the minority's proposals would have represented the end of both clubs and the provident or insurance principle and would have severely restricted GPs' private practice. A minority of doctors welcomed the idea of salaried state medical service, but most saw it as a major threat to their cherished goal of professional autonomy.[206] As it continued its efforts to develop its own scheme, the BMA responded to the Commission reports by stating some principles on which they believed any future state-funded service should be based, which it repeated during subsequent negotiations with the Liberal Government over National Insurance. These were that medical services rendered on behalf of the state should be paid for by the state; payment should be adequate and in accordance with the professional service required; and there should be adequate medical representation on all committees formed to control state medical provision.[207] As it happened, the proposals which emerged in the National Insurance Bill owed very little to the inquiry reports and took the debate about medical services for the poor in an entirely unexpected direction.[208]

Conclusion

By the end of the nineteenth century, GPs had achieved a measure of social acceptance if not respectability but a great many of them remained financially insecure. According to the editor of *The Spectator,* writing in December 1911, 'The profession of medicine in this country is unfortunately one which, as a whole, is distinctly ill paid. Of the general condition of the profession, it is scarcely too much to say that it is hard and precarious'.[209] Before the advent of the National Insurance Act in 1911, one-fifth of GPs were struggling to achieve a viable income.[210] This precariousness is evidenced by the establishment of a number of Medical Benevolent Societies aimed at the financial relief of doctors and their families who had fallen on hard times. H.N. Hardy notes in 1900 that 'the London societies' received 450–500 requests for relief each year and thus could not satisfy every request 'even for doles of £5 or £10 a year'.[211] Even critics of the profession agreed that this was not in the public interest. George Bernard Shaw commented that the ills of the medical profession arose from 'the doctor's position as a competitive private tradesman, that is out of poverty and dependence' and concluded that 'There is nothing more dangerous than a poor doctor'.[212] Fearing that their hopes of financial security and gentility were being jeopardised by the 'unethical' behaviour of a (largely impoverished) minority of doctors, an increasing number of GPs at the end of the nineteenth century began to adopt trade union-like tactics in defence of their collective interests. These tactics served to enforce the professional solidarity on which success in collective bargaining depended, and thus secure their professional autonomy and protect their individual freedom to deliver a proper standard of care to patients.

For those engaged in contract practice, this freedom was threatened by an intolerable workload, inadequate remuneration, and lay supervisory interference, all of which they believed were accentuated by the expanding power of the Medical Aid Societies. The desired alternative was a PMS run in each district by the doctors themselves. The BMA's reluctance to become a trade union owed much to the distaste which the grandees on its Council still had for any association between medicine and trade. Some of their number clung to an idealistic notion of medicine as a selfless, noble, and gentlemanly calling, seemingly above party politics, whereas others, embracing a Conservative ideology, viewed the idea of organised labour with alarm. Most of the medical elite of the BMA were, however, disinterested in the plight of the humble GP until the threatened emergence of a rival organisation, heralded by the Manchester conference in 1900, forced them to heed their GP members' complaints.

The reform of the BMA which this threat instigated rendered the Association better able to assert itself in the conflict that was to come over National Insurance. That conflict nevertheless served to underline how much the interests of GPs as a group differed from other parts of the medical profession and thereby kept alive the dream of a separate national body to represent GPs. The BMA was determined to create, through PMS, a means of delivering medical services to the working class which was as good as anything offered by the detested medical institutes but, crucially, under the control of the doctors themselves. The BMA's scheme relied on acceptance by the profession of a structure built around local committees of doctors. The BMA accepted that these committees should represent all local doctors not just members of the Association because the authors of the scheme maintained, 'The principle of collective bargaining of the profession must…be maintained at all costs'.[213] These committees would, *inter alia*, represent the 'courts of honour' which Sprigge, Hardy, and other commentators, inspired by German and other continental examples, felt were needed to inhibit the untoward effects of 'unethical' behaviour caused by unregulated competition. The Report of the Royal Commission on the Poor Law added emphasis to the need to finalise such a scheme. But the government's National Insurance Bill introduced in 1911 with its scheme for National Health Insurance took the profession somewhat by surprise. It represented an entirely new departure and posed an important question for the medical profession. They had to determine if what it offered was an opportunity, or a threat.

Notes

1 Irvine Loudon, *Medical Care and The General Practitioner, 1750–1850* (Oxford, 1986). p. 258. See also See Jacqueline Jenkinson, 'A 'Crutch to Assist in Gaining an Honest Living': Dispensary Shopkeeping by Scottish General Practitioners and the Responses of the Medical Elite, 1852 – 1911.' *The Bulletin of the Society for the Social History of Medicine*, 86 (1) (2012). pp. 1–36.

2 M. Jeanne Peterson, *The Medical Profession in Mid-Victorian London* (London, 1978). p. 215.

3 Anne Digby, *The Evolution of British General Practice, 1850–1948* (Oxford, 1999). p. 34.

4 Loudon, *Medical Care and the General Practitioner,* pp. 280–299. Peterson, *The Medical Profession in Mid-Victorian London,* pp. 135, 287. David B. Green, *Working Class Patients and the Medical Establishment: Self-Help in Britain from the Mid-Nineteenth Century to 1948* (Aldershot, 1985). pp. 15–21. For contemporaries' accounts, see Horatio Nelson Hardy, *The State of the Medical Profession in Great Britain and Ireland in 1900* (Dublin, 1901). pp. 29–31 and Alfred Cox, *Among the Doctors* (London, c.1949). pp. 57–60 and 71–77.

5 Loudon, *Medical Care and The General Practitioner*, p. 251.

6 This was enacted via the *Act for the Encouragement and Relief of Friendly Societies, 1793.* See Cosma Corsi, 'The Political Economy of Inclusion: The Rise and Fall of the Workhouse System.' *Journal of the History of Economic Thought,* 39 (4) (2017). pp. 466–474.

7 Martin Gorsky. 'Friendly Society Health Insurance in Nineteenth Century England', in Martin Gorsky and Sally Sheard (eds) *Financing Medicine: The British Experience since 1750* (Abingdon, 2006). ch.9. pp. 150–152.

8 Bernard Harris, 'Social Policy by Other Means? Mutual Aid and the Origins of the Welfare State in Britain during the Nineteenth and Twentieth Centuries.' *Journal of Policy History,* 30 (2) (2018). p. 205.

9 Gorsky 'Friendly Society Health Insurance in Nineteenth Century England,' p. 154.

10 *Ibid.,* p. 156.

11 See BMA Contract Practice Report, 'An Investigation into the Economic Conditions of Contract Medical Practice in the United Kingdom.' *BMJ,* 22 July 1905, Supplement, pp. 1–96.

12 *Lancet,* 22 January 1870, p. 126.

13 See Sidney and Beatrice Webb, *The State and the Doctor* (London, 1910). p. 138.

14 Cox, *Among the Doctors*, p. 56.

15 For an illustration of the doctors' problem with bad debts, see the *Lancet*, 18 February 1871, p. 239.

16 Gorsky, 'Friendly Society Health Insurance in Nineteenth Century England', p. 155.

17 Green, *Working-Class Patients and the Medical Establishment*, pp. 117–118.

18 *Ibid.,* pp. 75 and 28.

19 James C. Riley, *Sick not Dead: The Health of British Working Men During the Mortality Decline* (London, 1997). p. 49.

20 Sidney and Beatrice Webb, *The State and the Doctor,* pp. 140–141.

21 *BMJ*, 23 March 1895, pp. 657–658.

22 Green, *Working-Class Patients and the Medical Establishment,* p. 16.

23 *Lancet,* 11 October 1851, 'Vigilans' p. 359. Loudon, *Medical Care and the General Practitioner 1750–1850,* p. 258; Rosemary Stevens, *Medical Practice in Modern England: The Impact of Specialization and State Medicine* (New Haven, CT, 1966). p. 215.

24 Ernest Muirhead Little, *History of the British Medical Association 1832–1932* (London, 1932). p. 200.

25 Green, *Working-Class Patients and the Medical Establishment,* p. 20.

26 *Ibid.,* p. 15.

27 *Ibid.*

28 *BMJ*, 8 Feb 1868, p. 128.

29 *Ibid.*, 11 July 1868, 'The Sick Club Movement', p. 32. *Lancet*, 6 June 1868, 'The Profession in Southampton and the Club Question', p. 735; 8 August 1868, 'The Sick Club Question', p. 189.
30 *BMJ*, 11 July 1868, 'The Sick Club Movement', p. 32.
31 Green, *Working-Class Patients and the Medical Establishment*, p. 16.
32 Digby, *The Evolution of British General Practice*, pp. 96–97.
33 *BMJ*, 17 August 1867, 'A Poor Club Doctor', pp. 139–140.
34 Little, *History of the British Medical Association 1832–1932*, p. 200.
35 *Manchester University Medical Collections*, MMC 7/2/8.
36 A.S. (Arthur Strettel) Comyns Carr, W.H. (William Hubert) Stuart-Garnett, and J. H. (James Henry). Taylor, *National Insurance* (London, 1912). p. 75. Noel Parry and Jose Parry, *The Rise of the Medical* Profession: *A Study of Collective Social Mobility* (London, 1976). pp. 149–150.
37 Parry and Parry, *The Rise of the Medical Profession*', p. 149.
38 *Ibid.*, p. 150.
39 *BMJ*, 29 August 1936, T.A. Goodfellow, 'Medical Ethics', Supplement, p. 146.
40 For 'Courts of honour' see Samuel Squire Sprigge, *Medicine and the Public* (London, 1905), p. 234, and Hardy, *The State of the Medical Profession in Great Britain and Ireland in 1900*, p. 72.
41 Digby, *The Evolution of British General Practice*, p. 30.
42 *Ibid.*
43 *Ibid.*, p. 32.
44 *Ibid*, p. 101.
45 Francis Brett Young, *Dr Bradley Remembers* (London, 1938). p. 547.
46 Frank G. Layton, *The Old Doctor* (Birmingham, 1923). p. 10.
47 *Ibid.*, p. 17.
48 Cox, *Among the Doctors*, p. 30.
49 *Ibid.*, p. 57. See also E.S. (Ernest Sackville) Turner, *Call the Doctor: A Social History of Medical Men* (London, 1958). p. 251.
50 David B. Green, 'Medical Care in Britain before the Welfare State.' *Critical Review*, 7 (4) (1993). pp. 480–481.
51 Loudon, *Medical Care and the General Practitioner*, p. 222.
52 Hardy, *The State of the Medical Profession in Great Britain and Ireland in 1900*, p. 21.
53 *Ibid.*
54 Stevens, *Medical Practice in Modern England*, p. 32.
55 *BMJ*, 10 August 1872, 'Medical fees', p. 170.
56 Keir Waddington, 'Unsuitable Patients: The Debate Over Outpatient Admissions, the Medical Profession and the Late Victorian Hospitals.' *Medical History*, 42 (1998). p. 28.
57 Peterson, *The Medical Profession in Mid-Victorian London*, p. 228.
58 *Ibid.*, p. 258.
59 *Ibid.*, p. 272.
60 *BMJ*, 10 July 1886, 'Consultants and Practitioners', letter from Dr R. Rentoul, p. 89.
61 Loudon, *Medical Care and the General Practitioner*, p. 252.
62 *Lancet*, 4 July 1896, 'History of Coventry Public Medical Service', Letter from Dr Edward Phillips, pp. 56–57.
63 See, for example, the letter from Dr W. Strange, *BMJ*, 3 August 1889, p. 286.
64 Brian Abel-Smith, *The Hospitals 1800–1948: A Study in Social Administration in England and Wales* (London, 1964). p. 162.
65 *BMJ*, 12 June 1886, p. 1114 and 18 December 1886, p. 1190.
66 Second report para. 25517 (quoted in Abel Smith, *The Hospitals*, p. 166).

67 *BMJ*, 31 October 1896, p. 1350.
68 Waddington, 'Unsuitable Patients', p. 38.
69 *Ibid.*, p. 46.
70 *BMJ*, 9 November 1889, 'Hospital Dispensary and Outpatient Reform', pp. 1067–1069.
71 *Ibid.*, 28 September 1889, pp. 742–743; 29 June 1889, p. 1495, and 28 November 1889, p. 1194.
72 *Ibid.*, 10 April 1875, p. 484.
73 *Manchester University Medical Collections*, MMC/7/4/3/1, 'Provident Medical Aid', Report by the Manchester Medical Guild 1895, p. 9.
74 *BMJ*, 2 January 1909, p. 68.
75 James Mullin, *The Story of a Toiler's Life* (Dublin, 1921) UCD edn, 2000, p. 152.
76 *Ibid.*, 22 February 1896, pp. 489–490.
77 *BMJ* 32 March 1900, 'Scapula', p. 816.
78 *Lancet*, 30 January 1886, 'Fairplay', p. 235.
79 Turner, *Call the Doctor*, p. 250.
80 Mullin, *The Story of a Toiler's Life*, p. 152.
81 Peter Bartrip, *Themselves Writ Large: The British Medical Association, 1832–1966* (London, 1996). p. 136.
82 Comyns Carr, *National Insurance*, p. 56.
83 Turner, *Call the Doctor*, p. 251.
84 *BMJ*, 22 February 1896, pp. 489–490.
85 Green, *Working-Class Patients and the Medical Establishment*, p. 18.
86 *Ibid.*
87 Douglass W. Orr and Jean Walker Orr, *Health Insurance with Medical Care: The British Experience* (New York, 1938). p. 168.
88 John MacNicol, *The Politics of Retirement in Britain, 1878–1948* (Cambridge, 1998). pp. 129–131.
89 Herbert De Carle Woodcock, *The Doctor and the People* (London, 1912). p. 84.
90 *Lancet*, 3 March 1900, Dr C. Scott-Watson, p. 654.
91 Harry W. Pooler, *My Life in General Practice* (London, 1948). p. 484.
92 Winifred Stamp, *Doctor Himself: An Unorthodox Biography of Harry Roberts MD* (London, 1949). pp. 74–75.
93 *Manchester University Medical Collections* MMC/7/4/3/1, 'Provident Medical Aid', Report by the Manchester Medical Guild 1895, p. 2.
94 *Ibid.*, pp. 3–4.
95 *Ibid.*, p. 4.
96 Bernard Harris 'Social Policy by Other Means? Mutual Aid and the Origins of the Welfare State in Britain during the Nineteenth and Twentieth Centuries.' *Journal of Policy History*, 30 (2) (2018). p. 222 (table 3).
97 *BMJ*, Letter from Friendly Society Medical Officer, 7 December 1889, p. 1209.
98 Green, *Working-Class Patients and the Medical Establishment*, p. 21. See also Simon Cordery, *British Friendly Societies 1750–1914* (Basingstoke, 2003). p. 155.
99 Green, *Working-Class Patients and the Medical Establishment*, p. 22.
100 *Ibid.* p. 23.
101 *Lancet*, 'The Medical Work of Friendly Societies', 7 December 1889, p. 1209.
102 Green, *Working-Class Patients and the Medical Establishment*, p. 39.
103 *Lancet*, 16 April 1887, p. 809.
104 *Ibid.*, 22 October 1892, 'Verax', pp. 962–963.
105 Joan Lane, *A Social History of Medicine: Health, Healing and Disease in England, 1750–1950* (London, 2001). p. 78.
106 Green, *Working-Class Patients and the Medical Establishment*, p. 24.

107 *Ibid.*, p. 28.
108 Cox, *Among the Doctors*, p. 56.
109 Stamp, *Doctor Himself*, p. 72.
110 *BMJ*, 23 March 1895, pp. 657–658.
111 *Manchester University Medical Collections.* MMC/7/4/3/1 'Provident Medical Aid', Report by the Manchester Medical Guild 1895, p. 3.
112 Green, *Working-Class Patients*, p. 127.
113 A.J. (Archibald Joseph) Cronin, *The Citadel* (London, 1937). Vista edition 1996, p. 142.
114 *Manchester University Special Medical Collections*, Manchester Medical Guild Annual Report 1904 MMC/7/4/3, p. 2.
115 Little, *History of the British Medical Association*, p. 202.
116 *Ibid.*
117 See *BMJ*, 3 March 1900, letter from 'Rotherham GP', p. 546.
118 Squire Sprigge, *Medicine and the Public*, p. 232.
119 *Manchester University Special Medical Collections* MMC/7/4/3/1 'Provident Medical Aid', Report by the Manchester Medical Guild 1895, p. 7.
120 Hardy, *The State of the Medical Profession in Great Britain and Ireland in 1900*, p. 33.
121 *Ibid.*
122 *Ibid.*, pp. 33–34.
123 *Ibid.*, p. 34.
124 Green, *Working-Class Patients and the Medical Establishment*, p. 55.
125 Andrew Morrice, "Strong Combination': The Edwardian BMA and Contract Practice,' in Martin Gorsky and Sally Sheard (eds) *Financing Medicine: The British Experience since 1750* (Abingdon, 2006). pp. 168–169.
126 Norman R. Eder, *National Health Insurance and the Medical Profession in Britain, 1913–1939* (New York, 1982). p. 21 and *Lancet*, 'The Battle of the Clubs', Report by special correspondent, Adolphe Smith, 18 March 1905, p. 738.
127 See *BMJ*, 18 April 1896, p. 999; 16 January 1897, p. 168.
128 *Ibid.*, 18 April 1896, Dr James Dalgleish, p. 999.
129 Cox, *Among the Doctors*, p. 57.
130 *Ibid.*, p. 60.
131 *Ibid.*, p. 73.
132 *Ibid.*
133 *Manchester University Special Medical Collections*, MMC/7/4/6 *Manchester Medical Guild Quarterly*, no. XVII, July 1902. p. 9.
134 Cox, *Among the Doctors*, p. 73.
135 Squire Sprigge, *Medicine and the Public*, p. 235.
136 *Lancet*, 4 August 1895, pp. 476–477, and 4 July 1896, pp. 54–56.
137 Hardy, *The State of the Medical Profession in Great Britain and Ireland in 1900*, p. 30.
138 Ioan Gwilym Gibson, *Medical Benefit in Germany and Denmark* (London, 1912). p. 229.
139 *Ibid.*, p. 230.
140 *The Times*, 27 June 1911, p. 4.
141 Hardy, *The State of the Medical Profession in Great Britain and Ireland in 1900*, p. 31.
142 Clara Stewart, 'History of the Federation.' *Journal of the Medical Women's Federation*, 49 (1967). p. 70.
143 *Manchester University Special Medical Collections.* MMC/7/3/4, Official Report of the Conference on Medical Organisation 1900, p. 56.
144 Herbert De Carle Woodcock, *The Doctor and the People* (London, 1912). p. 94.

145 Sprigge, *Medicine and the Public*, p. 235.
146 Hardy, *The State of the Medical Profession in Great Britain and Ireland in 1900*, pp. 29–30.
147 *Ibid.*, p. 30.
148 Sprigge, *Medicine and the Public*, p. 232. Hardy, *The State of the Medical Profession in Great Britain and Ireland in 1900*, p. 30.
149 *Manchester University Medical Collections*, MMC/21/1/3/4, 'Presidential address by Samuel Woodcock MD', BMA Lancashire and Cheshire Branch correspondence.
150 *Manchester University Medical Collections*, MMC/7/4/3/4 'Official Report of the Conference on Medical Organisation 1900', pp. 8–9.
151 *Ibid.*, p. 8.
152 *Ibid.*
153 Cox, *Among the Doctors*, p. 74.
154 *BMJ*, 14 October 1899, Letter from Dr Samuel Crawshaw, pp. 1043–1044. However, the List of Manchester medical societies in the University Medical Collections compiled in 1901, MMC/7/2/8, says that it was established in 1892.
155 *BMJ*, 14 October 1899, Crawshaw, pp. 1043–1044.
156 *Manchester University Medical Collections*, MMC/7/4/2, Manchester Medical Guild Annual Report 1898.
157 *Ibid*, MMC/7/4/3, Manchester Medical Guild Annual Report 1903, p. 6.
158 *BMJ*, 6 September 1899, pp. 735 and 750.
159 *Manchester University Medical Collections*, MMC/7/4/3/4 Official Report of the Conference on Medical Organisation 1900, p. 1.
160 Bartrip, *Themselves Writ Large*, p. 142.
161 *BMJ*, 14 October 1899, pp. 1043–1044.
162 *Ibid.*
163 *Manchester University Medical Collections*, MMC/7/4/3/4 Official Report of the Conference on Medical Organisation 1900, p. 4.
164 *Ibid.*, pp. 18–19.
165 *Ibid.*, pp. 51–54.
166 *Ibid.*, p. 54.
167 *Ibid*, 2nd resolution, pp. 61–62.
168 *BMJ*, 12 May 1900, p. 1169 and Cox, *Among the Doctors*, p. 75.
169 *Ibid*, 12 May 1900 p. 1169 and *Manchester University Medical Collections*, MMC/7/4/3/4, Official Report of the Conference on Medical Organisation 1900, p. 56.
170 *Ibid.*
171 Cox, *Among the Doctors*, p. 75.
172 Bartrip, *Themselves Writ Large*, p. 144.
173 Cox, *Among the Doctors*, p. 76.
174 *Ibid.*
175 Bartrip, *Themselves Writ Large*, p. 145.
176 *Ibid.*
177 *Ibid.*
178 *BMJ*, 17 August 1901 p. 433.
179 *Lancet*, 8 June 1901, p. 29–30.
180 Bartrip, *Themselves Writ Large*, p. 148.
181 Cox, *Among the Doctors*, pp. 78–79.
182 *Ibid.*, p. 78.
183 Morrice, 'The Edwardian BMA and Contract Practice', p. 171.
184 Sprigge, *Medicine and the Public*, p. 234.

185 See Claudia Huerkamp, 'The Making of the Modern Medical Profession, 1800–1914', in Geoffrey Cocks and Konrad H. Jarausch (eds) *German Professions, 1800–1950* (Oxford, 1990). p. 78. See also Andreas-Holger Maehle, *Doctors, Honour and the Law: Medical Ethics in Imperial Germany* (Basingstoke, 2009). pp. 6–46.

186 Hardy, *The State of the Medical Profession in Great Britain and Ireland in 1900*, p. 72.

187 See *BMJ*, 6 June 1903, pp. 1339–1341, 13 June 1903, pp. 1380–1381.

188 In 1906 these warnings covered 22 such appointments. *BMJ*, 14 April 1906, p. 876.

189 Morrice, 'The Edwardian BMA and Contract Practice', p. 171.

190 *BMJ*, 6 June 1903, p. 1341.

191 Eder, *National Health Insurance and the Medical Profession*, p. 21.

192 *BMJ*, 22 July 1905 'An Investigation into the Economic Conditions of Contract Medical Practice in the United Kingdom', Supplement, pp. 1–96.

193 *Ibid.*

194 *Ibid.*

195 Morrice, 'The Edwardian BMA and Contract Practice', p. 175.

196 See Ray Earwicker, 'Miners' Medical Services before the First World War: The South Wales Coalfield.' *Llafur* (The Journal of the Society for the Study of Welsh Labour History), 111 (2) (Spring, 1981). pp. 39–52.

197 *BMJ*, 27 October 1906 Supplement, pp. 232–233.

198 *BMA Archive*, B/231/1, minutes of meeting of the Medico Political Committee on 7 April 1909. The continuation of this dispute is dealt with further in Chapter 4.

199 *Lancet*, 4 July 1896, pp. 56–57.

200 *BMJ*, Contract Medical Practice Report, 22 July 1905, Part V 'Special report on Provident Dispensaries' Supplement, pp. 30–31.

201 Eder, *National Health Insurance and the Medical Profession*, pp. 19–20. *BMA Archive*, Minutes of meetings of Medico Political Committee on 18 November 1908 and 22 September 1909.

202 *Ibid.*

203 *Report of the Royal Commission on the Poor Laws and Relief of Distress, Cmd.* 4499 (1909).

204 *BMJ*, 5 February 1910, Supplement, 'Interim Report of Special Poor Law Committee', pp. 41–43.

205 See Beatrice and Sidney Webb, The *State and the Doctor,* p. 233.

206 *BMJ*, 5 February 1910, 'Interim Report of Special Poor Law Committee', Supplement, pp. 41–43.

207 *Ibid.*, p. 43, para 20.

208 Chris Renwick, *Bread for All: The Origins of the Welfare State* (2nd ed., London, 2018). p. 58.

209 *The Spectator*, Editorial, 2 December 1911.

210 Digby, *The Evolution of British General Practice*, p. 14.

211 Hardy, *The State of the Medical Profession in Great Britain and Ireland in 1900*, p. 25.

212 George Bernard Shaw, Preface to *The Doctor's Dilemma* (London, 1906). Penguin Edition 1946, p. 86.

213 *BMA Archive*, B/231/1, Minutes of joint meeting between Special Poor Law Reform Committee and Contract Practice Subcommittee of 26 October 1910, Doc. 35.

4 'The political doctor is now born'

Lloyd George and the doctors' revolt, 1911–1913

In a book published in 1912, the specialist physician Herbert de Carle Woodcock wrote that 'Medical men are slothful in politics, prone to bear unfair treatment with just so much grumbling as falls short of revolt…They are not by nature rebels'.[1] This was the same year, however, in which a dispute between the medical profession and the Government escalated into a confrontation of monumental proportions which was to cast a shadow over their relationship for decades to come. The profession's battle with the Liberal Government over the introduction of National Health Insurance (NHI) in 1911–1913 has been analysed in great detail by historians interested in politics, state formation, and welfarism in Britain.[2] It has also been studied by those interested in the development of health services, and in the history of the medical profession, and featured in sociological studies of professionalisation.[3] But this conflict can also be seen as the most visible expression of the GPs' political consciousness which began to take shape during the 'battle of the clubs' at the end of the nineteenth century, and which increasingly affected the thinking and activities of the BMA and other representative groups during the first decade of the twentieth century. It was conditioned as much by the hopes and fears of ordinary GPs as by the personal ambitions and political prejudices of the profession's leaders. It was a conflict characterised by an unprecedented show of professional solidarity and decisive, yet ultimately ineffective, political action, the failure of which plunged the profession into a crisis of self-doubt and recrimination. While it may be seen as a continuation of the trade union-like activities taking place within the profession in the 1890s, the surprising militancy exhibited by many doctors and the ideological dogmatism of opposing professional factions in 1911–1913 may be symptomatic of a wider tendency affecting many areas of public life in Britain at that time. A broad spectrum of social and political groups, including Irish Republicans and Ulster Unionists, Trade Union syndicalists, and the more militant advocates of female suffrage, were observed to exhibit a form of political dogmatism underpinned by what G.R. Searle describes as a 'moral absolutism' which rejected the 'liberal culture of compromise' and 'government by discussion'.[4] Whether the doctors' fears justified the agitation which followed the enactment of National Insurance

DOI: 10.4324/9781003438274-4

in 1911 is debatable. But in what was seen by many of them to be an existential struggle for their profession, GPs could not be expected to be immune from such influences. While most doctors may have thought of themselves as members of a 'noble' and liberal profession, the conflict exposed a deep well of political conservatism fed by professional self-interest and fear of the unknown. It did little to improve the profession's image or win the trust and support of the wider public and left its representatives with a burdensome legacy of failed leadership which they were for decades after trying to live down.

The working classes, the state, and the provident principle

Historians agree that the reasons for the Liberal Government's social welfare legislation of 1906–1914 are complex and various. None would now suggest that the legislation should be viewed as a coherent social welfare programme as such, and certainly not part of a 'grand plan' to establish a welfare state. Lloyd George, the architect of many of the reform measures, and many in his party were influenced by the experience of social insurance in Germany from the 1880s.[5] The slower growth of the British economy relative to its rivals, Germany and the USA, after 1870 and the economic depression of the 1880s had a significant impact on the political classes in Britain.[6] Concerned that the decline in Britain's economic output might be inexorable and symptomatic of a more general decline in the strength and capability of its citizens, both Conservative and Liberal politicians looked to emulate Germany where social reform had been used by the state in an explicitly conservative manner – what Marxist historians have described, contemptuously, as 'social imperialism'.[7] Like their counterparts in Germany, British businessmen, in the Liberal party and outside it, supported social reforms on the grounds that they could contribute to the efficiency of the workforce. Recognising their value as 'human capital', progressive employers were increasingly concerned about the impact of health on the efficiency of their workers.[8] Health services were seen to aid efficiency by ensuring that the worker returned to the labour force as soon as possible after illness.[9] Both Conservative and Liberal imperialists also recognised that it would be impossible to defend the Empire without a healthy working class.[10] These concerns were given emphasis by studies of the physical and social conditions of the working classes by Booth and Rowntree and revelations from the interdepartmental committee report into physical fitness which emerged from concerns about army recruits for the Boer war.[11] Contemporary debates about 'racial degeneration' involved, on the one hand, the supposed merits of eugenics, and, on the other, recognition of the deleterious impact of environmental factors like inadequate housing, diet, and education, and of unemployment and disease. As the Prime Minister, Asquith, said:

> What is the use of talking about the Empire when here, at its very centre, there is always to be found a mass of people, stunted in education, a prey of intemperance, huddled and congested beyond the possibility of realizing in any true sense either social or domestic life?[12]

It was this thinking which lay behind the Liberal government's social legislation, which, among other challenges, sought to create a less fragmentary and more effective means of providing for the sick, disabled, elderly, and unemployed. There is widespread support, however, for the idea that politicians introduced social reform to boost electoral popularity or to prevent workers turning to extreme Labour, socialist, or syndicalist solutions (what T.H. Marshall called the 'class abatement' aspects of the reforms).[13] The Liberal Peer Lord Crewe warned Campbell Bannerman in 1905 that 'the Liberal party is on trial as an engine for securing social reforms. It has to resist the (Independent Labour Party) claim to be the only friend of the workers'.[14] As Martin Gorsky says, social reforms 'mediated the class tensions to which industrialisation gave rise' and could therefore be viewed as 'property's ransom for security'.[15] The proposition that the measures were introduced as a means of containing the socialist threat is evidenced by the fact that Conservatives and Unionists did not directly oppose them. Proof of a consensus on frustrating socialist ambitions can be found in the comments of A.J. Balfour that: 'Social legislation…is not merely to be distinguished from socialist legislation, but it is its most direct opposite and its most effective antidote'.[16]

The introduction of welfare measures was also influenced by a gradual change in attitudes towards poverty in the last decades of the nineteenth and the first decade of the twentieth centuries. Many enlightened thinkers recognised the link between sickness and poverty which the Webbs and other social scientists identified in their writings and which added weight to the arguments of those calling for a reform of the poor law system on humanitarian grounds.[17] The architects of the Liberal reforms were also influenced by the views of intellectuals like the Oxford philosopher, T.H. Green, who postulated an 'organic' view of society, and D.G. Ritchie, who made a case for a more collectivist approach by government towards social problems in what was still regarded essentially as an individualist society.[18] The new 'advanced Liberalism' which came into being was not, in the view of these authorities, an abandonment but a re-interpretation of individualism, as the state was encouraged to take steps to liberate the faculties of the individual, to remove obstacles to self-development and allow individuals to realise their personal potential. According to Pat Thane, 'advocates of state "collectivism" rarely wished government action to take the place of self-help, philanthropy and the duty to work, but rather wished to supplement and reinforce these attributes which were regarded as socially and morally desirable.'[19] James Vernon sees the Liberal 'revolution in government' as being grounded in the philosophy of laissez-faire and self-help. It was not just about creating a new kind of state, he says, but creating a new type of citizen who could govern themselves.[20] Making markets free demanded that the state develop new capabilities and responsibilities and the boundaries of the state were extended to new ways of governing and shaping the 'condition of England' and the 'social question'.[21] Recognising the practical difficulties and the economic and political cost of extending state power in this direction, the Liberal Government sought to involve private, charitable, and local government institutions to mediate its proposals for social welfare, devolving authority to administer these to a variety of agencies on the state's behalf.[22] In what Nikolas Rose describes as 'governing at a distance', the Government sought to implement its policy objectives by means of a public/private partnership with a variety of non-governmental institutions and was thus able to operate through networks or nexuses of authority (what the philosopher Michel Foucault calls 'modalities of power').[23] As Mary Poovey and Jose Harris have explained, there was a long tradition of voluntarism and charitable self-help in Victorian Britain which had produced many social institutions interested in and capable of delivering government-sponsored welfare programmes.[24] Foremost among these were the friendly societies whose role and functions were considered in the previous chapter. The path towards social welfare legislation was guided by a small number of prominent civil servants like Sir George Askwith, Sir Hubert Llewellyn Smith, and William Beveridge. By quantifying social problems and presenting them in a statistical rather than polemical manner, they succeeded in convincing other government officials as well as Ministers that social reform was consistent with ideas of scientific progress.[25] Studies of government papers and memoirs of civil servants point to the growth of a new type of determinism suggesting that extension of the role of government was a product of a bureaucratic process in which experts in the civil service, sometimes derided by critics as 'the boffinocracy', rather than politicians, were the prime movers of legislation.[26] These men were often motivated, just as many doctors were, by their own version of the 'professional social ideal'. Pat Thane describes experts exercising power on the state's behalf (what she calls 'bounded pluralism'), as an elite which conflated its personal interests with the national good.[27] Sir Robert Morant was a perfect example. In 1913, he stated: 'We can make work at the Government Department the most marvellous means for true social reform that the world has seen'.[28] Through these individuals, the authority of expertise became inextricably linked with the formal political apparatus of the state.[29]

Lloyd George's decision to introduce national sickness insurance was not based on an awareness of the inadequacies of British medicine. His scheme was a social, not medical measure designed to mitigate the effects of illness on workers and, indirectly, their dependants, and to help the breadwinner to return to work as soon as possible. While the Fabians argued that sickness was an inevitable consequence of poverty, for Lloyd George, poverty was 'the evil that sickness caused' and it was this that his scheme was designed to mitigate.[30] The choice of insurance as the method by which the Liberals sought to achieve this was driven by both ideology and pragmatism. The careful study which Lloyd George commissioned of the German Social Insurance model convinced him and his associates that it could be effective and affordable and they reasoned that it would be more acceptable to most of their supporters, and to the Treasury, to work through existing agencies in the field.[31] The adoption of the insurance principle was also influenced by Treasury fears that a future government might introduce tariff reform to pay for social legislation, while the alternative of leaving implementation in the hands of local government aroused fears of weakened financial discipline and geographical variation. The failure of local government attempts to solve social problems, evidenced in the response to Joseph Chamberlain's circular of 1886 and the Unemployed Workmen Act 1905, coupled with a clearer appreciation of the magnitude of social problems, increased the Liberals' desire for central rather than local government solutions.[32] Concluding that existing systems of relief and rehabilitation were inadequate, the Royal Commission on the Poor Laws (majority) Report of 1909 recommended that medical assistance for persons incapacitated from wage-earning should be provided on a provident basis, whereas the minority report favoured a much more radical approach, involving a non-contributory state scheme run by local authorities. These reports emboldened the Liberals to take decisive action in the way of social reform. Despairing of being able to deliver the necessary changes through a reformed poor law, however, due to the intransigence of the Local Government Board, they judged it politically expedient to bypass the problem and leave the poor law as it was, to 'wither on the vine'. They hoped that National Insurance would in time replace it with a more efficient and less stigmatising alternative.[33]

The 1911 Act was, according to John Turner, 'not a collectivist measure pushing out the boundaries of the state, but an umbrella for the extension of private welfare' which was 'at the limits of the state's competence'.[34] The government therefore relied on external interests to bridge the gap in capacity.[35] The easiest way to introduce NHI, Lloyd George decided, was to build on the existing system of sickness insurance operated by the friendly societies, making them, together with trade unions and insurance companies, 'Approved Societies' responsible for administering the scheme on the state's behalf. They would ensure that all qualifying workers paid into the scheme along with the state and their employers. The nature of the structures which emerged to form the administrative apparatus of the scheme was determined less by utility and idealism, however, than by the need to reach a compromise with competing vested interests, including the doctors who were to work under the Act.[36] It was for this reason that the passage of the Bill has been described as 'an almost classic history of lobby activity'.[37]

The medical reaction: fear, indignation, and defiance

Lloyd George and his officials had discussed his evolving proposals for health insurance at length with representatives of the friendly societies before the press and other interested parties, including the doctors, got wind of what was proposed. Although many friendly societies' representatives expressed concerns about a loss of independence, the Government's reforms offered them a potential lifeline. Many of the societies feared for their long-term stability in view of the increasing cost of sickness benefits claimed by a membership living longer than anticipated.[38] They feared 'an impending demographic crisis' as claims became 'long term, seasonal and chronic'.[39] However, more recent studies have shown that the main reason sickness rates increased with age was that when older people became ill, they remained off work for longer.[40] The societies' financial health was also threatened by increasing competition for younger workers from the commercial insurance industry. The majority of the smaller friendly societies were already threatened by insolvency. The MP Sir Leo Chiozza-Money opined that the scheme 'puts them on their feet again by giving them new reserve funds' and 'keeps them solvent by submitting them to an expert supervision'.[41] If the doctors were aware of these developments, however, they had no discernible effect on their views of National Health Insurance (NHI). While wary of state interference, many in the medical profession had begun to favour more systematic provision of medical services. As one medical observer wrote in 1912: 'National Health Insurance has long been overdue and a State medical church appeals to medical men as readily as to other people'.[42] Indeed, the BMA's proposals for 'The organization of medical attendance on the provident or insurance basis' (its blueprint for a national scheme of Public Medical Services run by doctors themselves), which the Association finally endorsed in March 1911, were more liberal and extensive than the Government's limited proposals for NHI.[43] In a memorandum considered at a meeting between the BMA's Special Poor Law Committee and Contract Practice subcommittee in 1910, Dr W. Gosse asked if the state scheme was to be limited to working men, stating that, 'Unless women and children are included it is impossible to see how an efficient national scheme can be carried out'.[44]

The Government's proposals for NHI largely caught the profession by surprise. Lloyd George had met with the BMA only briefly before his Bill was published and given little detail of his intentions. Bentley Gilbert notes the discrepancy between the three occasions Lloyd George claimed to have met with doctors' representatives and the single occasion noted by the BMA.[45] The initial response of the profession's leaders was understandably cautious.[46] Once they had learned of the friendly societies' role in it, however, their mood quickly darkened, and the BMA urgently sought meetings with the Chancellor to voice their concerns. The backbench Liberal MP Dr Christopher Addison was among those invited to advise the Chancellor on the doctors' reaction to his scheme. Addison informed him that, as currently formulated, the scheme 'simply stank in the nostrils of the whole medical profession'. If he tried to impose it on them, he said, he would 'find them solid to a man against it'.[47] For the GPs who, over several decades, had chafed at the constraints and humiliations imposed on them by the friendly societies, the Government's proposals represented the institutionalisation of lay control. Being national and likely to incorporate a sizeable percentage of the working population, moreover, the scheme threatened to alter irrevocably the market for working-class medical care. If constructed in the way the doctors wanted, it might prove a boon to the GPs as well as to their working-class patients but if the friendly societies had their way, it would result for the doctors in greater dependency, demoralisation, and permanently depressed levels of remuneration. Fortunately for the doctors, there were other powerful interests determined to prevent the friendly societies having a monopoly of control over the scheme. The commercial insurance companies (often referred to as 'the combine') were less keen to be involved in administering the scheme and wanted to restrict the influence it accorded to the friendly societies. They gradually threw their considerable weight therefore behind a proposal devised by Addison whereby the administration would be conducted not by the Approved Societies but by local 'health committees' answerable to central government commissioners.[48] To the consternation of the chief officials working on the scheme, W.J. Braithwaite and John Bradbury, Lloyd George was eventually dissuaded from vesting the power to administer the state-sanctioned scheme in the friendly societies' hands and, to appease the medical profession, he began to express sympathy for their concerns about the societies' failings. He wrote to the Cabinet on 30 March 1911 about this after interviewing 'a large number of doctors' about 'the medical side of the scheme'.[49] According to BMA official Alfred Cox, Lloyd George recognised that 'while a medical service is imaginable without Friendly Societies, it cannot be worked without doctors'.[50] The Chancellor was even persuaded to support the profession's demand for free choice of doctor, though it was anathema to the societies, and contrary to his previously expressed view that the experience of health insurance in Germany had shown that 'free choice of doctor promotes malingering'.[51] Thus, he told the House of Commons in 1911, 'No man who could afford to do otherwise would have a doctor prescribed for him by any club or society'.[52] His chief civil servant, Braithwaite, was greatly annoyed by this volte face, noting contemptuously that, 'The doctors had the whole house on the run with this specious cry of "free choice of doctor"'.[53] He tried and failed to ensure that the Approved Societies were able to select the scheme doctors, recording in his memoir, 'I did not realize what a pull the doctors had…I staved off the evil day, but only temporarily. We were doomed to have free choice of doctors thrust right upon us after all'.[54] In any case, the principle commended itself to the House, the authors of the first commentary on National Insurance claimed, because to compel the insured to 'have, as his medical attendant, one whom he might distrust, was unreasonable, especially as confidence in a medical adviser is an essential factor in the cure'.[55]

Mindful that the Conservative press was stirring up opposition among the medical portion of its readership, Lloyd George decided to meet the challenge head on by addressing the Special Representative Meeting called by the BMA on 11 June 1911 to debate the National Insurance Bill. It was an experience he later likened to being like that of 'Daniel in the lion's den'.[56] He had been well briefed about the doctors' concerns by, among others, Addison, who had been acting as an unofficial intermediary between the government and BMA officials at this time.[57] Following his speech, the BMA compiled a list of demands called 'the six cardinal points'.[58] These were an income limit of £2 per week for any participant in the service; free choice of doctor by the patient, subject to the doctor's consent to act; medical and maternity benefits to be administered by local health committees (later named Insurance Committees), rather than the Approved Societies, and all questions of medical discipline to be settled by Local Medical Committees (LMCs) composed entirely of doctors; the method of payment to the profession in the area of each Insurance Committee to be decided by the preference of a majority of local doctors; payment to the doctors to be 'adequate' (this was later defined as 8s 6d per patient per annum excluding the cost of medicines and other extras); adequate medical representation among the various administrative bodies working the Act and statutory recognition of the LMCs previously mentioned. As a member of one of the BMA's advisory committees, Addison may have contributed to the drafting of these points which clearly owe something to the BMA's response to the Royal Commission on the Poor Law.[59]

During his interrogation by the audience at the meeting, Lloyd George fielded questions on the cardinal points and gave affirmatory responses to all except the first and last of them. The question of remuneration was, he said, a matter to be further negotiated. On the question of an income limit to exclude the well to do from the scheme, he pointed out that the half a million miners currently enrolled in clubs were highly paid workmen. Were they to be excluded from the national scheme he asked, and if so, how could the legislation obtain parliamentary approval, given the considerable number of MPs who depended on their votes?[60] Gilbert states that Lloyd George's great political achievement was to turn opposition to himself to opposition to the friendly societies.[61] The Chancellor won rapturous applause at the BMA meeting when he told them that he would support a proposal to transfer responsibility for running the scheme from the friendly societies to local Insurance Committees.[62] But the BMA remained suspicious, even when the four cardinal points Lloyd George had conceded were incorporated by Addison into an amendment to the Bill which was passed with the Chancellor's support. Crucially, the amendment did not institute an income limit but left it to the local discretion of the Insurance Committees. However, it was later set at a rate of £160 per year for non-manual workers and there was no income limit for manual workers. There is some doubt as to whether Addison personally supported an income limit. He had asked for it to be included during the bill's first reading.[63] However, Alfred Cox claims that Addison thought the idea of an income limit was 'absurd'.[64] If Addison and Lloyd George thought that the amendment was enough to appease the Bill's opponents in the profession, however, they were soon disappointed. Conscious of the power their unprecedented show of unity appeared to have accorded them in negotiations with the government, many doctors urged the BMA to press home their advantage and demand the concession of the remaining cardinal points.

The BMA and professional resistance

Commenting on the agitation which followed the introduction of the National Insurance Bill, the specialist doctor Herbert de Carle Woodcock wrote: 'All those who desire the welfare of our profession as a means to its greater usefulness must welcome the changed attitude of the doctor upon political questions... medical men are ceasing to be Ishmaelites...The political doctor is now born'.[65] Taken together, the issue of remuneration and the income limit for the insured which, as previously demonstrated, lay at the heart of the profession's battle with the friendly societies, was for a great many doctors too important a matter to leave unresolved. As the newspapers reported, the income limit outlined in the Bill would, in the opinion of very many doctors, represent the end of private practice and had to be resisted at all costs.[66] The *Birmingham Post* reported one eminent professor saying that it 'would result in an immediate drop in the saleable value of their practices'.[67] A doctor wrote to the *Daily Mail* stating that the week before the Bill was introduced, his rural practice could have been sold for £2,000, but 'this week it would not sell at any price'.[68] At the BMA's representative meeting in June 1911, their president voiced the concerns of many when he referred to the need to compensate GPs for the expected loss in value of their practices.[69] The BMA eventually set out its case for 'adequate remuneration' stating that they wanted a minimum of 8s 6d per patient per annum exclusive of the cost of drugs. Were the BMA 'to entertain any suggestion of compromise upon this point', its medical secretary, James Smith Whitaker, wrote to Lloyd George, 'its action would undoubtedly be repudiated by the profession'.[70] Lloyd George had reason to be sceptical of the notion that the profession would refuse to accept anything less than this amount. During the second reading of the Bill, he had come across for the first time the BMA's 1905 Report on Contract Practice and 'was thrilled by it' as it proved that what he was offering was considerably more than what most GPs could expect to earn under existing club contracts.[71] He was recorded as saying, 'If any man had got them 5s he would have been a hero; I have arranged 6s and I am a villain'.[72] The BMA's report should, however, be viewed with scepticism given that, as Comyns Carr was later to point out, it may have seriously underestimated the number of patient attendances on which the average figure was based.[73] Whitaker assured his colleagues on the BMA's Council that, ultimately, the Government would have to concede their demands as no government could force the profession to serve under unacceptable conditions. The doctors had merely to refuse to serve en masse, he contended, and victory would be theirs.[74]

With the backing of the Association's Council, Whitaker set about mobilising the doctors. On 3 June 1911, he circulated a letter to every member of the profession, distributed through the BMA's new branch and division structures and advertised in the *British Medical Journal (BMJ)*, asking them to support BMA policy by joining the Association if not already members, pledging their refusal to enter the service other than when the BMA deemed it appropriate, and contributing to a fighting fund to meet the costs of opposing the Act. The fund was to be used 'for the direct pecuniary assistance of medical practitioners threatened with or incurring actual loss of income' by adhering to BMA policy.[75] A further circular letter of 21 June invited all doctors to sign an undertaking

> not to enter into any agreement for giving medical attendance and treatment to persons insured under the Bill, excepting such as shall be satisfactory to the medical profession and in accordance with the declared policy of the British Medical Association.[76]

The pledge of solidarity which had been wielded sporadically and, usually, ineffectively by GPs as a weapon in their battles with friendly societies in the second half of the nineteenth century was thus for the first time employed on their behalf systematically at a national scale by a highly organised and influential representative body. It was the first showdown between the Government and an organised medical profession the country had witnessed and was to set the pattern for conflicts that were to come.

The reaction to the call from the BMA was immediate and powerful. Old antagonisms were set aside as across the country doctors assembled in noisy and angry gatherings to express their fears and pledge support for the BMA in its quest to secure the guarantees set out in the 'six cardinal points'. One such gathering took place in Nottingham on 21 November 1911 at which the meeting resolved

> That the National Insurance Bill as at present drafted does not satisfactorily meet the demands of the profession as defined in the six cardinal points and that the scheme in its present form is unworkable, is detrimental to the medical profession and dangerous to the public health.[77]

Another GP wrote in his memoirs that the Act 'stirred up the medical profession like never before. Never before had so many GPs become acquainted with each other. Meetings galore, full of sound and fury'.[78] Significantly, a rider to the undertaking the GPs signed spoke of them joining NHI 'only through a Local Medical Committee representative of the district in which I practice'. Many local meetings thus resulted in decisions to establish provisional LMCs to coordinate resistance to the Act. The national and local press dutifully reported the increasing tally of doctors refusing to accept service under the Act. They published letters from anxious or irate doctors and reported on the doctors' meetings which resulted in the *Daily Mail* christening the affair 'The Doctors' Revolt'.[79] Eventually, some 27,400 signed undertakings were received by the BMA.[80] Though estimates of the composition of the medical profession at that time vary, it is assumed that there were only about 22,500 practising GPs, so the pledges were signed by a significant number of others, including Consultants, hospital staff doctors, and possibly even medical students. It demonstrated a surprising degree of professional solidarity.

Despite this, Lloyd George was not cowed. He believed that the benefits of the Act to the doctors had been poorly understood and doubted the ability of the BMA's leadership to properly represent the views of the many impoverished GPs he believed would benefit from working under it.[81] As early as June 1911, he estimated that the government could recruit a minimum of 7,000 doctors to offer a service as full-time salaried medical officers if the profession withheld cooperation.[82] As signed undertakings, letters of support and criticism, and accounts of opinions voiced at local meetings poured in to the BMA's headquarters, the voices of those in the profession who distrusted the Liberals, and Lloyd George in particular, or opposed NHI on principle, began to dominate the debate. Concerned that the BMA was wavering in its resolve, a group of doctors in Manchester formed a body called the National Medical Union (NMU) to oppose all talk of compromise with the government.[83] The Union denied that it was opposed to the Act or to the BMA. Its advisory committee recorded that its aim was 'to resuscitate' the BMA and 'make it a real mouthpiece for its members' and its opposition to the Act was based on the fact that 'the six cardinal points were not conceded or guaranteed'.[84] Some of the BMA grandees concealed their political party affiliations but others, like the BMA president Sir James Barr, did not. A 'tearing demagogue...with an aversion to all Liberals' according to Alfred Cox, he declared that, in removing the need for self-reliance, National Insurance would 'hasten the degeneracy of a spoon-fed race'.[85] Barr later showed his contempt for the Act by becoming one of the vice-presidents of the NMU when it reconstituted itself in 1913 as a 'rallying ground' for non-panel doctors.[86] While Liberal-supporting newspapers condemned such intransigence, others condemned the BMA's efforts to secure improvements in the government's offer through continued dialogue. Cox commented that the profession had thus become 'the shuttlecock of politics and the victim of press sensationalism'.[87] In the novel *Dr Bradley Remembers*, the narrator notes that, although doctors were among the least politically minded members of the community,

the colour of the profession as a whole (and particularly the men with big names who controlled the B.M.A.) was markedly Conservative. The opponents of the Bill realized this as well as he did and were doing their best to exploit it.[88]

Prominent among those 'big names' was the GP chairman of Council, the doughty Ulsterman, J.A. Macdonald. As the BMA's principal negotiator, Macdonald met the mercurial Welsh Chancellor several times, informing colleagues of his difficulty in suppressing the urge to throttle him![89] Lloyd George, however, remembered their encounters more affectionately, asking Ewen Maclean in 1928, 'How is Old Macdonald? He was against us but I liked him!'[90] Once the Bill became law on 6 December 1911, however, many GPs began to doubt the wisdom of antagonising the government and losing public sympathy. In a letter to the secretary of one of the newly formed LMCs, one Nottinghamshire doctor expressed a fear that the Conservative Party would 'use us as a stalking horse to upset the radicals'. He added: 'The Bill is law now and it is our business to get as much money out of it as we can'.[91]

The agitation of the profession was increased by two further developments. Firstly, while Addison's amendment had secured four of their six demands, an amendment sponsored by the recently elected MP for Luton, known as the Harmsworth amendment, secured an unexpected victory for the friendly societies and trade unions. It did this by allowing Medical Aid Institutes to continue to operate and be funded under National Insurance, though there was to be a moratorium on further such developments.[92] This was a bitter blow to those in the profession who had campaigned for their abolition or replacement by professionally run Public Medical Services. The second development was more of an 'own goal' by the BMA. Having agreed to include representatives of the profession in the administrative machinery of the Act, the government sought to test the resolve of the BMA by inviting their respected medical secretary, James Smith Whitaker, to become the Deputy Chairman of the new National Insurance Commission. Before responding, Whitaker placed the matter before the Council of the BMA which, after a lengthy debate, approved the appointment.[93] The resulting furore appeared to catch the Association by surprise and their attempts to rationalise the decision failed to placate the growing chorus of those who characterised it, publicly, as 'the great betrayal'.[94] One of the casualties of the backlash was the former chairman of the Representative Body, Sir Victor Horsley, a supporter of welfare reform and Liberal party member, who was heckled by angry doctors at a BMA meeting at the Queens Hall in December 1911 with cries of 'Traitor!' and 'Go to your Lloyd George!'.[95] The departure of moderates like Horsley and the diminishing influence of his successor as the chairman of the Representative Body, Dr Ewen Maclean, after he narrowly survived a vote of no confidence in him, left the BMA in the hands of uncompromising diehards egged on by Liberal-baiting newspapers like the *Daily Mail*.[96] The latter continued to praise the efforts of the 'no service' party at the expense of the moderates in the BMA, prompting a Dr Broadbent of Newark to complain to one of his colleagues that the *Mail* was 'inveigling the doctors' to reject the government's terms.[97]

In March 1912, the BMA's acting Medical Secretary, Alfred Cox, wrote to divisions and branches in England, Scotland, and Wales repeating his predecessor's instructions to establish provisional LMCs. The BMA knew that it could not act without the support of an overwhelming majority of GPs, a significant number of whom were not BMA members, so the divisions were told not to confine membership of or voting rights for LMCs to BMA members.[98] This was to prove significant in giving the LMCs, and subsequently Local Medical and Panel Committees (LMPCs), a democratic legitimacy which the BMA itself did not possess. In July 1912, the BMA's Council reported that 211 of these provisional LMCs had been established.[99] The militant stance which the BMA appeared to be taking in defence of GPs' interests, and the unified leadership it offered an otherwise disparate profession at that critical time boosted its membership (though its subsequent 'failure' was to result in the opposite effect).[100] Cox's letter also asked the provisional LMCs to coordinate collection from GPs of a 'pledge complimentary to the undertaking' (the undertaking not to serve under NHI without the concessions demanded by the BMA). This involved submitting post-dated letters of resignation from all existing forms of contract practice.[101] The supplemental pledges were to be placed at the disposal of the Association's State Sickness Insurance Committee but were deposited with the provisional LMCs who were to coordinate a collective refusal to accept locally inadequate terms of service. These totalled 33,000, that is they amounted to significantly more than the pledges to refuse service under the Act.[102] This decision was significant in setting the precedent for a course of action which GPs were later to use more decisively in the standoff with government in 1923. Cox also urged the LMCs to persuade their electorate to contribute towards the local and national 'defence trusts', the profession's political fighting funds. The idea of the pledge supplemental to the undertaking and the establishment of a national defence fund came from a motion to the representative meeting by the BMA's North Middlesex division.[103] Following this suggestion, LMCs began to collect local defence contributions, which were to be used to fund the expenses of the LMCs, and the national defence fund, which was administered by the BMA's State Sickness Insurance Committee and used to recompense doctors who suffered loss of income as a result of the dispute. Some 13,472 'guarantors' contributed £134,397 in total.[104] Reflecting on these events, Sir John Conybeare opined that this amount 'was quite insufficient...for its purpose of financing doctors who lost money by their refusal to accept service under the Bill'.[105]

The polarisation of medical opinion and collapse of professional unity

Cracks were already beginning to appear in the façade of professional unity, however, when in July 1912, the profession's case for a minimum remuneration of 8s 6d per patient was undermined by the publication of the Plender Report. Having decided to meet with the chancellor in June 1912 to press their case one more time, the BMA had agreed to the suggestion that a respected chartered accountant, Sir William Plender, undertake a co-sponsored investigation into GP incomes. The inquiry considered medical incomes in six towns: Cardiff, Darlington, Darwen, Dundee, Norwich, and St Albans. However, the Cardiff doctors largely declined to participate so their data had to be excluded. The data from the remaining towns showed that the ordinary GP received an average of 4s 5d per head per annum from all classes of patients out of which drugs had to be paid for, much less therefore than the 6s per head the Chancellor was offering for insured patients.[106] The BMA's State Sickness Insurance Committee had major doubts as to the accuracy of Plender's conclusions, doubts which have been partially vindicated by later investigations. Jeanne Peterson states that the five towns were 'clearly atypical'.[107] Moreover, the doctor/patient ratio was much lower than what later examinations showed to be the national average, and the arithmetic mean Plender used gave an average net income which was very different from that calculated later and more precisely by Guy Routh.[108] However, the report handed the Government a major propaganda victory. It allowed the chancellor to represent himself as the soul of generosity, especially when, in a final attempt to win over the profession, he succeeded in persuading the cabinet to increase the remuneration offered to 9s inclusive of the cost of drugs, which meant that the panel doctors could expect to receive between 7s and 7s 6d per patient.[109] Doctors in the poorest areas found that their income would be doubled, and large numbers consequently ignored BMA advice and joined the insurance panels.

Seeing that the BMA remained obdurate, Lloyd George also let it be known, via an interview with the magazine, *Nation*, that he was quite prepared to withdraw concessions already made and let the friendly societies resume the role he had originally intended for them. In areas where insufficient numbers volunteered to serve on the panels, he proposed to recruit a cadre of salaried doctors to serve the insured.[110] He later explained to the Insurance Advisory Committee the three options which were open to Insurance Committees to deal with insufficient panels, namely (1) allow the panel GPs to maintain high lists by employing a sufficient number of assistants; (2) invite outside GPs to form panel practices de novo; and (3) allow Insurance Committees to employ salaried GPs.[111] Conscious of the benefits which the Act would deliver to them and for their patients, GPs eager to work under the Act began to form their own pressure groups. In November 1912, a Liberal MP who was a also a GP of 25 years' standing, Dr John Esmonde, circulated an open letter to the profession urging GPs to serve under the improved conditions now offered and to communicate their names to him, stating, 'I am confident the work can be well done in both town and country and that a large majority of GPs wish to give the Act a trial'.[112] In early December, following a split vote in the BMA's Birmingham division, 26 GPs in the city issued a manifesto declaring their willingness to defy their leadership and work under the Act.[113] It was becoming clear to many GPs that many of those who were most vehement in urging the profession to stand firm and ignore the concessions won already from the Government were Consultants and specialists. These 'swell doctors' as Lloyd George had disparagingly called them, who were not likely to need to work under the Act, were guilty, according to Gilbert, of leaving behind 'the lowly, voiceless general practitioner for whom National Insurance promised a larger and steadier income than he had ever known'.[114] A prominent BMA Council member, Dr Lauriston Shaw, criticised those of his colleagues who put their own 'narrow and selfish interests' above 'the wider interests of the community'.[115] He was one of 300–400 doctors who formed the National Insurance Practitioners' Association in December 1912 to represent the doctors who were willing to work under the Act.[116] The fact that Shaw was himself a Harley Street Consultant was not lost on some of those attending a meeting of what the *Daily Mail* disparaged as the 'Work the Act League' where 'it was urged that there had been too much Harley Street domination'.[117] The secretary of the NMU, Dr J. Webster, engaged in a heated exchange of letters with Shaw in the *Manchester Guardian* in late 1912 when the latter suggested that GPs agree to join the panels as 'conditions had now changed'.[118]

Shaw and another prominent supporter of the government scheme, Dr Herbert H. Mills of Kensington, were subject to vitriolic attacks by BMA loyalists as was the unfortunate James Smith Whitaker, especially when he ignored the BMA Council's demand that doctors resign forthwith from any government employment.[119] Those who declared themselves willing to work under the Act were ostracised by the 'no service' party, labelled 'blacklegs' and found themselves subject to various sorts of pressure. The *Daily Mail* characterised them as 'the dregs of a great profession' and claimed that 'of the small minority who would apply for positions as insurance doctors, the wastrels will form a not inconsiderable portion'.[120] Consultants were urged to limit hospital house staff appointments, and GPs to confine assistant and locum tenens posts, to those who adhered to the BMA's undertaking.[121] In *Dr Bradley Remembers*, the eponymous hero resigns from the BMA and refuses to be cowed by comments that 'the position of a medical man who hasn't stood by his colleagues can be rather unpleasant'. The author subsequently notes that, 'The strength of the intimidation that had been used could be judged by the fact that even old Wills, a friend of twenty years' standing, refused to return his salute when they met in the high street'.[122] As divisions within the profession began to widen, the response from the press reflected their political allegiances. Government-supporting newspapers like the *Daily Chronicle* expressed dismay and incredulity at the BMA's apparent refusal to acknowledge that they had been granted substantially all they had asked for.[123] Despite the BMA's efforts to enforce solidarity, many of the provisional LMCs were pragmatically taking steps to prepare for the eventuality that GPs would work under the Act. They were conscious of the fact that the Act gave the Insurance Committees discretion over several aspects of the scheme and sought to negotiate the best terms they could while that discretion remained in place. In the County of Nottinghamshire, for example, the provisional Insurance Committee met a 'deputation of doctors' in December 1912, recording that a Dr Jacobs expressed a willingness to advise local GPs to serve on the panel 'if the committee would use its influence to obtain relief for the practitioners of regulations, they deemed grievances'.[124]

The BMA's Council published its assessment of what was seen as Lloyd George's final offer, concluding that it still fell far short of what they wanted. The anti-Liberal press lost no time in advising the profession to reject it yet again. Under the heading 'The Doctors' best courses', the *Daily Mail* prophesied that 'the doctor is to be mercilessly sweated in order to avert the financial collapse of the most unpopular Act of Parliament ever passed'.[125] The BMA called another plebiscite in December 2012. The result was 2,408 votes in favour of accepting the government's terms and 11,219 against. The *Daily Mail* carried the headline 'The Doctors say 'No!'', reporting that the vote was 7 to 1 against.[126] Significantly, however, nearly half the doctors who had signed the pledge had abstained from voting, a fact not lost on many in the profession or in the Liberal-supporting press.[127] The *Daily Chronicle* reported that six prominent members of BMA Council, including Lauriston Shaw, Ewen Maclean, and Victor Horsley, had resigned in protest at their colleagues' refusal to countenance a change in policy.[128] As the *Chronicle* confidently predicted the 'Inevitable collapse of BMA revolt', Whitaker's successor as the Medical Secretary, Alfred Cox, drafted a report for the BMA's Council which emphasised all the concessions that had been won in a vain attempt to secure a more conciliatory approach.[129] Reports were already reaching Cox and his colleagues, via despairing telegrams and letters from BMA branch secretaries that the panels were beginning to fill up in many areas.[130] In Bradford, where the GPs stood firm and refused to join the panel, the Insurance Committee advertised for salaried GPs to fill the vacancies. When they announced that they had three times as many applicants as required, many of whom were well-qualified doctors working as assistants to established GPs without means of advancement, the established doctors relented and agreed to join the panels en masse.[131] The same thing happened in Lancaster when Lord Ashton announced that he would personally ensure the appointment of a sufficient number of imported medical practitioners to fill salaried posts 'whatever it cost'.[132] Addison was pleasantly surprised to find a large meeting of doctors he had been asked to address in Birmingham entirely sympathetic to working under the Act.[133] A Birmingham delegate to the BMA's meeting in December acknowledged that he came a 'from an infected area' surrounded by districts in which GPs were joining the panels in great numbers.[134] Members of the BMA's Ealing division unsuccessfully picketed a meeting convened by the Middlesex Insurance Committee at Caxton Hall where 55 doctors agreed to accept service under the Act and the picture was similar in Enfield, Stepney, and Camberwell.[135] The *Daily Chronicle* noted that there were full panels in every part of Scotland.[136] Wales and the north of England had also 'rallied to Lloyd George', although doctors in many parts of the Midlands, the South, and much of the capital remained loyal to their pledges.[137] The *Daily Mail* kept up a steady stream of pro-doctor and anti-government rhetoric, maintaining that the number of 'backsliders' was insufficient to rescue Lloyd George's scheme and then denouncing the Government's press briefings about the number of panels that had been formed as 'Press

Bureau fictions' and the 'Failure of a big bluff'.[138] The growing desperation felt by the BMA's Council is evidenced by the fact that in late December 1912, it actually proposed that the provisional LMCs seek to bypass the Insurance Committees and negotiate terms for providing medical service to the insured directly with Approved Societies.[139] Addison was quick to point out that this represented a repudiation of one of the cardinal points.[140] Horsley concurred and included this among reasons cited in a statement he issued to the profession titled 'Why you should join the panels'.[141] Any thoughts of pursuing this proposal, however, were quickly dispelled when a meeting of 40 friendly societies unanimously rejected the idea.[142]

On 2 January 1913, Lloyd George announced that 10,000 doctors had now joined the panels, a number sufficient to cover three-quarters of the insured population.[143] Seeing the increasing numbers of doctors joining the panels in many areas, Government-supporting newspapers like the *Daily Chronicle* were now carrying headlines such as 'Stampede of the Doctors' and a sense of panic began to set in among the GPs.[144] Not one doctor in the New Forest had been prepared to join the panel, the GP Philip Gosse records, until a report reached them of 'an omnibus with drawn blinds' arriving at Lymington containing, it was believed, 'several scotch doctors sent there by Lloyd George to break the doctors' strike'. The result was 'an instant undignified scramble to get our names on the panel before it closed'.[145] A similar situation occurred in Sheffield.[146] In Liverpool, the Insurance Committee determined to overcome the boycott by appointing salaried doctors and was reported to have '200 men ready to import into the city'.[147] In Cardiff, the *Daily Telegraph* noted, 'there was a remarkable rush of doctors to join the panels'.[148] The diehards resorted to more desperate forms of persuasion and intimidation. A member of the National Insurance Practitioners Association, Dr Atteridge of Ladbroke Grove, London, awoke to find his house covered with posters warning the public that their 'so called choice of free doctor' would be limited to a small minority of 'men who have broken their pledge'.[149] A Willesden doctor told the *Daily Chronicle* that 'knowing he was a poor man', his GP colleagues had offered to pay him from their own pockets rather than 'see him go down' by not joining the panel.[150] A 'professional man' concerned at the tactics to which extremists had resorted to intimidate those joining the panels wrote to the *Daily Telegraph* claiming that 'the revolting doctors have gone to the length of employing sandwichmen to parade the streets in which the doctors live'.[151]

On 11 January, the *BMJ* acknowledged that the Government would be able to launch the scheme on the appointed day.[152] The BMA believed that it had another means, however, with which to frustrate the government's intentions. It pinned its hopes on a legal loophole in Section 15 of the Act which it felt would allow non-panel GPs to offer an alternative service to patients exercising their right to 'contract out' of the state scheme. This permitted persons, 'in lieu of receiving medical benefit under such arrangements as aforesaid, to make their own arrangements' and said that 'in such cases the Committee shall, subject to the Regulations, contribute from the funds…towards the cost of medical attendance and treatment…for such persons'.[153] However, the Government dashed that hope when Lloyd George made it clear in a speech to the Insurance Advisory Committee that the provision in question was intended to meet exceptional circumstances and stated, 'We will not allow it to be used to break down the Act in any area'.[154] In answering a question in parliament, C.G. Masterman confirmed that Insurance Committees would simply not approve such arrangements.[155] Undeterred, the self-appointed London Local Medical Committee was particularly keen to use this means to circumvent what they saw as the unwelcome control of the largely lay Insurance Committees. They persuaded a number of London GPs who had signed up to the panels to resign in anticipation of the large number of patients who would be entitled to choose them as their (non-panel) doctor.[156] They even circulated forms for GPs to give to patients for that purpose.[157] *The Times* reported that 1.5 million of these had been issued by the London LMC from its office inside BMA House.[158] Doctors in Middlesex who had attempted to resign were dismayed, however, at being told that their contracts were binding. Their names were 'starred' on the published panel list as having withdrawn from the list but 'not released by the committee'.[159] Although attempts to invoke this provision were subsequently made elsewhere during 1913, most notably in Kent, 'complex bureaucratic procedures' were used to discourage patients from contracting out and hopes of using the loophole were stymied.[160]

Provisional LMCs continued in some areas, however, to exploit opportunities to negotiate with Insurance Committees. The *Daily Mail* noted that, rather than accept the Government's terms as they stood, doctors in Salford

> had come to a temporary arrangement with the Insurance Committee under which the whole of the funds available for medical treatment…will be handed over to a representative committee of doctors who will distribute it among the practitioners attending insured persons in accordance with a scale of fees to be drawn up by the doctors themselves.[161]

This was to result in the adoption in Salford and Manchester of the method of payment by attendance rather than capitation. (This is dealt with further in Chapter 6.) An attempt to introduce this in the neighbouring county of Lancashire failed to materialise.[162] On 8 January, the *Daily Telegraph* reported that it was 'a safe estimate that more than 14,000 doctors have now come on the medical panels'.[163] The *Daily Mail* hinted at government manipulation of the figures signing up by pointing out that a large percentage of doctors were members of more than one list. They observed that some in London had registered on up to ten insurance panel district lists simultaneously, describing one such GP as 'ubiquitous'.[164] The fact remained, however, that, excepting a few lacunae where no GPs had signed up, the Government now had more than enough doctors to service the Act. On 17 January therefore, a gloomy yet still defiant BMA Special

Representative Meeting resignedly passed the resolution: 'That this meeting, recognizing the force of present circumstances and consulting the best interests of the profession now releases all practitioners from their pledges'.[165] Declining to comment on the inaccuracy of their predictions of the outcome of the dispute, the *Daily Mail* noted that 'the minority against release from the pledge was composed almost entirely of London doctors and the London Medical Committee will continue its campaign against working under the Act'.[166]

The revolt of the doctors had effectively ended. Many saw it as an ignominious defeat for the BMA and its membership suffered an immediate decline from which it took years to recover. As one Nottinghamshire GP put it, as a fighting machine for the profession, the efforts of the BMA 'had been simply futile'.[167] Alfred Cox was in no doubt as to where the fault for this lay. Referring to the grandees on the Council, he stated: 'It was a long time before I could forgive those who had led the Association into a humiliating debacle, when we might have claimed a substantial victory- and all, at the end, for the sake of sixpence'.[168] Cox later informed an American audience that the turning point in the battle was when the profession lost the support of public opinion by allowing the Government to portray the doctors as out to frustrate the will of parliament.[169] The doctors could hardly have expected to succeed where the House of Lords had failed. Several historians have accepted Cox's argument that 'the Harley Street leadership' of the BMA were to blame in being out of touch with their GP membership.[170] This is disputed, however, by Peter Bartrip.[171] Analysis of debates and letters to journals during the period of the dispute supports his conclusion by confirming that the 'diehards' were not exclusively Consultants and that the BMA was led astray not so much by Harley Street 'swells' than by its elected representatives, most of whom were GPs mandated by a mostly GP membership. But Cox's frustration is understandable. For the negotiations had in fact yielded significant benefits for the profession, prompting a National Insurance Commissioner to state in 1912: 'We are engaged in ramming down the doctors' throats the refreshing fruits of their own victory'.[172] The *Westminster Gazette* had observed a few months before the BMA's 'U-turn' that 'We all admire people who don't know when they are beaten. The trouble with the BMA is that it doesn't know when it has won'.[173] Cox was in no doubt as to the accuracy of this statement, concluding in his memoirs that 'We had in fact 'won on points'.[174] So, what exactly were the benefits British GPs enjoyed as the fruits of their disguised victory?

Material gain and reputational loss: the immediate impact of NHI on GPs

For many GPs, opposition to NHI had been about more than just remuneration, but it had been the principal bone of contention and the subject of the two cardinal points Lloyd George had been unable to concede. Experience of working under NHI soon demonstrated to the GPs, however, that much of the opprobrium heaped on the Chancellor by the profession in this regard was unjustified. Lloyd George proved to be correct in contending that the amount offered to the doctors would substantially increase their average income and provide them with much needed economic stability. It would be an exaggeration to say as Hermann Levy does that, 'The National Insurance Act was drafted with the explicit aim of improving the social and professional conditions of the doctor in order to improve the services rendered by him to the patient', but that it did have that effect is undeniable.[175] Sir Leo Chiozza-Money summed it up well when he wrote in 1912 that 'The effect of the Act from the doctor's point of view is to raise the status and pay of Society doctoring and to enlarge and make definite the medical income derived from working-class practice'.[176] The income limit remained a concern but, recognising that it was in the power of local Insurance Committees to adjust the limit if they saw fit after consultation with representatives of the profession, a number of LMCs made it their mission to try to secure the necessary adjustments, however unlikely that seemed to be.

In the weeks immediately following the launch of the new system, many doctors complained about the extra work and bureaucracy involved in accommodating an increased volume of patients anxious to test out the new system. An inquest in London into the death of a patient suffering from a perforated appendix heard that the deceased' overworked panel doctor from Battersea 'was having a perfectly dreadful time' and the jury added to the verdict of the patient's death by natural causes that the doctor had 'a scandalous amount of work to do'.[177] A Camberwell doctor reported that he had enlisted his wife and daughter to help him deal with the backlog of notes and medical cards.[178] Another 'overtired' panel GP complained of being 'deluged with day books, schedules, printed forms and literature of every description', describing it as a 'national scandal'.[179] However, panel GPs were pleased to find at the end of the first quarter after the 'appointed day' that their incomes had risen by an average of 40–60%.[180] In industrial areas of London like Bermondsey and Poplar, GP incomes increased by 100%.[181] Having become a salaried doctor, H.W. Pooler returned to being an independent contractor after noting that the Act had boosted his medical neighbours' income to three to four times what he was earning.[182] Doctors straight out of training who could previously have expected to earn no more than £300 a year could now expect to earn twice as much from a working-class panel practice which had become 'a worthy investment for the purchase of which a young doctor could now borrow money'.[183] Those 'unsaleable practices' turned out to be saleable after all and some fetched far bigger sums than they would have done before the advent of the panel.[184] NHI did not make GPs rich, but over the course of the three decades after 1912, it helped a great many of them achieve what they had always craved, that is, a comfortable middle-class existence. The panel doctors' reaction to their change of fortunes is perhaps best summed up by one of Pooler's colleagues who commented:

> When I see the queue at my surgery door and when I see the heap of papers on my consulting room table, all of which must be signed, I say 'Oh, damn Lloyd George', but when, at the end of the quarter, I handle the Insurance cheque, it is 'Well, here's to Lloyd George, the Doctors' friend!'[185]

Remuneration aside, the concessions which the BMA had wrung from the Liberal government had gone a long way towards securing some of the profession's most cherished ambitions. By negating the necessity for panel GPs to be full-time, NHI ensured that panel GPs would remain independent contractors not employees. GPs valued independent contractor status because it meant that they were effectively free agents, able to accept or refuse a variety of part-time work, including, if they had the time, capacity, and intention, other medical appointments and hospital work. The income limit on eligibility for the scheme ensured the viability of private practice in respect of those excluded from its benefits. By ensuring that all GPs could join the panel, it ended the friendly societies' control over entry to contract practice for the working classes by guaranteeing subscribers free choice of doctor and allowed GPs to compete on a more equal basis than before under what was, in many other respects, a continuation of the club system. Equally important, NHI offered GPs a means to protect their interests at the local level by ensuring that professional representatives sat as members of the Insurance Committees. These committees acted as a buffer between the GPs and the Approved Societies and were, from the GPs' point of view, a more objective arbiter of patients' complaints and of whether the terms and conditions of service were being fulfilled than the Approved Societies on their own would have been. At the national level, the GPs would be represented in due course in advisory committees and were able, through the BMA's Insurance Acts Committee, to articulate their wishes to the NHI Commissioners, while at the local level, they were to enjoy, through LMPCs, a share of the administration of the system in which they worked.

Conclusion

In the novel *The Old Doctor*, by the Walsall GP Frank Layton, the hero, Dennison, ruefully contemplates the outcome of the agitation preceding the commencement of NHI stating: 'Our leading men have put up a really Number One sized show. They've got for the G.P.'s of this land terms which are going to make General Practice very nearly worthwhile'. He expresses satisfaction that the new system 'will absolutely put the lid on the foul old cheap club system'.[186] Despite this positive prognosis, a significant minority of doctors were determined to remain outside NHI, and a large number had joined the panels with the utmost reluctance and had yet to be convinced that it would work to their benefit. The humiliation of their apparent defeat was to live long in the GPs' collective memory. While the GPs' opposition to NHI may be seen as, at best misguided, and at worst driven by selfish and irrational fears and prejudices, it was to create a mythology of noble sacrifice which affected the way GPs saw themselves in subsequent conflicts and determined the nature of political engagement with the governments of Britain for decades to come.

Herbert Woodcock may have been correct when stating that doctors were not by nature rebels. But when the flames of their professional indignation had been fanned by the Conservative press, they proved as willing to resort to extreme measures in pursuit of their political objectives as other politically marginalised groups had been. In the GPs' conflict with the Government over NHI, their opposition to friendly society control was a continuing political animus, and free choice of doctor, as an article of faith for the profession, had become a powerful propaganda weapon, which Lloyd George neatly sidestepped when he supported Addison's amendment. In this conflict, professional solidarity was tested to destruction and professional pride was severely dented by the spectacle of a humiliating public climbdown. In subsequent political battles, the spectrum of political opinion within the profession was just as wide, and the 'moral absolutism' of opposing wings was just as strong, as in 1911–1913. This should not, however, obscure the fact that many in the profession were supportive of a greater measure of state intervention in health services and desired a more systematic and less uneven system of healthcare for the poor, always provided that their professional autonomy and the rewards of private practice were vouchsafed. The 'professional social ideal' was never far from the minds of the GPs' leadership. Whether the struggle the GPs found themselves engaged in in 1912–1913 was really as 'life or death' as many believed it to be, it was one from which GPs emerged, from a material perspective, much stronger and more prosperous, and less socially insecure than they had ever been before, and from the political perspective more divided than ever, and more suspicious of central government. They had nevertheless obtained the means to exert a significant degree of influence over an increasingly important area of government policy and an opportunity to exercise a measure of power and self-government through the administrative apparatus of NHI. The challenge was how to make the new system work to their, as well as to their patients', advantage.

Notes

1 Herbert De Carle Woodcock, *The Doctor and the People* (London, 1912). p. 100.
2 Derek Fraser, *The Evolution of the Welfare State* (London, 1973). ch. 7; James R. Hay. *The Origins of the Liberal Welfare Reforms 1906–1914* (London, 1986). *passim*; Jose Harris, *Private Lives, Public Spirit: Britain 1870–1914* (London, 1993). ch. 7 and ch. 8;

Pat Thane, *Foundations of the Welfare State* (2nd ed., Harlow, 1996). ch. 3; Bernard Harris, *Origins of the British Welfare State: Society, State and Social Welfare in England and Wales1800–1945* (Basingstoke, 2004). pp. 150–166; Geoffrey R. Searle, *New Oxford History of England, A New England? Peace and War, 1886–1918, New Oxford History of England* (Oxford, 2004). pp. 361–371; Martin Daunton, *Wealth and Welfare: An Economic and Social History of Britain, 1851–1951* (Oxford, 2007). pp. 521–573; James Vernon. *Modern Britain: 1750 to the Present, Cambridge History of Britain* (Cambridge, 2017). ch. 4. Chris Renwick, *Bread for All: The Origins of the Welfare State* (2nd ed., London, 2018). ch. 2–5.

3 Bentley B. Gilbert, *The Evolution of National Insurance in Great Britain: The Origins of the Welfare State* (London, 1966). *passim* but especially ch.6 and ch. 7; Norman R. Eder, *National Health Insurance and the Medical Profession in Britain, 1913–1939* (New York, 1982). *passim*; Anne Digby, *The Evolution of British General Practice 1850–1948* (Oxford, 1999). ch. 13; Noel Parry and Jose Parry, *The Rise of the Medical Profession* (London, 1976). pp. 43–59, 83, 192–195; Margaret Stacey, *The Sociology of Heath and Healing* (London, 1988). pp. 104–121.

4 Searle, *A New England?* pp. 470–471.

5 Gilbert, *The Evolution of National Insurance*, pp. 291–293.

6 Hay, *The Origins of the Liberal Welfare Reforms*, p. 30.

7 Geoffrey Eley, *Modern Germany* (New York, 1998). vol. 2, 'Social Imperialism', *passim*. See also Bernard Harris, *Origins of the British Welfare State*, pp. 19–21.

8 Hay, *The Origins of the Liberal Welfare Reforms,* p. 54; See also Martin Gorsky, 'The Political Economy of Healthcare in the Nineteenth and Twentieth Centuries', in Mark Jacobs (ed) *The Oxford Handbook of the History of Medicine* (Oxford, 2013). p. 431.

9 Jose Harris, *Unemployment and Politics, 1886–1914* (Oxford, 1972). p. 218.

10 Gilbert, *The Evolution of National Insurance*, p. 61. Hay, *The Origins of the Liberal Welfare Reforms*, p. 18.

11 Charles Booth, *Life and Labour of the People of London* (London, 1892). *passim.* Seebohm Rowntree, *Poverty: A Study of Town Life* (London, 1901). *passim.* Renwick, *Bread for All*, pp. 93–103.

12 Quoted by Gilbert, *The Evolution of National Insurance*, p. 77.

13 Quoted in Hay, *The Origins of the Liberal Welfare Reforms*, p. 25. 'National Insurance was the Liberal Government's response to the threat of socialism.' Harris, *Origins of the British Welfare State*, p. 155.

14 Searle, *A New England?* p. 361. The Independent Labour Party (ILP) were among the most overtly socialist elements of the Labour movement.

15 Gorsky, 'The Political Economy of Healthcare in the Nineteenth and Twentieth Centuries', p. 431.

16 Quoted in Fraser, *The Evolution of the Welfare State*, p. 129.

17 Sidney and Beatrice Webb, *The State and the Doctor* (London, 1910). pp. 78, 81,123.

18 Harris, *Private Lives, Public Spirit*, pp. 228–229. Renwick, *Bread for All*, pp. 64–72.

19 Thane, *Foundations of the Welfare State*, p. 12. See also Searle, *A New England?* p. 394.

20 Vernon, *Modern Britain: 1750 to the Present,* p. 114. See also Michael Bentley 'Boundaries in Theoretical Language about the British State,' in S.J.D. Green and R.C. Whiting (eds) *Boundaries of the State in Modern Britain* (Cambridge, 1996). pp. 42–43.

21 Vernon, *Modern Britain: 1750 to the Present,* p. 115.

22 Harris, *Private Lives, Public Spirit*, ch.8.

23 Nikolas Rose, 'Government, Authority and Expertise in Advanced Liberalism.' *Economy and Society*, 22 (3) (1993) p. 292.

24 Mary Poovey, *Making A Social Body: British Cultural Formation 1830–1864* (Chicago, IL, 1995). p. 14; Harris, *Private Lives, Public Spirit*, pp. 220–250.
25 Hay, *The Origins of the Liberal Welfare Reforms*, p. 39. Renwick, *Bread for All*, pp. 110–115 and 178–180.
26 Renwick, *Bread for All*, p. 115.
27 Thane, *Foundations of the Welfare State*, p. 291.
28 Bernard M. Allen, *Sir Robert Morant, A Great Public Servant* (London, 1934). p. 280.
29 Nikolas Rose, 'Government, Authority and Expertise in Advanced Liberalism', p. 285. Thane, *Foundations of the Welfare State*, p. 291.
30 Gilbert, *The Evolution of National Insurance*, p. 315. John Grigg, *Lloyd George; The People's Champion 1902–1911* (London, 1978). pp. 316–317.
31 For a contemporary but contrary view suggesting that Lloyd George ignored or misinterpreted the evidence from the German experience, see William A. Brend, *Health and the State* (New York, 1917). pp. 213–214.
32 Hay, *The Origins of the Liberal Welfare Reforms*, pp. 40–41.
33 *Ibid.*, p. 42; Thane, *Foundations of the Welfare State*, p. 90.
34 John Turner, 'Experts and Interests: David Lloyd George and the Dilemmas of the Expanding State, 1906–19,' in Roy McLeod (ed) *Government and Expertise: Specialists, Administrators and Professionals, 1860–1919* (Cambridge, 1988). p. 211.
35 *Ibid.*, p. 204.
36 Hermann Levy, *National Health Insurance: A Critical Study* (Cambridge, 1944). p. 14.
37 Gilbert, *The Evolution of National Insurance*, p. 356.
38 James C. Riley, *Sick Not Dead: The Health of British Working Men During the Mortality Decline* (London, 1997). pp. 198, 106–110.
39 Gorsky, 'Friendly Society Health Insurance in Nineteenth Century England', p. 159.
40 Bernard Harris, Martin Gorsky, Aravinda Meera Guntupalli and Andrew Hinde, 'Long-term Changes in Sickness and Health: Further Evidence from the Hampshire Friendly Society.' *Economic History Review*, 65 (2) (2012). p. 744.
41 Sir Leo Chiozza-Money, *Insurance and Poverty* (London, 1912). p. 135. See also Bernard Harris, 'Social Policy by Other Means? Mutual Aid and the Origins of the Welfare State in Britain during the Nineteenth and Twentieth Centuries.' *Journal of Policy History*, 30 (2) (2018). pp. 207–213.
42 Woodcock, *The Doctor and the People*, p. 99.
43 *BMJ*, 4 March 1911, 'Report on the Organization of Medical Attendance on the Provident or Insurance Principle', Supplement, pp. 82–107.
44 *BMA Archive*, B/231/1, Minutes of meeting between the Special Poor Law Committee and Contract Practice Subcommittee on 26 October 1910, memorandum by Dr W. Gosse.
45 Gilbert, *The Evolution of National Insurance*, footnote to p. 363.
46 *The Times*, 22 May 1911, 'The State Insurance Bill – Action by the Medical Association', p. 9.
47 Christopher Viscount Addison, *Politics from Within, vol 1, 1911–1918* (London, 1924). p. 20.
48 Gilbert, *The Evolution of National Insurance,* pp. 368–382.
49 Sir Henry Bunbury (ed) *Lloyd George's Ambulance Wagon: The Memoirs of W.J. Braithwaite* (London, 1949). pp. 141–142.
50 Alfred Cox, *Among the Doctors* (London, circa 1950). p. 86.
51 Gilbert, *The Evolution of National Insurance*, p. 364.
52 *Hansard*, HC, 1 August 1911. col. 318.

53 Bunbury, *Lloyd George's Ambulance Wagon*, p. 198.
54 *Ibid.*, p. 182.
55 A.S. (Arthur Strettell) Comyns Carr, W.H. (William Hubert) Stuart-Garnett, and J.H. (James Henry) Taylor, *National Insurance* (London, 1912). p. 63.
56 Quoted in John Grigg, *Lloyd George: The People's Champion, 1902–1911* (London, 1978). p. 334.
57 Jane Morgan and Kenneth Morgan. *Portrait of a Progressive: The Political Career of Christopher, Viscount Addison* (Oxford, 1980). p. 12.
58 Peter Bartrip, *Themselves Writ Large: The British Medical Association 1832–1966* (London, 1996). p. 154.
59 Morgan and Morgan, *Portrait of a Progressive*, pp. 14–17
60 Paul Vaughan, *Doctors' Commons* (London, 1959). p. 200.
61 Gilbert, *The Evolution of National Insurance*, p. 367.
62 *BMJ*, 3 June1911, 'Report of Special Representative Meeting of 31 May, I June 1911', Supplement, p. 354.
63 Bunbury, *Lloyd George's Ambulance Wagon*, p. 171.
64 Cox, *Among the Doctors*, p. 91.
65 Woodcock, *The Doctor and the People*, p. 80.
66 *Daily Mail,* 5 June 1911, 'Doctor's Revolt...Income Limit in State Practice.' p. 6.
67 Professor J.T.J. Morrison, quoted in *The Birmingham Post*, 16 June 1911.
68 Quoted in E.S. (Ernest Sackville) Turner, *Call the Doctor: A Social History of Medical Men* (London, 1958). p. 255.
69 *The Times*, 27 June 1911, p. 4.
70 Bartrip, *Themselves Writ Large*, p. 156.
71 Bunbury, *Lloyd George's Ambulance Wagon*, p. 167.
72 *Ibid.*, p. 172.
73 Comyns Carr, *National Insurance*, p. 56.
74 Bartrip, *Themselves Writ Large*, p. 155.
75 *BMA Archive*, B/231/1, Medico Political Committee circular 112, 1 May 1911 'Professional Defence Appeal for £5,000'.
76 *BMJ*, I July 1911, 'National Insurance, Action of the British Medical Association, The Undertaking and the Memorial', Supplement, p. 2.
77 *Nottinghamshire County RO*, DD/1440/23/1;1911–1913, 21 November 1911.
78 Dr M.F. Taylor quoted by F.E. Lodge, 'Reminiscences from a Fenland Practice.' *BMJ*, 22 December 1984, p. 1760.
79 For example, *Daily Mail*, 9 January 1912, p. 8; 10 January 1912, pp. 5–6.
80 Vaughan, *Doctors' Commons*, p. 202.
81 He declared that 'a Deputation of Doctors is always a Deputation of swell Doctors.' Gilbert, *The Evolution of National Insurance*, p. 363.
82 Bartrip, *Themselves Writ Large*, p. 155
83 *Manchester University Medical Collections*, NMU 1, minutes of Advisory Committee meeting on 28 December 1911, p. 3.
84 *Ibid.*, minutes of Advisory Committee meeting on 19 January 1912, p. 1.
85 *The Times,* 14 October 1911.
86 *Manchester University Medical Collections*, NMU 1, minutes of Executive Committee meeting on 20 February 1913.
87 Cox, *Among the Doctors*, p. 86.
88 Francis Brett Young, *Dr Bradley Remembers* (London, 1938). p. 709.
89 Cox, *Among the Doctors*, p. 87.
90 Macdonald Obituary, *BMJ*, 5 May 1928, p. 782.

91 *Nottinghamshire County RO*, DD/1440/23/20–43, LMC correspondence. Letter 17 December 1911 from Dr F. Broadbent of Collingham to Dr Ernest Ringrose, Secretary, Newark Local Medical Committee.
92 See Simon Cordery, *British Friendly Societies, 1750–1914* (Basingstoke, 2003). p. 168. Comyns Carr, *National Insurance*, pp. 61–63.
93 Vaughan, *Doctors' Commons*, p. 204.
94 Letter from Dr Frederick James Smith, *The Times*, 6 December 1911.
95 Sir John Conybeare, 'The Crisis of 1911–1913: Lloyd George and the Doctors.' *Lancet*, 15 (May 1957). p. 1033.
96 For the *Mail's* account of the meeting see report dated 21 February 1912, p. 7.
97 *Nottinghamshire County RO*, DD/1440/23/20–43, LMC correspondence, February 1912.
98 *BMA Archive*, B/231/1, Memorandum D46 accompanying letter (D47) from Dr A. Cox to BMA Divisional Secretaries 18 March 1912.
99 John H. Marks, *The History and Development of Local Medical Committees, Their Conference and Its Executive*, Edinburgh University MD Thesis, 1974, p. 28.
100 Cox, *Among the Doctors* p. 99. The high-water mark of BMA membership in 1912 was 26,568. Bartrip, *Themselves Writ Large*, p. 162.
101 The supplemental undertaking was issued in a further letter from Cox, *BMA Archive*, B/231/1, Memorandum D49, dated 29 April 1912.
102 Marks, *The History and Development of Local Medical Committees*, p. 26.
103 *Ibid.*, 19 February 1912, p. 6.
104 Vaughan, *Doctors' Commons*, p. 203.
105 Conybeare, 'The Crisis of 1911–1913', p. 1033.
106 Gilbert, *The Evolution of National Insurance*, p. 408.
107 M. Jeanne Peterson, *The Medical Profession in Mid-Victorian London* (London, 1978). p. 218.
108 Guy Routh, *Occupation and Pay in Great Britain, 1906–1979* (2nd ed., London, 1980).
109 Gilbert, *The Evolution of National Insurance*, pp. 411–412.
110 *Nation*, 3 August 1912, 'Medical Supplement', pp. i–ii.
111 *Daily Chronicle*, 3 January 1913, p. 5.
112 *Ibid.*, 22 November 1912, p. 5.
113 *Ibid.*, 'Doctors Coming Round', 12 December 1912, p. 4.
114 Gilbert, *The Evolution of National Insurance*, p. 407.
115 Bartrip, *Themselves Writ Large*, p. 160; *Daily Chronicle*, 6 December 1912, p. 4.
116 Vaughan, *Doctors' Commons*, p. 209. *Daily Mail*, 14 December 1912, p. 8.
117 *Daily Mail*, 14 December 1912, p. 8.
118 *Manchester University Medical Collections*, GB 133 MMC/7/1/3 and 7/18/1, Extract from *Manchester Guardian*, 21 December 1912.
119 Addison acknowledged their bravery in his memoirs, *Politics from Within*, vol.1, p. 23.
120 *Daily Mail*, 16 December 1912, p. 9.
121 Conybeare, 'The Crisis of 1911–1913', p. 1034.
122 Francis Brett Young, *Dr Bradley Remembers* (London, 1938). pp. 709–713.
123 *Daily Chronicle*, 23 December 1912, 'The BMA and the Doctors', p. 4.
124 *Nottinghamshire County RO*, SO NHI /1–3, Report of the Medical Benefit Subcommittee, 29 December 1912.
125 *Daily Mail*, 2 November 1912, p. 4.
126 *Ibid.*, 23 December 1912, p. 5.
127 *Daily Chronicle*, 'The BMA and the Insurance Act', 21 December 1912, p. 5.

128 *Ibid.,* 'Severe Criticism of Association's Policy', 24 December 1912, p. 1.
129 *Ibid.,* 25 December, p. 1. Cox, *Among the Doctors*, p. 96.
130 Cox, *Among the Doctors*, p. 97.
131 Turner, *Call the Doctor*, p. 259. Gilbert, *The Evolution of National Insurance,* p. 415.
132 Marks, *The History and Development of Local Medical Committees*, p. 31.
133 Addison, *Politics from Within*, vol. 1, p. 24.
134 Bartrip, *Themselves Writ Large*, p. 161.
135 *Daily Mail*, 26 December 1912, p. 5.
136 *Daily Chronicle*, 27 December 1912, p. 1.
137 Turner, *Call the Doctor*, p. 259.
138 *Daily Mail*, 27 December 1912, p. 3; 30 December 1912, p. 5.
139 *Daily Chronicle*, 27 December 1912, p. 1.
140 *Ibid.*
141 *Ibid.*, 28 December 1912, p. 5.
142 *Ibid.*
143 *Daily Mail*, 3 January 1913, p. 5; *Daily Chronicle*, 3 January 1913, p. 1.
144 *Daily Chronicle*, 8 January 1913, p. 1.
145 Philip Gosse, *An Apple a Day* (London, 1948). pp. 8–9.
146 Turner, *Call the Doctor*, p. 259.
147 *Daily Mail*, 7 January 1913, p. 4.
148 *Daily Telegraph*, 7 January 1913, p. 9.
149 *Daily Chronicle*, 8 January 1913, 'Scandalous Outrage at Doctor's House', p. 1.
150 *Ibid.,* 9 January 1913, 'Curious Story from Willesden', p. 7.
151 *Daily Telegraph*, 16 January 1913, p. 11.
152 *BMJ*, 11 January 1913, Editorial, p. 83.
153 *National Insurance Act 1911,* Section 15, subsection 3.
154 *Daily Chronicle*, 3 January 1913, p. 1.
155 *Daily Mail*, 7 January 1913, p. 4.
156 *Ibid.*, 9 January 1913, p. 5.
157 *Daily Telegraph*, 20 January 1913, p. 8.
158 *The Times*, 10 January 1913, p. 8,
159 *Ibid.*, 13 January 1913, p. 5. See also *Daily Chronicle*, 8 January 1913, p. 1.
160 Eder, *National Health Insurance and the Medical Profession*, pp. 52–53.
161 *Daily Mail*, 6 January 1913, p. 9.
162 *BMJ*, 11 January 1913, Editorial, p. 83.
163 *Daily Telegraph*, 8 January 1913, 'More Panels Formed', p. 9.
164 *Daily Mail*, 15 January 1913, 'The Insurance Muddle-Farcical Position of the Panels', p. 3.
165 *BMJ,* 25 January 1913, Supplement p. 97.
166 *Daily Mail*, 20 January 1913, p. 7.
167 *Nottinghamshire County RO*, DD/1440/23//20–43, LMC correspondence, Letter from Dr W.B. Hallowes of Newark to Dr Ernest Ringrose.
168 Cox, *Among the Doctors*, pp. 98–99.
169 Alfred Cox, 'Seven Years of National Health Insurance in England.' *Journal of the American Medical Association*, LXXVI, 7 (May 1921). p. 1310.
170 See Gilbert, *The Evolution of National Insurance*, pp. 407 and 409. Eder, *National Health Insurance and the Medical Profession*, p. 45. Morgan and Morgan, *Portrait of a Progressive*, p. 12.
171 Bartrip, *Themselves Writ Large*, pp. 163–164.
172 Allen, *Sir Robert Morant*, p. 282.

173 Quoted by Vaughan, *Doctors' Commons*, p. 209 (no citation).
174 Cox, *Among the Doctors*, p. 99.
175 Levy, *National Health Insurance*, p. 122.
176 Sir Leo Chiozza-Money, *Insurance and Poverty* (London, 1912). p. 97.
177 *Daily Mail*, 22 January 1913, p. 7.
178 *Ibid.*, 25 January 1913, p. 3.
179 *Ibid.*, 10 February 1913, p. 4.
180 Eder, *National Health Insurance and the Medical Profession*, p. 56.
181 *Ibid.*
182 Harry W. Pooler, *My Life in General Practice* (London, 1948). p. 57.
183 Gilbert, *The Evolution of National Insurance*, p. 44.
184 *Ibid.*, p. 440, quoting survey by the *National Insurance Gazette* 13 December 1913.
     See also Turner, *Call the Doctor*, p. 264.
185 Pooler, *My Life in General Practice*, p. 57.
186 Frank C. Layton, *The Old Doctor* (Birmingham, 1923). pp. 140–141.

5 Inauspicious beginnings

Medical trade unionism, the
Great War, and early attempts
at 'bargained corporatism',
1913–1919

In 1913, the credibility of the BMA and its right to represent the interests of NHI panel doctors were both open to question. During the course of the First World War, however, the Association managed to turn this situation around and lay the foundations of a relationship with government based on what Harold Perkin would have described as 'bargained corporatism'. This he defines as 'a tacit entente between government officials and putatively representative organisations offering themselves as intermediaries in negotiating with the state outside parliamentary channels, while regulating their membership within a wider system of order'.[1] The BMA did this by means of two parallel developments. Firstly, they established, through a not-always-obvious or deliberate process of alliance-building, a mutually beneficial relationship with the Conference of LMPCs. This gave them the necessary mandate with which to negotiate and collectively bargain on the panel GPs' behalf. Secondly, they succeeded in establishing a positive working relationship with the officials responsible for NHI which was focussed on improving both patients' and doctors' experiences of the scheme. This process was accompanied, however, by continued attempts by rival professional interest groups to challenge the BMA's authority. The advent of war did not curtail the arguments about the panel doctors' pay and service requirements, about who could best represent their interests, or about the future development of NHI and its relationship with other medical services. Indeed, the longer the war continued, the louder and more vituperative the arguments became.

The GPs sacrificed much during the war years and counted themselves among its long list of victims. However, the BMA was an unexpected beneficiary of the conflict. The patriotic impetus of the call to arms allowed the BMA to demonstrate the merits of professional self-government, and their willingness to work in partnership with the state was in stark contrast to the truculent self-interest demonstrated by the profession's trade union lobby. While consolidating its representative credentials, however, the BMA's Insurance Acts Committee (IAC) did not find it easy to rid itself of the threat of rival organisations. In fact, the IAC's right to represent the panel GPs was subjected to repeated challenges both during and after the war. Thus, while battles raged in Flanders, the annual

DOI: 10.4324/9781003438274-5

conferences of LMPCs taking place during this period proved the backdrop for an ideological conflict of a similarly unforgiving kind. Crucial decisions were taken during this period which affected the future character and status of British general practice, its relationship with government, and the nature of its representative structures.

Before the war: negotiating machinery and the mandate of the Conference of LMPCs

In 1913, the BMA found itself being pulled in opposite directions. Pragmatists within its ranks recognised the need to accept that NHI was a reality and to make it work for the public and the insurance doctors. However, the 'diehards' were not completely vanquished and, recognising that a still significant minority of GPs remained unreconciled to the Act, encouraged the Association to establish a 'non-panel doctors committee' to represent their interests.[2] The position of the extremists at opposite ends of the debate over NHI had begun to harden. On the left, an organisation calling itself the State Medical Services Association (SMSA) was already talking of NHI as the first step towards a more comprehensive state medical service centred on salaried doctors. It numbered among its executive notable figures such as Addison, the Fabians Sidney Webb, and George Bernard Shaw, and Labour activists like Dr Alfred Salter and Ramsay MacDonald.[3] At the other extreme, the National Medical Union (NMU) had confirmed its implacable opposition to any state-sponsored scheme and in December 1913 committed itself to becoming an association of non-panel doctors.[4] Between these positions, there were many insurance doctors who, though weary of the conflict which had blighted their reputation with the Government and the public, wanted stronger representation than the BMA appeared to give them. The BMA's defeat reignited the arguments put forward at the Manchester Guild conference in 1900. It helped resurrect the idea that the interests of GPs would be best served by an organisation representing their interests alone and an increasing number of GPs believed that to be effective, such an organisation had to be a registered trade union.

A Public Medical Service (PMS) had been established in Leicester in December 1912 when the local doctors had seized the opportunity to take over the local provident dispensary. The organisation set up to run it called itself the Union of Medical Practitioners and was duly registered under the Trade Union Act. When writing to the *BMJ* about this initiative in January 1913, its chairman, R. Wallace Henry, clearly hoped that it might serve as the basis of a national organisation.[5] His announcement elicited little enthusiasm but proved the catalyst for a long running debate in the letter pages of the *BMJ* over the summer of 1913 about the merits of a medical trade union and a new organisation to champion the interests of insurance doctors. In March 1913 under the heading 'Trade unionism and medicine', Dr A. George Bateman, the Secretary of the Medical Defence Union, reiterated the familiar argument that trade unionism was incompatible with medicine.[6] His comments were dismissed by Dr Henry Cardale, future chairman of the London Panel Committee, who contended that it was perfectly possible to establish a medical trade union that acted ethically and in a manner consistent with the honour and interests of the profession.[7] In April 1913, Dr Gordon Ward, a member of the Kent County Medical Committee, set out the case for a trade union to work alongside the BMA, declaring himself as 'an enthusiastic advocate of the National Medical Guild'.[8] The Guild was established as a trade union sometime in early 1913. Writing to the *BMJ* in May 1913, Dr E.H. Worth explained that the Guild 'was really the old London Medical Committee which… helped the London men stick to their pledge'.[9] Though praised by prominent non-panel GPs like Dr Charles Buttar, the Guild was explicitly supportive of panel doctors and was buoyed by the views of GPs like Dr R.W. Innes Smith who informed *Medical World* in January 1914 that a postal vote of practitioners in Sheffield showed them to be 20–1 in favour of a trade union.[10] Buttar congratulated the Guild for its efforts in mounting a legal challenge to the NHI Commission's ruling that non-panel doctors' certificates could not be recognised for insurance benefit purposes.[11] In the *BMJ* in December 1913, Dr Russell Combe proposed that a new defence fund be set up and registered under the trade union act. He suggested that this be independent of the BMA but managed by trustees appointed by the Association and organised by officers of BMA divisions.[12] The idea seems to have taken root as a report on it was included in the annual report of BMA Council in May 1914.[13] The report proposed that the fund be established as a trust rather than a trade union, citing once again the example of the National Union of Teachers which, it pointed out, was an unincorporated body which had deliberately refrained from seeking legal incorporation either as a company or as a trade union. In the ensuing debate in the *BMJ* under the heading 'The Special Fund: Trade Union or Trust?', R. Wallace Henry argued strongly in favour of a trade union.[14] However, he found himself subject to a withering rebuke by fellow BMA Council member E. Rowland Fothergill and 'tit for tat' responses rumbled on over the summer of 1914 concluding with Wallace Henry decrying Fothergill's imagined 'nightmare of medical syndicalism'.[15] The correspondence was punctuated by a contribution from London GP Dr Percy Raiment, the General Secretary of the National Medical Guild, who pointed out the legal jeopardy faced by an organisation not registered as a trade union, particularly if subjected to a charge of malice. This was a judgment which, as will be seen, was to prove remarkably prescient as far as the BMA was concerned.[16]

In his memoirs, the BMA Secretary Alfred Cox recorded that, 'If the controllers of the National Health Insurance Commission had been small minded people they would have treated the Association as a defeated and discredited body and would have encouraged attempts…to side-track it in dealing with insurance affairs'.[17] The GPs were fortunate, however, that the civil servant Lloyd George had entrusted to implement the scheme, the highly capable Sir Robert Morant, was broadly pro-doctor and keen to enlist the BMA's support in making NHI a success both for the insured and for the panel GPs.[18] He was supported by the commission's Deputy Chairman James Smith Whitaker who, despite the rancour shown towards him by many of his erstwhile colleagues in the profession, was anxious to foster harmony between the commissioners and the Association. The new leadership of the BMA was equally keen to establish a constructive working relationship. In May 1914, the annual report of the BMA's Council noted that:

> It is obvious that with the large numbers of practitioners who are now giving service under the Insurance Act…it is to the interest of the profession that the Association acting on behalf of the profession generally, should be on good terms with the commissioners.[19]

Norman Eder states, 'Exhausted by its three-year adversary relationship with the government, the BMA quickly tried to move to a new position of partnership with the Health Insurance administration'.[20] When in April 1913 the Government announced its intention of introducing clarifying amendments to the Act, the BMA's State Sickness Insurance Committee set to work compiling a list of what they considered sensible and reasonable amendments. Almost all of these were overlooked in the amending Act published in July 1913 apart from the reaffirmation of the £160 income limit for non-manual workers. However, the Act made provision for regulations to be drawn up by the Joint Insurance Commission which quickly found itself fielding competing suggestions from the profession and from representatives of the Approved Societies, who still harboured a desire to exercise greater control over the scheme.[21]

At the BMA's annual meeting in Brighton in July 1913, the Representative Body reflected on the Association's recent failings. A proposal that the Association become a trade union was heavily defeated but the meeting approved the recommendation from its Council which stated that 'no system of reorganisation of the Association can be effective which does not take into consideration the position of Local Medical Committees and devise some means of coordinating their work with that of the Association'.[22] This message set the tone for discussions which took place immediately after the annual meeting at a conference of Local Medical Committees (LMCs) instigated not by the BMA Council, which had declined, on grounds of cost, a request to host the conference, but by the local BMA division and its secretary, E. Rowland Fothergill.[23] Fothergill was to play a major part in relations between the BMA, LMPCs, and other bodies. Although he frequently exasperated BMA colleagues and their opponents, Cox describes him as a 'devoted worker for cooperation amongst doctors'.[24] The conference was a modest affair attended by less than a full complement of LMC representatives. It was most notable for the fact that a motion calling for 'fusion' between the BMA and the LMCs was rejected but a resolution was passed that 'as far as possible there should be cooperation between the LMCs and the BMA'.[25] The BMA's Representative Body had decided to replace the State Sickness Insurance Committee with a new Insurance Acts Committee (IAC) as a standing committee of the Association. The IAC's remit was 'to deal with all matters arising under the National Insurance Act that are dealt with by the National Insurance commissioners, insurance committees and local medical committees'.[26] Members were to be elected by Council and the Representative Body on a territorial basis, with reserved seats for representatives of women doctors, public health doctors, and poor law medical officers. All were required to be BMA members, though at least one-fifth were to be panel doctors. The GP obstetrician Mabel Ramsay was appointed to the IAC as a representative of women doctors 'in her own right' but was duly appointed the Medical Women's Federation (MWF) representative when it came into being in 1917 and remained their IAC representative until 1937.[27] An amendment requiring that four seats on the committee be reserved for LMC officers was rejected.[28] The chairman, appointed at its first meeting later that month, was the respected chairman of the BMA Council, J.A. Macdonald. Much of its first meeting was taken up with a discussion about the need to establish a special defence fund for the organisation of the profession, but at its second meeting in September 1913, the committee appointed an LMC subcommittee comprising the chairman and four members of the committee and five others 'co-opted to represent other interested parties'. It thereby allowed for input into the committee's business from doctors involved in LMCs (and, subsequently, Panel Committees).[29]

As will be more fully explained in the next chapter, the National Insurance Amendment Act 1913 included the provision to establish separate Panel Committees.[30] The IAC therefore began discussions with the commissioners about a model constitution for LMCs and Panel Committees and persuaded the BMA to convene, in March the following year, a conference in London of 'Local Medical *and* Panel Committees'. By then, the benefits and the deficiencies of the NHI scheme from the doctors' viewpoint had become obvious and the steps which the BMA had taken to raise concerns with the NHI Commission were the subject of agitated debate and argument. While most of the representatives present at the Conference recognised the need for good working relationships with Government, there were many who felt that the Association's response was too conciliatory and believed that an entirely new organisation would be more effective. The Conference therefore debated a proposal to establish an Association of LMPCs. This was opposed by those who felt that it would prove a rival to the BMA.[31] The Conference ultimately resolved to establish a *Federation* of LMPCs which would be associated with the BMA and to establish a voluntary levy of panel practitioners' remuneration to support its operation. A provisional committee was appointed to devise an appropriate constitution for this new body which was also instructed to consider its potential relationship with the National Medical Guild.[32] The provisional committee wrote to all LMPCs about the Federation and found the majority to be in favour of its proposed links with the BMA.[33]

In May 1914, the IAC met with the provisional committee and proposed to the BMA Council that the Federation be able to appoint seven additional members of the IAC, and that accommodation, facilities, and staff be provided for it at the BMA's headquarters and space given in the *BMJ* Supplement to report on its activities.[34]

The advocates of trade unionism in the medical profession were largely but not exclusively supporters of independent contractor status. Most GPs at this time believed that salaried service was at odds with their desire for autonomy, and many still feared that NHI would prove the first step towards the development of a state medical service in which doctors would become government employees. In a lecture in early 1914, one of the leading lights of the SMSA, Sir John Collie, set out their case for a full-time salaried service as the logical extension of the panel scheme.[35] Other SMSA stalwarts supportive of the salaried service idea, Professor Benjamin Moore and Dr Charles Parker, set out their views in the *Lancet*.[36] Similar proposals were advocated in the *BMJ* by Dr Milson R. Rhodes, echoing ideas he had voiced in 1912.[37] His comments aroused an impassioned response from defenders of independent contractor status and free choice of doctor. One commentator, Dr J. Charles, stated that such proposals would 'break with a system of practice which has long and adequately served its purpose' and, as an illustration of the extent to which both the insurance doctors and their patients had already become acclimatised to the new system, he added 'and departs from a system which had already found widespread favour with the public and general acceptance by the medical profession'.[38] Even some left-leaning doctors wanting a more comprehensive service for the population balked at the idea of doctors becoming civil servants, or worse, subordinates of local authority Medical Officers of Health. Writing to *Medical World*, Lauriston Shaw urged his colleagues to allow the existing panel service to develop and evolve rather than initiate radical changes to which doctors would be even more vehemently opposed. This was to be preferred, he said, as 'the British way of doing things'.[39] The maverick East-end GP Harry Roberts echoed Shaw's comments, suggesting that the panel system was working well and that all it needed to offer a complete service to patients was access to specialist treatment.[40]

A number of doctors involved in setting up of the London Panel Committee, including its Chairman, Henry Cardale, and Secretary, Alfred Welply, were enthusiastic supporters of the panel system and questioned the BMA's right, based on its record, to champion the interests of the panel GPs. Unimpressed by other medical organisations, they decided to establish their own trade union to represent panel doctors. The inaugural meeting in July 1914 of what they named the Panel Medico Political Union (PMPU) was chaired by Christopher Addison and founding members included a number of socialist doctors such as Alfred Salter.[41] Henry Brackenbury, the chairman of the Middlesex LMPC, was among a minority of doctors attending the meeting who opposed the establishment of a new representative body. His suggestion that it was unnecessary to establish a new organisation as the BMA was now pro-panel was met with derisive contempt.[42] The IAC was clearly fearful of the influence of the anti-BMA lobby and, when surveying LMPCs in November 1914 about their constitution, membership, and funding, asked each committee if they were in favour of 'entering into a close and steady relationship' with the BMA.[43] It was not until March 1915 that, in a letter to all insurance practitioners headed 'What the Association has done for panel practitioners', Alfred Cox reported that the response from LMPCs to this question was 'very favourable', citing 162 out of 192 supporting the close relationship described.[44]

By this time the PMPU had distanced itself from the Federation of LMPCs, which the London Panel Committee pointedly refused to join when denied what it regarded as a proportionate number of seats on its executive.[45] The extent to which opinion was divided on this matter is illustrated by the debate reported in *Medical World* in December 1914 in which London Panel Committee member H.G Cowie commented sarcastically that 'the close and steady relationship' between the BMA and LMPCs implied that 429 Strand (the BMA's headquarters) 'should be recognised as the Mecca for all panel pilgrims and especially for secretaries of panel committees'.[46] His Panel Committee colleague Dr Angus further objected to 'the temerity of the BMA in claiming representative authority when not one of 8,000 GPs who were not BMA members were eligible to serve on the IAC'.[47] In July 1915, *Medical World* became the official organ of the PMPU and from then on its editorials and commissioned articles became increasingly strident in their criticism of the BMA which it felt was not up to the task of defending the panel GPs against existential threats. An article in February 1915 described these as including 'the menace of the approved societies wishing to hold us as "bondslaves", and politicians, commissioners and civil servants wanting to reduce the GP's pay'.[48] By then, however, the profession, like the rest of the British public, was preoccupied with matters of a less parochial nature.

The profession and the war: self-government, self-sacrifice, and a system under strain

On the eve of the BMA's Annual Representative Meeting in Aberdeen in July 1914, Dr Mark Taylor of the National Medical Guild wrote to the *BMJ* arguing that the BMA be affiliated to the Guild, which, with the Association's support and sponsorship, could, he said, take on the task of defending medical interests. Referring to the recently reported success of the *Leipziger Verband* in its battle with the German insurance funds, he said that for evidence to support the virtues of medical trade unionism, British GPs need only look to Germany.[49] At the close of the representative meeting, all eyes were indeed fixed on Germany, but for entirely different reasons. Alfred Cox noted that during the meeting, 'we noticed that the national and territorial medical officers silently disappeared' and on the Monday following the BMA officials' return to London, their suspicions were realised when war was officially declared with Germany and its allies.[50] Due to the popular belief that it would be over by Christmas, there was no immediate concern about the impact of the war on civilian medical services even though within the first few months, some 10% of the country's medical practitioners had either volunteered or been called up as reservists.[51]

The patriotic response of the medical profession reflected that of the professional and managerial classes generally, which showed a far greater willingness to serve the war effort than the general population. The percentage of the 'the professions' volunteering during 1914–1916 (41.7%) was the joint highest of occupational groups.[52] An article in August 1914 in *Medical World* noted the recent decision by the London Panel Committee to treat gratuitously families of enlisted men who had volunteered for service in the forces. This, it said, 'exemplifies the self-sacrificing tradition of the medical profession and will doubtless be followed by other medical committees'.[53] LMPCs were equally concerned, however, to protect the interests of the GPs who had volunteered to serve their country. Thus, Lancashire LMPC's Honorary Secretary wrote to its constituents in September 1914 urging them to 'loyally safeguard the interests of those of their colleagues who are called to leave their practices in the service of their country and to undertake any medical duties entailed for the sole benefit of the absentees'. He reported that they had requested the local Insurance Committee to rule that no transfer takes place of the patients of any doctor absent on military service for the duration of the war.[54] It quickly became apparent, however, that unless recruitment from the ranks of the medical profession was organised in some way, large and potentially destabilising gaps could appear within the fabric of civilian medical services.

The BMA had already resolved to support the war effort by 'placing the whole resources and machinery of the Association at the disposal of the government'.[55] In the month following the outbreak of war, the BMA's Scottish Committee had voted at a meeting in Edinburgh to establish a Scottish Medical Service Emergency Committee which quickly set about organising a network of local medical war committees, linked to BMA divisions, to supervise substitution arrangements for doctors who had enlisted and arrange provision of free medical attendance for soldiers' families.[56] This offered a model for the rest of the country to follow and in January 1915, the Association set up a Central Medical War Committee (CMWC) which the Annual Representative Meeting endorsed in July.[57] The establishment of the CMWC was broadly welcomed by the government and seen as 'part of the general tendency towards planning for a protracted war'.[58] Sir Alfred Keogh, Director General of the army medical service, subsequently agreed to devolve to the CMWC the whole responsibility for recruiting doctors. He did this, according to Cox, 'because he believed it was the only way to avoid the risk of depleting the profession in those areas in which essential munitions work was being done'.[59] Though the doctors were unaware of it, the government's reliance on the BMA and its CMWC was consistent with the way in which it harnessed the expertise of industrialists and trade unionists in the service of the war effort and was a form of corporatism which government officials proved only too willing to embrace.[60] Cox was the central figure behind the CMWC's work.[61] He benefited from a constructive relationship with Morant who lent the committee a number of civil servants to supplement the large staff ('mainly girls') supporting its work.[62] One of the committee's first tasks was to establish an accurate register of where practitioners were based. A survey showed that by July 1915, 25% of the profession had joined up and it was apparent that 'certain areas are already depleted and cannot spare more men'.[63] The committee's main task, therefore, was 'to find the men who could be spared and make it easier for them and others who might wish to join by arranging for voluntary substitution by older men'.[64] Divisional secretaries were instructed to help set up local medical war committees to supply information about the local medical workforce and, in consultation with the LMPCs, provide early warning of any problems with civilian services. Women were denied opportunities to serve at the front though many undertook supplementary roles as civilian medical practitioners and eventually as members of the Women's Army Auxiliary Corps, the Women's Royal Naval Service, and Women's Royal Air Force.[65] The suggestion by the President of the MWF, that vacant positions in Local Authority medical services could be met by women made was ignored but eventually the demand for women as GP locums exceeded supply.[66] Racial prejudice prevented better use being made of non-white doctors until late in the war.[67] By 1918, however, Indian, Chinese, Portuguese, and Egyptian doctors were performing locums in various British cities.[68]

The CMWC recognised that unrestricted recruitment would compound pre-existing problems caused by the maldistribution of panel GPs. An editorial in *Medical World* at the start of the war stated: 'The profession at the moment is seriously undermanned' adding, 'We require at least 8,000 more doctors to cope with the normal amount of sickness and ill health that may be expected each year'.[69] In fact, as the CMWC were to find out, some areas were actually comparatively over-provided with doctors, whereas others had barely enough to service the insured population. Ensuring that there were a sufficient number of doctors to serve the needs of the Army and the civilian population was made more difficult by the fact that the pattern of civilian need in wartime was different to that preceding the war due to the concentration of large parts of the economy on war work. This saw a huge expansion of industries related to munitions concentrated in certain areas, and the replacement of much of the existing industrial workforce by women and boys.[70] At the start of the war, it was expected that the shortage of medical manpower within the civilian population would be offset by the demands of the armed forces for new recruits. Indeed, the insured population initially fell by 12.5% but this was counterbalanced by the entry into insured employment of hundreds of thousands of mainly female munitions workers.[71] By October 1916, 1.2 million men, 200,000 boys, and 400,000 women were engaged in munitions work.[72] The existence of previously undiagnosed and untreated illness among insured women may explain the disproportionately high use made by female patients of the panel doctors' services acknowledged by the commissioners.[73] In addition to catering for their needs, the panel GPs were expected to provide the often extensive medical care needed by discharged soldiers previously eligible for NHI who had been invalided out of the forces as casualties of war. Thus, the proportion of persons who were considered 'poor insurance risks' within the insured population rose and with it the workload of the panel doctors, who felt constrained by their patriotic duty and recognition of the ultimate sacrifice made by others from complaining too loudly about their situation. By the end of 1915, over 70 doctors per week were being recruited into the Royal Army Medical Corps (RAMC).[74] The continued demand for doctors by the war office meant that cuts in the civilian medical workforce were beginning to bite. The Secretary of the Leicester Medical War Committee reported that 'local men are working to their utmost capacity, as 68 out of 247 in practice in 1914 have joined up' and 'There was now a serious risk of men breaking down under the strain if more work is put on them'.[75] The attitude among those left to cover their colleagues began to change the longer the strain of substitution arrangements continued. In August 1915 in an article in *Medical World*, a Dr W.F. Copley-Woodhead wrote that, 'There are certain medical men in Blackpool with large panels eligible to join his majesty's forces. Why should I, with a small panel, attend their panel patients for nothing?'[76]

In November 1915, Morant circulated a memorandum to the war cabinet in which he declared that the point of dangerous depletion of medical manpower may already have been reached in certain areas.[77] At a joint CMWC/NHI Commission meeting later that month, the CMWC accepted his proposal that exemption from recruitment of medical personnel be accorded to those in rural areas where the population to GP ratio was over 1,500:1, in 'semi-rural' areas 3,000:1, and in urban areas 5,000:1.[78] At the same meeting, the CMWC submitted proposals for the order in which different categories of doctors should be called up, taking account in particular of their marital status. At the head of the list of those liable to be called up were 'all newly qualified men without practices', followed in descending order by 'junior medical men employed by local authorities, hospital registrars and assistants, and partners in general practice'. At the bottom, single-handed GPs in private practice were considered more worthy of exemption that single-handed GPs in panel practices.[79] An indignant Morant objected that this ranking proved that the committee had been thinking entirely about medical interests and not those of the public.[80] The CMWC was forced to give ground and thereafter effectively had to negotiate with the commissioners over every panel doctor considered for enlistment. The GPs' absence caused escalating problems. In Salisbury, the local war committee reported that 'it was absolutely impossible to lose another doctor'.[81] Many working-class areas of London were also struggling and the impact on remaining doctors was considerable. In parts of Scotland, GPs were working 15–16 hours a day.[82] On returning to her Plymouth practice after two years caring for wounded soldiers in Red Cross Hospitals in Belgium, Mabel Ramsay found herself covering patients in three other practices. Though working 16 hours a day, she states phlegmatically that it was preferable to being under shellfire.[83] A correspondent to the *BMJ* complained that GPs across the country were overworked and 'threatened with physical breakdown'.[84] 'The strain on older doctors was terrific', Cox noted, 'and some of them died under it'.[85]

Up until this point, the authority of the CMWC and its Scottish equivalent was unchallenged. They had somehow managed to deliver all the doctors the war office demanded. The Government was therefore happy to recognise them as statutory professional organisations with powers to act as appeal tribunals for doctors claiming exemption.[86] However, some within the profession were not happy with the way these powers were wielded. They objected to the fact that the age limits for medical service were higher than that of the civilian population. Under the Military Conscription Act, the age limits for medical conscription were set at 45 for overseas duty and 55 for home duty.[87] In January 1916, the CMWC instituted an enrolment scheme whereby GPs willing to serve in the RAMC allowed their names to be entered onto a list of those eligible to be called up when required.[88] The same month, *Medical World* quoted 'a recent article in *The Times*' which referred to 'mutterings…against the authority of the central war committee' which it considered to be 'the outcome of the bitterness…experienced during the passage of the National Insurance Act'.[89] In February 1916, an unattributed article in *Medical World* entitled 'More work and less pay for panel doctors' complained that:

> The panel doctor, unlike some businessmen, has not gained but lost by the war. He has had to face the increased cost of living and receives no war bonuses and has done a vast amount of gratuitous work for the dependants of those fighting for the empire.[90]

In a rather unsentimental commentary on the actuarial basis of the panel system it continues, 'It has taken from us the healthy lives who gave us no trouble and left us with the unhealthy ones'. This view was echoed in the minutes of the London Panel Committee which in September 1916 noted that the work performed by panel doctors now exceeded that of before the war and 'The men who have been removed from the panel lists were among the best lives (sic) and were unlikely to be any serious charge on the services of practitioners for many years' and that 'many of these men are now returning permanently damaged in health'.[91]

Civilian GPs' contributions to the war effort were not confined to tending the sick. The military relied on them rather than RAMC officers to medically examine the thousands of volunteers and conscripts for the forces, but their recommendations were often ignored or overridden. A 'civilian examiner of recruits' complained that the RAMC had discharged a man with a mild case of flat feet...even though he was a professional footballer![92] Contemporary comments suggest that the exercise was often perfunctory. 'Another examiner of recruits' complained in the *BMJ* that he was obliged to examine up to 120 recruits an hour.[93] By the end of the war, the author of *The Old Doctor* notes, 'the examination of recruits was increasingly left to local doctors who performed the work practically every day of the week when not attending to their patients'.[94] As further testament to the inequity of the recruitment process, GPs were outraged to discover that they were only paid in respect of recruits they passed as fit for service and received no payment for those they rejected.[95] The additional responsibilities heaped on civilian GPs did not end there. Francis Maylett Smith states in his memoirs that 'civilian doctors had their work cut out in writing, or refusing to write, bad medical histories for men called up against their will'. There were 'troublesome interviews', he says, 'with men who had some abnormality of possible exemption value such as round shoulders, bowlegs or a bunion'.[96] Soldiers on leave posed problems of another kind. The nearest he ever came to being assaulted, he said, was when he refused to certify that a soldier's mother was so ill that he should be excused from re-joining his unit at the appointed time.[97]

In August 1916, in order to reach the latest recruitment quota, the CMWC felt obliged to alter the exemption limit, increasing the ratio of patients to doctor in rural areas to 3,000 and in semi-urban to 4,000.[98] However, doctors were now more reluctant to come forward, recognising that RAMC officers' skills were not being utilised efficiently and were left with little to do in between offensives except administrative duties. In *Dr Bradley Remembers*, the elderly John Bradley is left with one other colleague to manage all the patients of panel colleagues who have been called up and notes begrudgingly that while he was working all hours, 'they led the only intermittently strenuous life of medical officers in military hospitals far removed from danger'.[99] The CMWC was well aware of this situation and felt obliged to complain about it to the military. The letters pages of the *BMJ* cited numerous examples.[100] However, Keogh adamantly refused to respond to the CMWC's complaints which he seemed to regard as a personal insult.[101] Moreover, allegations of poor organisation were disputed in the *BMJ* by one 'official observer'.[102] By 1917, mounting casualties increased the military need for doctors but the Germans' decision to torpedo hospital ships meant that more had to be treated in field hospitals in France. The government therefore decided to include the medical profession within the General Mobilisation order and on 21 April 1917 enlistment notices were sent to every civilian medical practitioner in the country.[103] Morant had warned the war office that mass conscription of doctors would endanger civilian health if there were no means to compel redistribution of medical manpower. The CMWC concurred with Morant and his officials that the 'tipping point' had now been reached and threatened to take no further part in medical recruitment.

The message struck home, and the mobilisation order was rescinded a few days later.[104] Despairing of how to solve the problem, Keogh escalated the problem to Sir Auckland Geddes, the minister of National Service. Although a doctor himself, Geddes was equally unsympathetic to the CMWC's complaints. His irritable comment to them that 'A great many medical men in the army get the complaints put up for them by outside bodies, statutory committees or something like that' suggests that LMPCs were involved in articulating the complaints of GPs both at home and in the armed services.[105] The burden of gratuitous work relating to ex-servicemen and their families was beginning to become irksome to many GPs. By 1917, Kent LMPC's discontent was evident from their resolution that 'The attention of the Kent Insurance committee be called to the waste of medical men in the district on military duties'.[106] Panel GPs returning from war service complained that substitution arrangements had not prevented patients leaving their lists and joining those of the deputising doctors.[107] But patients and the Approved Societies were not always happy either with the substitution arrangements in place to cover the absent GPs, as is evident from the complaint referred to the Lancashire LMPC from the Independent Order of Rechabites in February 1915. They stated that patients of a Dr Carrell believed the service they received during his absence, from Dr Monks of Wigan and Dr Fletcher of Ince, was inadequate. They complained that Dr Monks' surgery was open only once a day, whereas Dr Carrell's had been open three times a day. The committee authorised its secretary to identify some more satisfactory arrangements for the patients.[108]

Determined to resist the war office's latest demand for medical recruits, Morant wrote to Geddes in December 1917 warning him that meeting the quota 'would occasion a row in parliament'.[109] Services were at a breaking point and the CMWC concurred with Morant in stating that 'should an epidemic occur the consequences for the civilian population would be grave'.[110] Morant backed up his campaign with statistics showing that the army now had six to eight times the number of doctors available to civilians.[111] Throughout the war, the CMWC had considered a variety of forms of collective substitution arrangements. Many successful schemes were developed as local initiatives. The Manchester medical war committee developed one in 1916 involving a rota to cover depleted practices and pooling of fees so as to provide doctors in uniform with half the sum they had earned in the last full year prior to their enlistment. In 1916, the Glasgow Committee proposed the creation of district centres to concentrate panel work and by 1918 similar arrangements had been set up by Nottingham, Leicester, Birmingham, and Oxford.[112] By 1918, the CMWC were considering an altogether more radical idea suggested by Morant, namely a compulsory system of medical transfer whereby doctors from 'overstocked' areas like Bournemouth could be directed to go and work as panel doctors in 'understocked' areas like Shoreditch in London. Cox expressed doubts as to whether this could be implemented. However, by the summer of 1918, a Treasury guarantee and a standard contract for substitution had been agreed whereby each doctor would be paid £525 per annum plus a share of the earnings of the practitioner they were covering for above that level.[113] The fact that this did not take place was due to a change in the Allies' fortunes following the U.S. entry into the war and a commitment by the Ministry of National Service to make more efficient use of the existing RAMC establishment and rely on medical school graduates to replace those killed or discharged from duty.[114]

By the time of the armistice in November 1918, some 14,700 doctors, approximately half the profession, were in uniform and 574 had been killed or died on active service.[115] The medical profession prided itself that it had 'done its bit' and gone the extra mile in its service to the country. It was due to the hard work and sacrifice of the mainly older doctors left at home that medical services for the civilian population had not broken down. Research into the health of the civilian population suggests that for a good proportion of the civilian population, general health and life expectancy actually improved during the war.[116] This was due to the rise in family incomes resulting from the availability of well-paid war work and near full employment, the increase in wages relative to prices, the imposition of rent controls, and improved nutrition despite shortages of certain foodstuffs. Restriction of alcohol consumption under wartime licencing laws also brought health benefits as did workplace canteens available to over one million workers.[117] But, Jay Winter states, 'It would be a mistake to suggest the medical profession played no part in the successful defence of public health' during 1914–1918, adding, 'The achievement of the medical community in Britain was basically to prevent worse things happening'.[118] The workload of GPs did not immediately improve following the cessation of hostilities, however, as the presence of displaced soldiers increased the spread of Spanish flu across Europe. This added to the strain on the returning doctors struggling to rebuild their practices after the war. A first-hand account of what GPs faced in dealing with the pandemic is provided by Francis Maylett Smith in the first volume of his memoirs. Smith caught the flu himself and was critically ill for six days before recovering.[119] Harry Roberts' biographer also offers a harrowing description of the devastation wrought by the virus in the overcrowded slums of the east end of London.[120] Mabel Ramsay witnessed the spread of the outbreak as it decimated the military hospital where she was working in Plymouth and into the general population. During the remainder of the outbreak, she found herself in consequence working 18 hours a day.[121] The huge numbers dying from the flu during the pandemic prompted the NHI commission to question if enough had been done by insurance committees and the panel GPs to prevent the spread of infection. A letter from NHI official L.G. Brock in January 1919 requesting Insurance Committees to 'take stock of and address inadequacies in the handling of the influenza epidemic in consultation with panel committees' led one LMPC to respond in high dudgeon, commenting that, despite the depletion of their numbers by one-quarter due to the war effort, 'the County Profession...had done their utmost to cope with the exceptional needs of the public'.[122] Another NHI official sought to allay their anger by writing two months later to explain that 'no criticism' of the GPs' efforts had been intended.[123]

After the war: the demand for recompense and debates about improvement and expansion

Reflecting on the profession's contribution to the war effort, and its many sacrifices, Alfred Cox wrote that

> The war did much to re-establish my faith in the integrity and good sense of my profession, a faith that had been somewhat shaken by the manifestations of the 'mob' complex during the insurance struggle... In the war one saw the profession at its best.[124]

Indeed, the government and the nation had reason to be grateful for the doctors' many sacrifices and the remarkable way in which the BMA managed to organise medical manpower and balance the competing demands of the military and civilian populations. The BMA could also congratulate itself on having ensured, through support for substitution arrangements, that, barring a few exceptions, the panel doctors who had gone away to war still had viable practices to come home to. This was not always the case for those in private practice. But it would be wrong to suppose that GPs generally, both those returning and those who stayed behind, were happy with their lot. The level of prosperity enjoyed by many owners of businesses supporting the war effort and by the workers whose earnings far exceeded pre-war levels did not escape the notice of GPs whose workload increased while their income remained largely static.[125] In August 1916, Dr E.H.M. Mulligan wrote to the *BMJ* complaining that, 'Our capitation fee of 7s is now only worth about 4s 2d due to the increased cost of living'.[126] The parlous situation faced by the country had not prohibited a number of successful strikes by organised trade unions who saw it as a perfect opportunity to press their case for improved working conditions and wages. Foremost among these were miners and dockworkers, but engineers, typographers, and even teachers threatened strikes and were rewarded with pay rises, though a few trade unionists were arrested and prosecuted under the Munitions of War Act.[127] The GPs, however, had been constrained by middle-class mores and their sense of patriotism from taking extreme action in support of their case for better pay and conditions. Now that the war was over, they looked for signs that their selflessness was to be rewarded.

Despite the pressures facing the practitioners during the war, panel GPs still found time to register concerns and complaints about the way NHI was administered and to press their representatives at local and national levels to obtain improvements in the scheme and their remuneration. Dr J.A. Bell, Chair of the

Gloucestershire LMPC, complained that the IAC had failed to seize an opportunity to address the multiple grievances of panel doctors.[128] He subsequently recorded receiving postcards from 'scores of panel committee officers' sympathising with his views.[129] Surprisingly, the minutes of LMPCs and the IAC during this period contain only passing references to the war. They are almost entirely taken up with the same matters which concerned them before the war began, and although their membership was depleted by the call to arms, Insurance Committees and LMPCs continued to meet and conduct routine business, as did BMA divisions and committees, including the IAC. Nor did the war curtail political infighting between supporters and opponents of the BMA, the latter now adding dissatisfaction with the CMWC to their list of complaints about the Association. While the PMPU used this to support their claim to supplant the IAC as the authentic voice of the panel doctors, even those sympathetic to the BMA believed that they had much to prove before they could hope to secure the unqualified support of anything like a majority of panel doctors and/or LMPCs. Following the outbreak of war, the idea of a Federation of LMPCs to work with or under the BMA seems to have fallen into abeyance, as did the National Medical Guild of whom little more is heard, although they were still in existence in 1917, as shown by correspondence with Kent LMPC about the unsuccessful attempt to register the Kent Medical Guild as a trade union.[130] But while the PMPU sought to promote itself as a more effective alternative to the BMA, individual LMPCs in York, Cheshire, and Kent tried unsuccessfully to register local representative bodies as trade unions.[131] In Kent, Gordon Ward's attempts to register the Kent Medical Guild as a trade union were stymied when the GMC declined to consent to the proposal.[132]

The PMPU membership was at that time almost exclusively London-based. In 1915, 18 of its 30 council members were from London and a further seven were from southeast England.[133] But after it had acquired the ownership of *Medical World*, the union succeeded in gaining new members in areas as far apart as Glasgow and Bournemouth and began to target LMPCs where it found individuals sympathetic to its cause.[134] After failing to establish an independent medical trade union in Kent, Gordon Ward became a zealous convert to the PMPU and one of its most vociferous and effective spokesmen, writing a regular column in *Medical World* using the nom de plume *Hereward*. After lengthy discussion of legal advice on challenging the GMC decision involving correspondence with the National Medical Guild, and a decision to join the Association of Panel Committees (APC), the Kent LMPC eventually decided to form themselves into a branch of the MPU.[135] Although the PMPU's Combative Secretary, Alfred Welply, openly disparaged LMPCs, his London Panel Committee colleagues recognised that to have any hope of supplanting the BMA, they would need to attend and seize control of the annual LMPCs Conference. At the annual Conference in June 1915 therefore, they sought to eliminate the BMA from panel politics by moving an amendment to a motion on future panel contract negotiations stating that 'No action of the British Medical Association shall be deemed to interfere with the right of panel committees to make representations to the commissioners on their own initiative'.[136] The amendment was overwhelmingly lost and a resolution passed whereby the Conference urged LMPCs to view the BMA as their 'voice' in central contract negotiations.[137] They sought to further strengthen their links with the IAC by resolving that six Conference representatives be nominated to serve alongside BMA nominees on that committee.[138] The Conference nominees subsequently elected included Henry Brackenbury, the chairman of the Middlesex LMPC and Ridley Bailey, the chairman of Staffordshire LMPC. While dismissing the need for any other representative body, the Conference invited the IAC to come up with a scheme for collective bargaining for consideration at the following year's Conference. Norman Eder views this Conference as marking the point at which the IAC's authority became unassailable.[139] But this conclusion is open to question. The obvious frustration occasionally shown by even the most ardent BMA supporters at the IAC's failure to ameliorate the panel doctors' concerns meant that the IAC could never completely rely on the support of the Conference with any certainty, and the spectre of a rival organisation emerging to take its place was never entirely laid to rest.

The endorsement which the IAC received from the Conference in 1915 was strengthened by the adoption the following year of its scheme for collective bargaining which involved defeating an alternative proposal devised by Kent LMPC by which responsibility for industrial action could be devolved to LMPCs.[140] This was sufficient to convince the NHI commissioners that it was the IAC alone with whom they should consult on insurance matters. In a Commission memorandum undated and unsigned but most likely written by James Smith Whitaker sometime in 1916 entitled 'Is the Insurance Acts Committee representative?' the commissioners were advised of the status of LMCs and Panel Committees and the Conference of LMPCs which 'has come to adopt the IAC as virtually an executive committee'.[141] The IAC, it concludes, 'may thus fairly be regarded as representative of the Local Medical and Panel committees throughout Great Britain; and is so accepted by them, and therefore also by the insurance practitioners and the medical profession generally'. Showing his understanding of the political manoeuvrings within the profession at that time, the author notes 'dissentient voices' in some recent conferences 'as to the representative character of the IAC coming from three or four committees, namely Chester, Kent and York'.[142] Now the NHI commissioners were satisfied as to their representative credentials, the form of corporatism which the BMA had exercised when recognised as the government's industrial partner in managing the supply of doctors for the war effort was now extended, by association, to the IAC in the resolution of the panel GPs' grievances.

The annual report of BMA Council in May 1916 noted that, 'The Representative Body will be glad to know relations between the Association and the large majority of Local Medical and Panel Committees…continue to be close and mutually beneficial'. It continued that 'Head office is being used as a clearing house for passing on to local committees the expertise gained and forwarded by other committees' and that 'The addition to the IAC of representatives of Local Medical and Panel Committees has greatly strengthened that body'.[143] Despite this, the IAC's enemies still had plenty of ammunition with which to castigate them. The controversial inclusion within the Administration of Medical Benefit (Amendment) Regulations 1915 of a provision permitting Insurance Committees to abolish 'rep mist' prescriptions and another requiring prescriptions be person-ally signed by panel doctors provided one example.[144] The IAC was embarrassed to report that they had not been consulted about either of these measures but compounded the fault in the eyes of many GPs when in circular M7 they 'urged that the new regulations might well be accepted' by LMPCs.[145] The reaction to this in Kent and Cheshire can be gauged by the fact that the LMPCs went so far as to collect undated resignations in a vain attempt prevent the abolition of 'rep mist' being enacted.[146] A Surrey GP was outraged that his LMPC had supported the IAC which he felt had done a disservice to GPs in urban areas with large numbers of patients, his views being echoed by Cardale, the chair of the London Panel Committee.[147] The BMA was accused of even greater dereliction of duty when, for reasons not altogether clear, it agreed to a reduction in the notification fee for measles from 2s 6d to 1s following an epidemic in 1916, a decision which earned them the opprobrium of not just the PMPU but also the NMU, and even the Medical Protection Society.[148]

Medical World reserved its most excoriating diatribes for the Association's Medical Secretary, Alfred Cox and the GP chosen to replace Macdonald as the chairman of the IAC in July 1916, Henry Brackenbury. Both these men believed in reasoned argument rather than table-banging threats as the best means to se-cure improvements in the panel doctors' remuneration and regulations govern-ing the scheme. They hoped to win the trust and sympathy of the commissioners by proving themselves to be reasonable, responsible, and ethical intermediaries, anxious to bring about improvements in the service to the insured and, if pos-sible, extend the benefits of the scheme.[149] The longer the war went on, how-ever, the more discontented and angry the overworked and unappreciated panel doctors became. In September 1916, Dr Dennis Sheehan decried the 'chronic medico-political inertia with which the profession was gripped' alleging that it was 'seething with discontent'.[150] He stated that 'sporadically as in Kent and Cheshire men are prepared to take matters into their own hands' and were 'pre-pared for resignation from the panel'. Brackenbury found himself on the back foot in defending the IAC's decision to accept an arrangement to compensate GPs for the extra work of attending to discharged servicemen through an attendance payment rather than a general increase in capitation. His critics alleged that the money for these attendance fees would, like temporary residents fees, be taken from the existing insurance fund 'pool' and was not therefore 'new money'.[151] Brackenbury denied this and justified the IAC's agreement on the basis that the arrangement was temporary and would allow the profession time to gather more compelling data to support a claim for a general increase in remuneration.[152] The aforementioned Dr Sheehan castigated the IAC's 'meek acceptance' of this arrangement as 'the very negative of virile leadership'.[153] In May 1917, dissatisfaction with the IAC led the London Panel Committee to write to LMPCs about the desirability of establishing a new organisation directly representative of their interests.[154] With the support of Kent LMPC, they organised a conference in London in July at which representatives agreed to establish a new organisation calling itself the Association of Panel Committees (APC).[155]

The BMA and collective bargaining: South Wales, Coventry, and the GPs' war bonus

In answering those who questioned its effectiveness in representing doctors' interests, the BMA could point to its success in using, when required, trade union-like tactics. In an article in the *BMJ* in 1919, Alfred Cox described how the Association had bested the miners' Medical Aid Institutes in South Wales following a dispute which in his memoirs he admitted 'occupied much of my time and attention when I was Medical Secretary'.[156] The dispute, noted in Chapter 2 as having begun in 1905, escalated in 1912–1913 when GPs were locked out of some of the South Wales Institutes after refusing to accept the unilateral decision to introduce fixed salaries for medical officers in place of the previous 'poundage' arrangement. The BMA had responded by 'blacklisting' those appointments. Francis Maylett Smith offers a first-hand account in his memoirs of the bitterness caused by this dispute.[157] Cox observed that these disputes, which continued during 1914 and 1915, were 'in the nature of a class conflict'. The miners took the unjustified view, he said, that the doctors were generally 'masters men' and the miners 'wanted to be sure that they would be *their* men and could be dismissed if not found satisfactory'.[158] The miners' medical institutes were strongly opposed by local doctors, 'many of whom were as a result brought almost to the point of ruin', he noted. Cox states that he 'enjoyed addressing the miners in the disturbed areas and they enjoyed heckling me'.[159] As a trade unionist himself in all but name, a sometime socialist and friend of Keir Hardie, Cox felt sure of his ground and was later tickled by the description of him by a Welsh colleague as 'the A.J. Cook of the medical profession'.[160] (Cook was a contemporary miners' Union leader famed for his belligerence.)[161] As a result of the BMA's efforts, the institutes struggled to find suitable candidates for their medical officer posts and in early 1915 responded to a suggestion of a meeting with representatives of the BMA's medico-political committee which, in a BMA Council report, had set out a series of conditions for withdrawing their boycott.[162] The meeting took place at the BMA's headquarters on 18 July 1915.[163] It resulted in a compromise by which, in return for the BMA's agreement to recognise existing schemes, the Welsh societies agreed to participate in a joint deputation to the Welsh NHI commissioners to ask that the body approve no further medical institutes as part of the scheme.[164] The agreement was sufficient to bring a temporary halt to the conflict.[165] In 1917, however, the BMA's freedom to employ its by-now-familiar tactics in disputes of this kind was seriously challenged in what became known as the 'Coventry case'.

The success of the Coventry Dispensary Friendly Society to which 50% of the working population of that city belonged had long been a source of consternation to the BMA. While its rival PMS, established in 1907, failed to attract the same following, the local BMA division determined to use every means at its disposal to make life uncomfortable for doctors who agreed to work for the Dispensary.[166] Not only did they ostracise these doctors, but they also pressurised Consultants in hospitals in Coventry and Birmingham to cut all ties with them and, even more shockingly, to decline to accept their patient referrals. Even local dentists and members of the nursing profession were pressurised into withholding treatment from the dispensary's patients.[167] In 1914, four dispensary doctors instituted legal proceedings against the BMA division and its officers alleging that they were victims of libel, slander, and conspiracy and the Association itself was joined as co-defendant. The hearing of the case was delayed by the war but in a lengthy judgment published in the *BMJ* in October 1918, the judge, Mr Justice McCardie, subjected what he described as the 'menacing possibilities' of the *Bradford rules* to forensic examination.[168] He noted that the 'humiliation and bitterness of the campaign fell not only on the dispensary doctors but on their wives and families to whom other GPs and consultants were enjoined not to offer medical treatment'.[169] In one particularly egregious instance, one of the defendants, Dr Kenderdine, declined to attend to a dying patient whom the dispensary GP, Dr Burke, being ill himself, could not attend, until the patient's husband signed a resignation letter renouncing Dr Burke as their medical attendant. After noting that Kenderdine inspected the letter as the patient lay unconscious, the judge commented laconically that the patient 'expired the next day and the boycott ceased to affect her'.[170]

The judge was clearly troubled by the fact that the boycott was employed against non-members of the Association and concluded that 'the uncontested power to bring ruin on any medical men was... void of any statutory sanction'.[171] He deduced that the 'infamous conduct' of which the dispensary doctors were accused was financial rather than moral in character and said that the question of ethics, as the word was popularly understood, had nothing to do with the matter.[172] He thus found the defendants, both the BMA division officers and the Association itself, guilty of restraint of trade and actual malice, declared that the wording used in the blacklist was defamatory, and awarded significant damages. This damning verdict was a catastrophic blow to the BMA which immediately set up a committee to consider its implications and necessary changes to its policies and procedures. On legal advice, they issued new guidance to divisions which, *inter alia*, discouraged unilateral action. The wording of 'warning notices' in the *BMJ* was also altered significantly.[173] It marked a turning point in determining how far the BMA, and any group of medical professionals, could or should go in the legitimate pursuit of professional interests. The effects of the case were not lost on the advocates of trade union status, however, and reignited the debate about whether the political fighting fund to support action in support of collective bargaining could be wielded by any organisation that was not a registered trade union. In a memorandum considered by the committee and attached to the minutes of its first meeting, Alfred Cox complains of being cross examined continuously by 'those who believe trade unionism offers a short cut out of our legal difficulties'. The Coventry judgment, he said, 'will accentuate this belief'.[174]

When the Annual Conference of LMPCs met in October 1917, Brackenbury, the IAC chairman, was once again forced to defend his committee's negotiating record. To the accusation of Dr Genge of Croydon that the IAC were 'ever anxious to find favour with the commissioners' Brackenbury said that it was true that they did not go seeking a fight but to present a case 'which would bear investigation on its merits'.[175] Henry J. Cardale proposed that the regulations recently agreed be withdrawn because the Conference had never authorised payment by attendance for discharged servicemen and claimed that the IAC's actions 'infringed the statutory privileges of the panel committees'. The motion was lost by 133 votes to 20.[176] Brackenbury was aware that earlier that month the London Panel Committee had endorsed the establishment of the new APC, under the chairmanship of the York GP Peter Macdonald.[177] It came as no surprise therefore when the London representative Dr Cowie proposed an amendment stating that 'the time has now arrived when negotiations affecting the panel service should be carried on with direct representatives of the panel committees'. He was supported by PMPU members Stanscombe of Southampton and Coke of Kent who said that in his area, 'they distrusted the IAC which had given the birthright of panel practitioners away'. Dr Major Todd of Durham, the GP who had previously been elected to chair the short-lived Federation of Panel Committees, pointed to the anomalous position the IAC found itself in as a BMA Committee, but Brackenbury responded that the IAC was 'a more or less independent committee of the BMA' whose remit gave it powers to 'deal independently with all matters relating to the interests of insurance practitioners'.[178] The London amendment was lost and a motion of confidence in the IAC passed by a substantial majority. Brackenbury then moved a new proposal for collective bargaining which included for the first time an explicit provision for mass resignation from insurance contracts should negotiations with the commissioners break down irretrievably. His proposal was opposed by PMPU spokesmen on the grounds that IAC was not an appropriate body to direct such action but also by the moderate Lauriston Shaw who described it as 'a declaration of war on the commissioners without any accompanying plan as to what the profession was to do after the war'.[179] Once again, the Conference endorsed the recommendations of its executive, increasing the range of sanctions available to it to wield on their behalf.

In June 1916, the Faculty of Insurance, a lobby group representing the friendly societies and the insurance companies, published a report which advocated the extension of NHI in a way which would give the Approved Societies more responsibility.[180] The IAC responded by attempting to draw up its own list of improvements. In January 1917, it wrote to BMA divisions and LMPCs about the future nature of insurance practice enclosing a questionnaire (D9) in which doctors were invited to evaluate the clinical, social, and political aspects of the scheme.[181] These were brought together in a report which was presented to the LMPCs' Conference later that year.[182] An example of one LMPC's reply can be found in the minutes of the Staffordshire LMPC executive committee meeting on 20 February 1917. While stating that the feeling of the medical profession in their area towards NHI was 'Generally satisfied', they reported that they did not consider the remuneration to be fair and that they required 'a 30% increase on the present rate'.[183] The report subsequently published notes that

> Many politicians, the press and public may hold that the service is inadequate in extent and in quality and that it carries with it the taint of cheapness and semi-charity which should have no place in a system…for which the state is responsible.[184]

It concludes that, 'The profession entirely agrees that medical benefit is inadequate in extent and all are agreed that the present system is imperfect and requires modification'. The report found that GPs wanted:

- inclusion within NHI of consultant and specialist services, institutional facilities, diagnostic and laboratory services, dental, mental, physiotherapeutic, and nursing services;
- exclusion of certain services, to be paid for separately, e.g., anaesthetics, or provided separately by specialists, e.g., venereal disease treatment;
- relief from the burden of clerical work and a ban on Approved Societies demanding clinical details as a condition for payment of benefit;
- an independent national medical referee service to adjudicate on medical questions within the scheme;
- a Ministry of Health to oversee the working of the Act and coordinate state-sponsored health services under the National Insurance, Poor Law, and Education Acts;
- an increased capitation fee to reflect the increased usage of the scheme and wartime inflation.[185]

The report agreed that an attempt should be made to include all classes of workers and their dependants in the scheme and an income limit not exceeding £160 per annum applied to all workers, both manual and non-manual.[186] The authors of the report noted that in respect of replies received 'the degree of unanimity... is remarkable'. What is also remarkable is the correlation between the profession's thoughts and those of the NHI Commission's medical advisory committee. An undated memorandum from around this time prepared at the direction of the chairman of the NHI Joint Commission contains a list of proposed improvements which are almost identical to those featured in the BMA's report.[187]

In the summer of 1917, however, discussions with the commissioners focussed on the more immediate issue of a war bonus for panel GPs and in February 1918, the IAC's conditions of service subcommittee met with the Commission chairman, Sir Edwin Cornwall MP. Cornwall was dismissive of their entreaties and his 'insults' attracted great opprobrium in the medical journals and at the subsequent LMPC conference. E.H. Stanscombe claimed that the IAC's ineffectiveness resulted in a reply (from Cornwall) 'that would not have been given to a bricklayer's union'.[188] Having failed to win over one influential member of the government, the IAC then sought and obtained a meeting with the Chancellor of the Exchequer, Andrew Bonar Law. The Chancellor received them courteously but respectfully explained that war bonuses had been given to 'those whose income was so low that the increased cost of living was intolerable'. With regard to civil service bonuses, these had been confined to those earning less than £500 a year and it wasn't the case, he said, 'that those of middling income were to be brought up to the level of income they had enjoyed pre-war'.[189] He eventually agreed, however, to consider the idea of a war bonus and urged the IAC to collect evidence to support their claim for an increased capitation fee. The committee responded by drawing up a questionnaire to send to LMPCs (M36 1917–1918). In correspondence with Cox about a draft of this document in early 1918, the civil servant R.W. Harris advised that it would suffice as 'preliminary information' but would lack validity unless supported with confirmatory information such as practice receipts.[190] In August, Cox sent the commissioners the tabulated results of the rather limited response from LMPCs comprising six urban, six semi-urban, and ten rural districts.[191] The commissioners responded that there was insufficient detail, and that further supportive information was required.[192] Seeing that the civil service bonuses had now been extended to those earning below £1,000 a year, however, a Commission memorandum noted that an extension to the panel GPs of the allowance for increased costs of living 'cannot now be resisted'.[193] To the GPs' consternation, however, the Treasury did succeed in restricting the amount of the bonus awarded. It was limited to 12.5% for practitioners earning below £500 a year and 10% for those earning between £500 and £1,000 per year, subject in each case to a maximum increase of £60 per GP per year.[194]

In April 1918, a special Conference of LMPCs was held to consider the outcome of the IAC's latest negotiations. The mood was sombre and quickly turned to a debate about mass refusal to sign contracts from 1919.[195] Brackenbury explained that the IAC had written to individual LMPCs about this, but a number had misunderstood what was asked, stating that they could not contemplate a strike during wartime, which he said was not what was being proposed.[196] In a surprising move, given their previous stance on this issue, the London Panel Committee then proposed a motion that, 'while in no way relinquishing the justice of the profession's demand for improved remuneration...it was right to postpone action given the perilous situation of the country at the present time'.[197] Cardale then once again called on the IAC to promote the formation of an organisation 'directly representative of various sections of the profession', meaning no doubt the APC. Brackenbury reminded the Conference that in the previous October, it had strongly deprecated the formation of other representative bodies and the motion was defeated overwhelmingly.[198] The call to panel doctors to follow their patriotic duty was opposed by representatives from Lancashire and Southampton but was carried by a large majority. At the Annual Conference of LMPCs later that year, Brackenbury described further meetings which had taken place with the commissioners.[199] The Conference was generally supportive of the IAC's efforts but was fearful that the profession was being played with. When Cardale moved a motion that the requirement for Conference's nominees to the IAC to be BMA members be withdrawn, it may have surprised him to find the motion 'heartily supported' by Brackenbury himself.[200]

In explaining this action, the IAC chairman stated that his LMPC 'wanted to have partnership between the Panel Committees and the British Medical Association as wholehearted and unsuspicious as possible'. Brackenbury had clearly prepared the way for this momentous change to the constitution of one of the BMA's most important committees by consulting BMA Council members beforehand. At the BMA's Annual Representative Meeting in 1919, he reminded the Representative Body of their agreement the previous year that 'those things which were matters of interest to insurance practitioners only should be dealt with by the Conference (of LMPCs)'.[201] However, it was insufficient to quell the feelings of distrust among his opponents who complained that 'panel practitioners were the only body of people in the country who had withheld their hand from fear of embarrassing the government'.[202] A heated debate followed in which Brackenbury urged the Conference not to support a motion requiring the IAC to reject the Government's offered bonus and 'break faith with the commissioners' lest the government seek to suspend the NHI scheme altogether.[203] The motion was lost but significantly by only 53 votes to 29. The conference ended with a discussion of proposals to establish a new defence fund, which prompted MPU council member Dr Stanscombe, with reference to the Coventry case, to ask what would happen if the use of the fund were ruled to be in restraint of trade.[204] This was a question which the MPU and its supporters would continue to ask and which bedevilled for years to come the IAC's attempts to establish a uniform support structure for its political activity on behalf of panel doctors.

Conclusion

Before the war began, GPs, like their patients, were just beginning to appreciate the benefits of NHI. However, the bitterness surrounding the BMA's 'defeat' in 1913 continued to colour the way GPs and the plethora of interest groups vying for their attention viewed the situation of panel doctors and ideas about how the scheme could be improved. The BMA leadership had learned a hard lesson in 1912–1913 and was quick to adapt to the new reality. The First World War gave the Association an unprecedented degree of autonomy in the organisation of medical services but its achievements, though impressive, were not always appreciated by the rank and file. By 1918, the Annual Conference of LMPCs was recognised by the profession and government officials as the fount of panel GPs' political authority. This provided the basis for the IAC's use of what might legitimately be called 'bargained corporatism' but the somewhat fragile accommodation between the Conference and its 'executive' was to prove for the latter to be at once both its main source of strength and an effective constraint on its ability to consider and support radical ideas.

The war temporarily negated any chances of expanding the service to include specialist treatment or dependants of the insured. Debates about these matters and about the need to integrate NHI with other organised health services continued, however, throughout the conflict which saw the capacity of a diminished GP workforce stretched to breaking point as medical services were subsumed within an economy dedicated to the promulgation of 'total war'. During the war, the GPs' workload was greatly affected by the increased incidence of chronic ill health experienced by disabled servicemen and by women workers whose health problems had previously often gone undiagnosed and untreated. Many panel doctors continued to look at this, like the Approved Societies, from an insurance point of view in terms of the balance between 'healthy' and 'unhealthy' lives and complained that the 'bargain' they had entered into with the government was based on assumptions which no longer held true. In the coming decades, panel GPs continued to be obsessed about the level of their remuneration. A significant number of them had begun to look beyond the limitations of what NHI offered in response to evolving professional and societal expectations of what medicine and the state should provide. But increased workload compounded the growing feeling that their services and many sacrifices during the war years were insufficiently appreciated and that, without a significant increase in remuneration and professional morale, standards of medical care were destined to fall as it proved increasingly difficult to retain and recruit the best doctors to work under the scheme. The 'professional social ideal' was still far from being realised.

Notes

1 Harold Perkin, *The Rise of Professional Society; England since 1888* (2nd ed., Abingdon, 2002). pp. 287. Perkin attributes this phrase to the social scientist Colin Crouch.
2 *BMJ*, Supplement 6 December 1913, p. 513. Its first meeting took place on 19 November 1913. *BMA Archive*, B/251/1/1, minutes of the Non-Panel Doctors Committee, 1913–1914.
3 The constitution and membership of the SMSA are described in *Medical World*, 21 August 1913, p. 118.
4 *Medical World*, 4 December 1913, p. 693.
5 *BMJ*, 25 January 1913, Letter from Dr R. Wallace Henry, 'Union of Medical Practitioners', p. 194.

6   *Ibid.*, 15 March 1913, Letter from Dr A. George Bateman, 'Trades Unionism and Medicine', p. 581.
7   *Ibid.*, 29 March 1913, Letter from Dr Henry J. Cardale, p. 687.
8   *Ibid.*, 19 April 1913, Letter from Dr Gordon Ward, p. 852. For more on the subject of doctors as MPs, see Roger Cooter, 'The Rise and Decline of the Medical Member: Doctors and Parliament in Interwar Britain.' *Bulletin of the Society for the Social History of Medicine*, 78 (1) (2004). pp. 59–107.
9   *BMJ*, 3 May 1913, Letter from Dr E.H. Worth, p. 406.
10   *Medical World*, 15 January 1914, Letter from Dr R.W. Innes Smith, p. 18.
11   See his letter to *Medical World* of 10 May 1913 p. 1030.
12   *BMJ*, 27 December 1913, Letter from Dr Russell Combe, p. 1644.
13   *Ibid.*, 2 May 1914, Annual Report of BMA Council, Supplement, Appendix X, p. 319.
14   *Ibid.*, 9 May 1914, Letter from Dr R. Wallace Henry, 'The Special Fund: Trade Union or Trust?' p. 1045.
15   *Ibid.*, 27 June 1914, p. 1451.
16   *Ibid.*, 23 May 1914, Letter from Dr Percy C. Raiment, pp. 1155–1156.
17   Alfred Cox, *Among the Doctors* (London, c.1949). p. 101.
18   Norman R. Eder, *National Health Insurance and the Medical Profession, 1913–1939* (New York, 1982). p. 118.
19   *BMJ*, 2 May 1914 Supplement, p. 285, para 125.
20   Eder, *National Health Insurance*, pp. 67–68.
21   *Ibid.*, p. 63. The Approved Societies' efforts were spearheaded in parliament by the Conservative MP Godfrey Locker-Lampson.
22   *BMJ*, 26 July 1913, 'Report of the Annual Representative Meeting on 18 July 1913', Supplement p. 124.
23   *Ibid.*, 5 July 1913, 'Supplementary Report of Council', Supplement, p. 9 para 232. Cox, *Among the Doctors*, p. 100.
24   Cox, *Among the Doctors*, p. 100.
25   *BMJ*, 2 August 1913, Supplement p. 168.
26   *Ibid*, 26 July 1913, Report of the Annual representative Meeting on 18 July 1913, Supplement p. 127.
27   Mabel Ramsay, *The Doctor's Zig-Zag Road* (Unpublished autobiography,1953). Royal College of Physicians archive, p. 117. Joyce Cockram, 'The Federation and the British Medical Association.' *Journal of the Medical Women's Federation*, 49 (1967). p. 76.
28   *BMJ*, 26 July 1913, 'Report of the Annual Representative Meeting on 18 July 1913', Supplement p. 127.
29   *Ibid.*, 30 September 1913, 'Report of meeting of IAC on 11 September 1913', Supplement, p. 250.
30   *National Insurance (Amendment) Act 1913* (enacted 15 August 1913). Section 32.
31   *BMJ*, 21 March 1914, 'Conference of Local Medical and Panel Committees on 13 March 1914', Supplement p. 163.
32   *Ibid.*, pp. 165–166.
33   *Ibid.*, 23 May 1914, Supplement, p. 383.
34   *Ibid.*, 27 June 1914, 'Supplementary Report of Council', Supplement, p. 478, recommendation J.
35   *Medical World*, 15 January 1914, 'The Medical Man and National Health Insurance' Lecture by Sir John Collie, and 'Defects in the Act and their Remedy', pp. 94–99. See also *BMJ*, 8 August 1914, 'Discussion on a State Medical Service: A Panel System', pp. 286–291.

36 Bernard Harris, *The Origins of the British Welfare State: Social Welfare in England and Wales, 1800–1945* (Basingstoke, 2004). p. 225.
37 *BMJ*, 24 January 1914, 'A State Medical Service', Supplement, pp. 38–39, and 20 April 1912, 'A National Medical Service', Supplement, pp. 402–404.
38 *Ibid.*, 14 February 1914, Supplement, p. 82.
39 *Medical World*, 25 December 1913, p. 821.
40 *Ibid.*, 1 January 1914, p. 18.
41 *Ibid.*, 16 July 1914, pp. 88–95.
42 *Ibid.*, p. 91.
43 *BMA Archive*, B/203/1/2, Minutes of the Insurance Acts Committee meeting on 12 November 1914, Doc M2.
44 *Ibid.*, Minutes of the Insurance Acts Committee's LMPCs subcommittee meeting on 6 May 1915.
45 *Medical World*, 29 October 1914, 'The Panel Doctor and his interests', pp. 511–513.
46 *Ibid.*, 17 December 1914,' Report on London Panel Committee', p. 688.
47 *Ibid.*, p. 689.
48 *Ibid.*, 11 February 1915, 'What We Have to Fight', pp. 298–304.
49 *BMJ*, 4 July 1914, Letter from Dr Mark Taylor, pp. 44–45. See also the editorial 'The organization of the profession in Germany' *BMJ*, 28 March 1914, p. 726 which offers an accurate account of the status and activity of the *Verband*.
50 Cox, *Among the Doctors*, p. 109.
51 Jay Winter, *The Great War and the British People* (2nd ed., Basingstoke, 2003), pp. 155–159.
52 *Ibid.*, p. 34. Table 2.3.
53 *Medical World*, 13 August 1914 'The Medical Profession and the War', p. 259.
54 *Lancashire and Cumbria LMCs archive*, Letter from Dr Thomas Campbell, Hon. Sec of Lancashire LMPC, 10 September 1914.
55 Cox, *Among the Doctors*, p. 110.
56 *Ibid.*, Winter, *The Great War*, p. 156. See also J.R. Currie, *The Mustering of Medical Service in Scotland 1914–1919* (Edinburgh, 1922). pp. 5–6.
57 *Ibid.*
58 Winter, *The Great War*, p. 157.
59 Cox, *Among the Doctors*, p. 112.
60 James E. Cronin, *The Politics of State Expansion: War, State and Society in Twentieth Century Britain* (London, 1991). p. 67.
61 Winter, *The Great War*, p. 157.
62 Cox, *Among the Doctors*, p. 111.
63 *BMA Archive*, B/67/1/1, minutes of Central Medical War Committee meeting on 30 July 1915.
64 Winter, *The Great War*, p. 157.
65 Letitia Fairfield, 'Women Doctors in the British Armed Forces, 1914–1918', *Journal of the Medical Women's Federation* (MWF), 49 (1967). pp. 99–100.
66 Winter, *The Great War*, p. 171.
67 See *BMJ*, letters from C. Muthu, 21 August 1915, p. 312, and Dr H. Khoras, 28 August 1915, p. 348.
68 Winter, *The Great War*, p. 170.
69 *Medical World*, 13 August 1914, 'The Medical Profession and the War', p. 259.
70 Winter, *The Great War*, p. 159.
71 Eder, *National Health Insurance*, p. 91.
72 Winter, *The Great War*, p. 207.

73 Jane Lewis, *The Politics of Motherhood: Child and Maternal Welfare in England 1900–1939* (London, 1980). pp. 44–47. Helen Jones, *Health and Society in Twentieth Century Britain* (London, 1994). pp. 62–63.
74 Winter, *The Great War*, p. 158.
75 *Ibid.*, p. 160.
76 *Medical World*,19 August 1915, p. 249.
77 Winter, *The Great War*, p. 160.
78 *BMA Archive*, B /67/1/1, minutes of CMWC meeting on 19 November 1915.
79 *Ibid.*
80 *Ibid.*, minutes of CMWC meeting on 6 December 1915.
81 *Ibid.*, minutes of CMWC meeting on 31 December 1915.
82 Currie, *The Mustering of Medical Service in Scotland*, p. 23.
83 Ramsay, *The Doctor's Zig-Zag Road*, p. 90.
84 *BMJ*, 30 September 1916, Letter from J. Cuthbertson-Walker, pp. 476–477. See also *BMJ*, 17 February 1917, letter from 'Scarified', p. 245.
85 Cox, *Among the Doctors*, p. 112.
86 Winter, *The Great War*, p. 165.
87 *Ibid.*
88 Currie, *The Mustering of Medical Service in Scotland*, p. 52.
89 *Medical World*, 7 January 1916, 'Doctors on War Service', p. 20.
90 *Ibid.*, 4 February 1916, p. 149.
91 *BMA Archive*, LMC/1/2, minutes of the London Panel Committee meeting on 28 September 1916, min 6.
92 *BMJ*, 1 January 1916, p. 33.
93 *Ibid.*, 28 April 1917, p. 565.
94 Frank G. Layton, *The Old Doctor* (Birmingham, 1923). p. 158.
95 *Medical World*, 21 January 1916, 'Medical Examinations of Recruits', p. 81.
96 Francis Maylett Smith, *A G.P.'s Progress to the Black Country* (Hythe, Kent, 1984). p. 91.
97 *Ibid.*
98 Winter, *The Great War*, p. 165.
99 Francis Brett Young, *Dr Bradley Remembers* (London, 1938). p. 718.
100 *BMJ*, See letters from 'GP', 17 July 1915, p. 117, and A. Macbeth Elliot, 16 October 1915, p. 588.
101 Winter, *The Great War*, p. 165.
102 *BMJ*, letter from J. Lynn Thomas, 26 February 1916, p. 325.
103 Currie, *The Mustering of Medical Service in Scotland*, pp. 111–112.
104 Winter, *The Great War*, p. 166.
105 *Ibid.*, p. 168.
106 *Kent LMC archive*, Minutes of the Kent LMPC on 2 May 1917.
107 *Cheshire County PRO*, NHL 7135/ 1, Minutes of meeting of the County Palatine of Chester LMPC on 28 October 1917, p. 3.
108 *Lancashire and Cumbria LMCs archive*, Minutes of meeting of the Lancashire LMPC on 10 February 1915.
109 Winter, *The Great War*, p. 169.
110 *BMA Archive*, B/67/1/5, minutes of CMWC meeting on 29 December 1917.
111 *National Archives/Public Records Office, Kew*, MH 79/7. 'The Question of Further Withdrawals of Doctors from Civilian Practice for Recruitment of the Army Medical Services,' memorandum by Sir Robert Morant, 5 March 1918.
112 Winter, *The Great War*, p. 171.
113 *BMA Archive*, minutes of CMWC meeting on 18 June 1918.

114 Winter, *The Great War,* pp. 171–172.
115 Cox, *Among the Doctors*, p. 109.
116 Winter, *The Great War,* pp. 105–115.
117 *Ibid.,* pp. 209–216.
118 *Ibid.,* pp. 154–155.
119 Smith, *A G.P.'s Progress to the Black Country*, pp. 111–116.
120 Winifred Stamp, *Doctor Himself: An Unorthodox Biography of Harry Roberts MD* (London, 1949). pp. 77–78.
121 Ramsay, *The Doctor's Zig-Zag Road*, p. 95.
122 *Cheshire County PRO*, NHL 7135/ 1, minutes of meeting of the County Palatine of Chester LMPC on 4 January 1919, pp. 87–88.
123 *Ibid.*, minutes of meeting of 15 March 1919, letter from E.J. Maude, NHI Commission.
124 Cox, *Among the Doctors*, p. 120.
125 See *Medical World*, 4 February 1916 (editorial) 'More work and less pay for Panel Doctors', p. 149, and 11 February 1916, J. Nelson 'The Effect of the War on Civil Practice', p. 167.
126 *BMJ*, 26 August 1916, Letter from E.H.M. Mulligan, p. 309.
127 See Hugh A. Clegg, *A History of British Trade Unionism since 1889, vol ii, 1911–1933* (Oxford, 1985). pp. 119–160 and 168–170.
128 *BMJ*, 1 September 1917, p. 305.
129 *Ibid.,* 15 September 1917, p. 374.
130 *Kent LMC archive*, minutes of the Kent County LMPC meeting on 21 May 1917.
131 *BMJ*, 30 September 1916, letter from Dr Denis Sheahan, p. 476. See also his letter to the *BMJ*, 21 October 1916, p. 572, and *Kent LMC archive*, minutes of the Kent County LMPC meeting on 1 November 1916.
132 *Kent LMC archive*, minutes of the Kent County LMPC meeting on 1 November 1916. See also the letter from Gordon Ward to the *BMJ*, 21 October 1916, p. 572.
133 *Medical World,* 29 July 1915, p. 210.
134 Glasgow panel GPs formed a Scottish branch of the MPU in 1915. *Medical World*, 22 April 1915, p. 490. A Bournemouth branch was established in 1919. *Medical World*, 2 May 1919.
135 *Kent LMC archive*, minutes of Kent County LMPC meeting on 14 November 1917.
136 *BMJ*, 26 June 1915 Supplement, p. 329.
137 *Ibid.*
138 *Ibid.,* 6 May 1916, Supplement, p. 97, s.120.
139 Eder, *National Health Insurance*, p. 101.
140 *BMJ*, 4 November 1916, 'Report of Conference of Local Medical and Panel Committees', 19 October 1916, pp. 128–129.
141 *National Archive*, MH 62/116. Undated, unsigned memorandum, p. 1, point 3.
142 *Ibid*, MH 62/116, p. 2, point 5.
143 *BMJ*, 6 May 1916, Supplement, p. 98, s.125.
144 *Ibid.,* p. 99, s.134.
145 *Ibid.*
146 *Kent LMC Archive*, minutes of LMPC meeting on 17 November 1915. *Cheshire County PRO*, NHL 7135/1, Minutes of meetings of the County Palatine of Chester LMPC on 14 November 1915, mins 1 & 2, 3 September 1916, mins 3 & 4, and 24 September 1916, min 4.
147 *Medical World,* 17 March 1916, pp. 341–343 (Dr A. Gordon Ede). *Medical World,* 23 June 1916, Henry J. Cardale 'The Present Position of Insurance Practice- Its Difficulties and Possible Development', pp. 785–786.

148 *Ibid.*, 19 May 1916 p. 627; 22 May 1916, p. 66. See also *BMJ,* 15 April 1916, letter from E. Surridge, Supplement, p. 67.
149 A summary of the points discussed with the commissioners was published in the *BMJ,* 14 October 1916, 'Medical Remuneration under the Insurance Act', Supplement, pp. 102–107.
150 *Ibid.*, Letter from Denis Sheahan, 30 September 1916, p. 476.
151 *Ibid,* Letter from Brackenbury, 19 September 1916, p. 437 and replies from J.A. Bell et al., 22 September 1916, p. 403.
152 *Ibid.*, 22 September 1916, Supplement, p. 61.
153 *Ibid.*, 14 October 1916, p. 342.
154 *Kent LMC archive*, minutes of the Kent LMPC meeting on 2 May 1917.
155 *Ibid.*, minutes of 25 July 1917. *BMA Archive,* minutes of the London Panel Committee meeting on 25 September 1917, min.11.
156 *BMJ,* 22 March 1919 'Why should the medical profession be organised and how should it be done?' Supplement, pp. 39–40; Cox, *Among the Doctors*, p. 172.
157 Francis Maylett Smith, *The Surgery at Aberffrwd: Some Encounters of a Colliery Doctor Seventy Years Ago* (Hythe, Kent, 1981). ch.19 'The doctors' halfpenny strike.'
158 Cox, *Among the Doctors,* p. 173.
159 *Ibid.,* p. 174.
160 *Ibid.,* p. 176.
161 See Peter Clarke, *Hope and Glory: Britain 1900–2000* (2nd ed., London, 2004). p. 139.
162 *BMJ,* 8 May 1915, 'Annual Report of BMA Council, Report of Medico Political Committee 28 April 1915', Supplement p. 188, recommendations L and M.
163 *Wellcome Collection* (BMA files) SA/BMA/C.102 Box 54, 'Friendly Societies and Medical Aid Institutes 1910–1948', Minutes of Conference between representatives of Medico Political Committee Contract Practice Subcommittee and representatives of the Friendly Societies Medical Alliance and the South Wales and Monmouthshire Alliance of Medical Aid Societies, 18 July 1915.
164 *Ibid.,* p. 6.
165 *BMJ,* 31 July 1915, Report of BMA Annual Representative Meeting 23–24 July 1915, Supplement, pp. 61–62.
166 *Ibid.,* 26 October 1918, 'The Coventry Case', Supplement, pp. 53–60.
167 *Ibid.,* pp. 55–56.
168 *Ibid.,* p. 54.
169 *Ibid.,* p. 55.
170 *Ibid.,* p. 56.
171 *Ibid.,* p. 58.
172 *Ibid.,* p. 59.
173 *BMA Archive,* B/158/1/1, minutes of Special Committee on Position Arising out of the Coventry case. The Committee met twice, on 4 December 1918 and 14 March 1919.
174 *Ibid.,* p. 4, para 6.
175 *BMJ,* 28 October 1917, 'Report of Annual Conference of Local Medical and Panel Committees', Supplement, p. 77.
176 *Ibid.,* p. 80.
177 *BMA Archive,* LMC/1/2, Minutes of the London Panel Committee meeting on 9 October 1917, min 3.
178 *BMJ,* 28 October 1917, 'Report of Annual Conference of Local Medical and Panel Committees', Supplement, p. 81.

179 *Ibid.*, p. 85.
180 Eder, *National Health Insurance*, p. 102.
181 *BMJ*, 27 January 1917, 'The Future Policy of the British Medical Association as regards National Health Insurance', Supplement, pp. 13–14.
182 *Ibid.*, 23 June 1917, Supplement, pp. 143–147.
183 *North Staffordshire LMC archive*, minutes of the Staffordshire LMPC meeting on 20 February 1917.
184 *BMJ*, 23 June 1917, Supplement, p. 144.
185 *Ibid.*, p. 146.
186 *Ibid.*, p. 143.
187 *National Archives*, MH 62/116, Memorandum, undated and unsigned, prepared for the Joint Insurance Commission – 'Developments Necessary for the Provision of a Complete Medical Service for Insured Persons.'
188 *Medical World*, 19 April 1918, p. 246. See also comments of Dr Modlin of Sunderland at the Conference of LMPCs in October 1918, *BMJ*, 2 November 1918, Supplement, p. 65.
189 *National Archives*, MH 62/125, Verbatim report of meeting between Andrew Bonar Law and IAC deputation on 15 March 1918, p. 11.
190 *Ibid.*, Undated memorandum to National Health Insurance Commissioners.
191 *Ibid.*, Letter from Cox dated 6 August 1918.
192 *Ibid.*, Letter from NHI Commission Secretary dated 23 August 1918.
193 *Ibid.*, Undated and unsigned memorandum I.C. 151/617, p. 2.
194 *Ibid.*, Unsigned letter from HM Treasury to NHI Commissioners dated 5 December 1918.
195 *BMJ*, 20 April 1918, Report of Special Conference of Local Medical and Panel Committees 11 April 1918, Supplement, p. 41.
196 *Ibid.*, p. 43.
197 *Ibid.*, p. 42.
198 *Ibid.*, p. 43.
199 *BMJ*, 2 November 1918, 'Report of Conference of Local Medical and Panel Committees, 24 October 1918', Supplement, pp. 62–63.
200 *Ibid.*, p. 65
201 *BMJ*, 2 August 1919, Supplement, p. 45.
202 *Ibid.*, comments by Dr Modlin of Sunderland.
203 *Ibid.*, p. 66.
204 *Ibid.*, p. 67.

6 'Statutory bodies with martial attitudes'

The role of Local Medical and Panel Committees, 1913–1948

According to an article in *The New Statesman* in 1917, the National Insurance Act 1911 had set up a 'supplementary constitution' for the GPs who had accepted service under National Health Insurance (NHI). This was a reference to the Local Medical and Panel Committees (LMPCs) established as professional representative bodies under the Act in 1912–1913. These committees, the article maintained, vouchsafed the doctors 'a measure of self-government' and exercised a significant influence over the way local Insurance Committees administered the government's scheme.[1] The report of the Royal Commission on National Insurance in 1926 echoed this assessment, acknowledging that LMPCs were 'a valuable element in the medical side of the Insurance scheme'.[2] Two decades later, the civil servant R.W. Harris claimed that the major share of administration which these committees afforded the profession was unique in comparison with their continental counterparts.[3] Despite these endorsements, LMPCs, and their role in the administration of NHI, have been almost completely ignored by historians. As noted in the Introduction, important works by Peter Bartrip and Anne Digby make little or no mention of LMPCs, while they are relegated to a footnote by Frank Honigsbaum.[4] Norman Eder is more generous, making use of the unpublished MD Thesis on the history of Local Medical Committees (LMCs) by former BMA chairman, Dr John Marks, though he regretted that the records of LMPCs had 'not been located'.[5] This chapter aims to redress this deficiency and, using hitherto unresearched archival material, accord to LMPCs some recognition of their importance as co-authors of the regime under which the insurance doctors operated. By examining how the LMPCs were formed and functioned, and the contribution they made to the day-to-day operation of NHI, it is possible to assess the extent to which they could be viewed as agents of the government in two principal respects. Firstly, in using the delegated authority they enjoyed in mediating between GPs and the state apparatus; and secondly, in their attempts to fulfil the profession's cherished aim of self-government in the exercise of professional discipline.

According to John Turner, Liberal governments relied on professional expertise to bridge the gap in their administrative capacity and professions became

DOI: 10.4324/9781003438274-6

in certain cases government 'constituencies', due partly to the expertise they offered and partly to the political power they exercised through their influence over their members.[6] Recognition of this in the doctors' case led Lloyd George to make a series of concessions guaranteeing them both a share in the administration of his scheme and considerable latitude to self-govern through their elected committees. This reflects what James Vernon sees as a refinement of the principles of laissez-faire within the Liberals' governing philosophy.[7] For Tom Crook, 'governance' at this time relied on the interplay of plural localised hierarchical 'systems'.[8] The LMPCs that consequently came into being can be viewed as one such system, mediating between GPs and the state. Evidence of this may be found in the role they played in the policing of prescribing and certification, in determining the scope of what insurance GPs were meant to provide under their contracts, and in the adjudication of complaints about GPs by patients, and by GPs about other GPs. As will be shown, LMPCs made it their business to relieve GPs of as much of the bureaucratic burden of insurance practice as possible while at the same time ironing out the rough edges of the scheme and seeking improvements which, in accordance with 'the professional social ideal', they believed to be in the public's interest as much as their own.[9]

However, as local defenders of GPs' professional interests and guarantors of their deep-seated desire for self-determination, LMPCs were, paradoxically, the means through which the profession could mobilise resistance to the government whenever those interests were deemed under threat. Consequently, their relations with the instruments of government authority at both local and national levels involved alternating periods of cooperation and conflict. If this dichotomy seems surprising, it is nonetheless consistent with what some European researchers have recently described as 'regulated self-regulation', that is, a system of rule in which mutually beneficial cooperation between the state and professional bodies is deemed to be founded in a 'tense relationship' in which state and society 'wrestle with each other'.[10] It also echoes the ideas of Michel Foucault, who characterised the relationship between a sovereign power and those with whom it decides to share or delegate power as 'a perpetual struggle', which he termed an 'agonism'.[11] Although they were not identified as such at the time, LMPCs may also be looked upon as the reification of the 'associational independence' which socialist pluralists like Harold Laski and G.D.H. Cole believed professional representative and quasi-governmental institutions needed to demonstrate in order to keep the powers of an expanding central state in check.[12]

In a letter to *Medical World* in 1919, the BMA loyalist Rowland Fothergill stated: 'the panel practitioners have gradually become convinced that Local Medical and Panel Committees have been formed to safeguard their interests only and are taking the next step of looking on them as fighting units'. He continued that they 'would do well to look elsewhere. Statutory bodies would hardly be allowed to take up martial attitudes to the government'.[13] However, as will become clear, the LMPCs' status as key stakeholders in a government-sponsored scheme did not preclude them from challenging government and its local officials and acting at times in a combative manner. As will be shown in subsequent chapters, the LMPCs provided the authoritative foundation for collective bargaining by the BMA's Insurance Acts Committee (IAC) but were far from passive participants in their campaigns. While made up of individuals whose political leanings were largely conservative, they were occasionally demanding of action defying government authority, including the threat of mass resignation from the insurance service, which would rival that of the most militant trade unionists.

State agency, representation, and self-regulation

The collapse of the medical profession's opposition to the introduction of NHI in 1912–1913 was seen by many as an ignominious defeat. But as the BMA's medical secretary Alfred Cox observed, the outcome was really a disguised victory for the doctors.[14] Under Section 62 of the National Insurance Act 1911, the doctors were granted seats on the Insurance Committees which acted as a buffer between them and the Approved Societies, thereby inhibiting lay interference in GPs' work. Just as important, Insurance Committees were obliged to consult 'local medical committees representative of practitioners operating in the area of insurance committees' on all matters affecting the administration of medical benefit under the Act. 'Addison's amendment', as it was called, thereby established for the first time a universal network of recognised representative bodies, through which the medical profession, locally, was to play a part in the administration of state-sponsored social policy. Addison reasoned that the best way of getting the profession to fully embrace NHI was to allow them to play a central part in its administration and envisioned local doctors' committees working alongside Insurance Committees and supporting them in their work.[15] Being aware of the debates which continued to take place in medical circles about intraprofessional etiquette and the need for 'courts of honour', he also saw them as a means by which a responsible profession could police itself and raise standards of practice through authoritative leadership and peer review. Believing that self-government was more compatible with the Liberal traditions of laissez-faire than bureaucratic control, he helped persuade Lloyd George that statutory recognition of LMCs would meet many of the profession's immediate concerns while enabling them to fulfil a variety of functions on the state's behalf.[16]

The reason this suggestion appealed to Liberal politicians and civil servants is not difficult to fathom. Committees were an essential part of central government apparatus and, as a means of harnessing necessary expertise from a wider community of interests, were a tried and tested means of extending and validating government authority.[17] They were also an essential and familiar part of how the medical profession conducted its professional business. The BMA and the Royal Colleges were structured around committees, and when training and working in the voluntary hospitals, GPs would have been familiar with the medical committees which helped administer the hospitals while representing the views of hospital doctors.[18] As the BMA's medical secretary, Charles Hill, was later to observe, 'the committee is the most efficient instrument I know for the crystallizing of decisions from the pool of people's knowledge and experience'.[19] Before NHI, there was, as has been shown, no national network of GP representative committees. Medical guilds and local practitioner associations were scattered and diverse in nature and attempts to organise a national structure based on them had failed.[20] The Manchester conference on medical organisation in 1900 had identified the need for 'Local district associations formed to discuss medical ethical or medico political topics *to which all practitioners in the locality have the right to belong*' (added emphasis).[21] The BMA's attempts to reform itself after 1902 had created new local representative structures, the divisions, which facilitated a greater amount of engagement with and between its membership. But, in keeping with its claim to represent a unified profession, the divisions comprised doctors from every rank and craft and were not solely concerned with the interests of GPs.[22] Moreover, the divisions comprised BMA members only and the BMA's membership comprised nowhere near a majority of GPs. They were even less representative after 1913 when so many doctors resigned from the BMA in protest at what they saw as the failure of the Association's leadership in the dispute with government over NHI.[23] By insisting that the medical committees recognised under the Act were representative of all local practitioners *in the area of the Insurance Committees*, 'Addison's amendment' ensured that the new representative structures were based on and tied to the administrative boundaries of NHI. They were therefore, crucially, independent of the BMA with whose local 'divisions' they were not geographically coterminous, and, being elected by and accountable to all local GPs, they enjoyed a democratic legitimacy to which the BMA itself could not lay claim.

When some LMCs, most notably in London, declined to seek recognition under the Act, the government authorised Insurance Committees to appoint, where necessary, separate 'Panel Committees' which comprised doctors serving on the NHI panels, and to give them the authority to recognise these as LMCs.[24] This provision, contained in Section 32 of the Amendment Act 1913, was urgently needed in London, where medical opinion remained polarised and where there were at one time three separate committees contesting the right to speak for local GPs.[25] The confusion was not abated however as, while it was open to local GPs to make the Panel Committee and their LMC one body, the statutory responsibilities of each remained distinct and there were certain functions reserved to LMCs which the government neglected to transfer to the new Panel Committees. These were the intraprofessional disciplinary functions and 'scope of service' functions described later in this chapter. As proof of its desire to establish a business-like relationship with the NHI Commissioners, in March 1914, the BMA's newly established IAC jointly agreed a model scheme for LMPCs offering two main options: Scheme A provided for areas where all GPs had joined the

Panel so the membership of the LMC and Panel Committee was identical, while Scheme B provided for the LMC to consist of a locally determined mix of panel and non-panel doctors, which would operate separately from but in parallel with the local Panel Committee.[26]

The model scheme set out arrangements for elections which were invariably conducted via electoral 'districts' usually coterminous with Insurance Committee administrative districts, but the GP committees exercised a degree of latitude in determining their size and composition, often co-opting non-panel GPs, Consultants, and public health doctors who could bring valuable experience or insights to their deliberations. The previously mentioned Dr Lauriston Shaw, a Harley Street Consultant, was co-opted onto the London Panel Committee and served it faithfully as its treasurer for nearly a decade. The Bermondsey GP Alfred Salter was a scathing critic of the committee, however, stating that in elections to the committee, 'in too many cases the wrong man has been returned'.[27] His attacks seem strange considering that the London Panel Committee was packed with supporters of the left-leaning Panel Medico-Political Union (PMPU) which he helped found in 1914. It is not clear also whether he included among 'the wrong men' either of the two women GPs on the 67-strong committee, Elizabeth Baker and Ethel Bentham. Dr Bentham was a fellow socialist who played a prominent part in the committee, representing them at successive Annual Conferences of LMPCs from 1918 and was eventually elected to parliament in 1929 as one of the Labour Party's first female MPs.[28] Another female GP to play a prominent role in their LMPC was the GP obstetrician Mabel Ramsay. She represented the Plymouth Panel Committee at the LMPCs Conference in 1916 where she was the only woman present.[29] She 'greatly enjoyed' attending the Conference and found that, in medico-political work at least, she was treated with professional courtesy and respect by her male colleagues. Although she ceased to be a panel GP when becoming a full-time obstetrician and gynaecologist, she continued her association with the committee, she reports, serving as its Honorary Treasurer and Chairman for two years (though she neglects to say which two!). She remained the Honorary Secretary of the LMC until 1948.[30]

In October 1914, the BMA's newly established IAC surveyed LMC and Panel Committees and reported that 110 out of 136 that replied said their LMC and Panel Committee membership was 'practically identical'.[31] From that point onwards, they were generally referred to as LMPCs. Where membership was not identical, the profession and Insurance Committees were obliged to acknowledge their separate identity and functions. Despite the existence of a number of 'non-panel associations' in London, the body eventually recognised as the LMC for the capital was not dominated by doctors antagonistic to NHI. The Panel Committee actually worked closely with the LMC and as early as May 1914 recommended that membership of both bodies be identical.[32] They proceeded to meet jointly for the first time in July 1916. The Insurance Committee then reminded them that the two committees still had separate functions and thenceforward they continued to meet separately and maintain separate minutes.[33] In Staffordshire, the fact that the two committees ran in harness was illustrated in the agenda for the first meeting on 21 April 1914 which showed the LMC meeting at 2.30 pm and 'the Panel Committee subsequently about 3.15'.[34] The Staffordshire LMPC's members' frustration with the requirement for separate elections is evident in their demand in May 1914 that the tenure of the existing membership of the committees be extended for another year

> in view of the fact that three times already in the past 15 months the practitioners of the county area have elected them, substantially the same persons, and have employed machinery …which is…in all essentials that set forth in the model scheme.[35]

In Kent, the Insurance Committee questioned the membership of the Panel Committee as only two-thirds of it were panel doctors and in July 1914, it was agreed that the LMC and Panel Committee remain separate.[36] In Cheshire, the membership of the two committees was from the outset identical and only rarely did its members feel the need to meet in a separate session as the LMC.

While requiring Insurance Committees to consult medical committees on a range of issues, Addison's amendment had ensured that up to five members of each Insurance Committee were to be drawn from the medical profession. Of these, two were to be 'medical members resident in the area, elected in a manner provided by regulations by an association of qualified medical practitioners within the locality', plus up to two medical members appointed by the local authority, and one by the Insurance Commissioners.[37] In practice, the LMPCs served as the 'local association' in this context. Complaints were made occasionally by LMPCs that more doctors were needed on Insurance Committees to counterbalance the influence of the Approved Societies. Herman Levy maintained that in both the Insurance Committees and the Insurance Commissioners, the doctors had expected to get a larger share of representation.[38] However, the reduction in the number of members of Insurance Committees brought by regulatory changes in 1921 meant that the influence of medical representatives increased proportionately. The Royal Commission in 1926 noted that the average attendance at Insurance Committee meetings was as low as 15–20 persons.[39] This is reflected in the minutes of the Nottinghamshire County Insurance Committee. While in 1913 there were five doctors out of a total membership of 54, by the mid-1920s, only 16–20 members attended regularly of whom three were GPs.[40] Despite these changes, LMPCs still felt 'underrepresented'.[41]

The interchange of bureaucratic instruction and 'expert' advice between Insurance Committees and LMPCs formed the basis of a relationship on which the local operation of the NHI scheme functioned effectively for 35 years. Much of this took place in the standing subcommittees through which most of the Insurance Committees' business was conducted. These comprised the Medical

Benefits subcommittee, which dealt with issues around the scope of service, allocation of patients, certification and record keeping; the Medical Service subcommittee, which dealt with disciplinary matters arising from complaints about alleged breaches of contract; and the Pharmaceutical Services subcommittee, which scrutinised prescribing, determined whether specific drugs could be provided under the scheme or not, and oversaw creation of local drug formularies.[42] The medical members of these groups were almost always LMPC nominees but Insurance Committees also consulted with LMPCs directly on the matters they discussed. Reflecting the importance accorded to these interactions, the LMPCs often set up their own subcommittees to coordinate the advice given, which in practice was seldom ignored. The London Panel Committee appointed seven subcommittees, each comprising up to 20 members, listed as 'finance, general purposes, administration, organisation, pharmaceutical, ethical, and parliamentary'.[43] Following the introduction of mileage allowances in 1914, Insurance Committees also set up mileage subcommittees which were later allowed to use a proportion of their funds to meet 'special claims' from practitioners such as expenses associated with postgraduate education courses.[44] LMPC representatives played a major part in the work of these subcommittees.[45] In Kent in 1920, the Insurance Committee established an allocations subcommittee to which the LMPCs were invited to nominate three representatives.[46] Other subcommittees on which the Kent LMPC was represented included the finance and rural dispensing subcommittees.[47]

How LMPCs functioned was influenced by how they were funded. When the provisional LMCs were established during the 'doctors' revolt' in 1912, the BMA set the precedent of inviting GPs to support the committees' running costs and contribute to a central 'National Insurance Defence Fund' to coordinate the national campaign of resistance, via a voluntary 'levy' of their remuneration.[48] The amount practitioners were invited to contribute to the latter was set nationally. Once recognised by the Insurance Committee, the LMPCs were entitled to request from them an amount needed to support local activities, derived from the insurance GPs' remuneration, within a statutory limit of 1d per patient per annum. LMCs, where separate, enjoyed no such right. A motion to the LMPCs' conference in 1921 calling for the Ministry of Health to meet LMC members' travel expenses was rejected at the request of the IAC which 'had always believed these should be financed by the profession'.[49] In March 1914, the Lancashire LMPC asked the Insurance Committee to allot ⅜d per patient of which the Local Pharmaceutical Committee were to receive ⅛d.[50] In May 1914, the London Panel Committee noted the receipt of £500 for administrative expenses but later that year complained that the total received was £700 less than they had asked for.[51] Being statutory, deductions from GPs' remuneration to cover the LMPC's administration costs were compulsory, whereas the additional or alternative contributions recommended by the LMPCs to meet their costs and contribute to the BMA's central defence fund were not. Voluntary contributions would only be taken from the practitioners' remuneration by the Insurance Committee on submission of a written form of consent. An example of this can be found within the records of the Lancashire County Panel Committee which shows that a Dr W. Clegg-Newton agreed on 18 June 1914 to contribute ⅛ per patient per quarter.[52]

Not all practitioners were compliant, however, and much time and effort were expended by LMPCs in trying to cajole constituents into paying. In June 1913, the Kent Panel Committee viewed with regret 'the feeble response to the appeal for subscriptions towards the expenses of the Committee'. Only 250 had agreed out of 800 doctors.[53] In July 1914, the Lancashire LMPC 'deprecated' the decision of GPs in one of its constituent electoral districts not to pay the amount requested.[54] In August 1914, the Staffordshire LMPC obtained a list of 160 GP 'defaulters' and in 1921 enjoined each member of the committee to 'induce' non-payers to sign the necessary forms.[55] Occasionally, objections to levies were ventilated publicly. In an article in the journal *Medical World* in 1915, Alfred Salter openly questioned what the London Panel Committee did with the voluntary levy payments it received. A Panel Committee member, Dr C.W. Hogarth, responded defensively citing the 'countless hours spent on committee work' and listing specific projects which had occupied his and other Panel Committee members' time.[56] Having no obvious source of income, LMCs relied on the goodwill of their membership and cross subsidisation of costs by Panel Committees. In Kent in October 1921, the Panel Committee voted to grant the LMC £20 to cover its expenses but this was vetoed by the Insurance Committee. This prompted the Panel Committee to propose that it be officially recognised as the LMC for the county and the Ministry of Health acceded to their request.[57]

What did the expenses incurred by LMPCs consist of? A Statement of Accounts for the Staffordshire LMPC for the year ended June 1921 shows expenses for meeting room hire (the Swan Hotel), printing costs, members travelling expenses, payments for scrutinising prescriptions, and expenses paid to the chairman, Dr Ridley Bailey.[58] In 1933, the expenses of the North Riding of Yorkshire LMPC included *inter alia* the 'half cost' of surgery inspections, scrutiny of mileage claims, and donations to medical charities.[59] Some LMPCs paid members for attending meetings. In 1920, Kent LMPC increased its fee for attending meetings from half a guinea to one guinea.[60] It increased it to two guineas per day in 1924.[61] The Lancashire LMPC offered locum costs to its representatives attending the Annual Conference of LMPCs.[62] Committees were not always generous when it came to expenses as is evident in Staffordshire where they only agreed to reimburse third-class travel costs for members' attendances.[63]

Evidently, the Staffordshire LMPC was able to function without a paid Secretary at this time, whereas for a great many LMPCs, this was a major and necessary expense. In the autumn of 1914, an IAC survey revealed emoluments ranging from £10.10s per annum in Nottingham to £250 per annum in London, the same amount being offered in Lancashire, and in Essex where the Secretary was a medical practitioner.[64] Being self-employed, GPs were acutely conscious of the value of their time spent on representative activities. In January 1921, the secretary of Kent LMPC, Dr Salisbury, resigned from the Insurance Committee when the latter decided not to pay for his time while he received an honorarium from the LMPC.[65] Disputes with the Insurance Committee about expenses continued in the following year when another Kent LMPC member, Dr Gordon Ward, sought to resign from various subcommittees after the Insurance Committee's auditor 'refused to pass any fees paid to medical members other than those of the panel committee or its subcommittees'.[66] The same doctor was chastened when in 1923, 'on auditor's advice', the LMPC itself rejected his claim for expenses for attending a Medical Practitioners Union meeting.[67] In 1925, the Kent LMPC set up a subcommittee to investigate its secretarial and administrative expenses taking evidence from other committees such as Manchester. Concluding that the costs were 'extravagant', it resolved to terminate existing arrangements, following which its Secretary, Dr Salisbury, promptly resigned.[68]

In general, it appears that relations between LMPCs and Insurance Committees were courteous and business-like. This may seem surprising, given the major part the provisional LMCs played in the BMA-led opposition to the Act, but, as one GP put it in 1913: 'We are getting on well with the Insurance Committee...We believe we shall, by tactful and diplomatic dealing, obtain more than by adopting an antagonistic attitude'.[69] Norman Eder talks of the professional understanding which the LMPCs had with the Insurance Committee clerks as being based on a 'shared sense of goodwill' and describes the Insurance Committees management of the scheme as 'operating like an informal affair among gentlemen'.[70] Flexibility was the key to this relationship. The Insurance Committees had wide powers but were expected to exercise them with reasonability and tact. Where they failed to do so, the LMPCs could be relied upon to resist, and any lack of trust quickly escalated into conflict. In London in 1915, for example, a proposal by the Insurance Committee to institute a wholesale reduction in the capitation fee to reflect the enlistment of large numbers of insured persons in the armed forces led to a 'strong protest' at a mass meeting of insurance doctors. GPs present bemoaned 'the chaos at Chancery Lane', the Committee's 'incompetent staff', their 'disgraceful lack of courtesy', and attempted 'breach of contract'.[71] The chairman of the Insurance Committee, Mr F. Coysh, was subsequently forced to resign after the Panel Committee felt unable to support his actions.[72] In Bristol the same year, the LMPC was angered by the decision to withhold payment of 'unallotted funds' from 1913 pending a dispute over the costs of excessive prescribing.[73] The matter was only resolved in 1916 following the intervention of local MPs Sir Philip Magnus and Charles Roberts.[74] In Kent in 1915, the LMPC was enraged by the Insurance Commissioners' decision to ban the dispensing of 'rep mist' or repeat prescriptions issued more than a month after the original. The LMPC chose the extreme response of encouraging GPs to submit undated resignations from the panel. One hundred were received but 'held over' by the LMPC pending resolution of the dispute.[75] In Cheshire, the LMPC felt equally strongly about the same matter and about other changes to the conditions of service announced by its Insurance Committee. They matched the degree of militancy shown by Kent by requesting 'pro forma' resignations of which a significant number were received but ultimately not acted upon.[76]

Another rare example of a breakdown in working relationships occurred in Dorset in 1927 when the GPs' unhappiness with the attitude and behaviour of the Insurance Committee clerk, Mr Henry Moore, resulted in an outright refusal to cooperate with the local administration. The dispute was only resolved following Ministry of Health intervention.[77] In striking contrast to this, the mutual respect between the clerks and LMPCs in other areas is evidenced by the fact that in 1925, the Kent LMPC sought to appoint the Insurance Committee clerk, Mr Lloyd, as their secretary, and Staffordshire LMPC appointed his counterpart, Mr Hodgens, as their secretary in 1933.[78] The idea that there could be a conflict of interest seems never to have occurred to them. The generally cordial relationship between the LMPCs and Insurance Committees in the 1930s is further illustrated by the inclusion in the North Riding of Yorkshire LMPC's accounts of the cost of 'entertaining the Insurance Committee to luncheon'.[79]

The assertion of professional expertise and autonomy

LMPCs were quick to assert their rights to be consulted about all aspects of medical benefits under the Act. Remuneration had proved to be the chief sticking point in the profession's dispute with the Government in 1911–1913 and the method of payment was the first matter to be decided. All LMPCs supported the adoption of capitation fees except Manchester and Salford, which experimented with a system based entirely on fees for attendance and items of service.[80] This was eventually abandoned in 1928 after the NHI Commission concluded that it was unsustainable.[81] GPs favoured capitation as it was the easiest system of payment to understand and administer and the one with which they were most familiar, due to its use in friendly society sickness insurance schemes. Under this system, the number of attendances called for by chronically sick patients was balanced by the absence of demand from those in generally good health. However, GPs could still claim a number of separate 'item of service' payments for operations, anaesthetics, and emergency treatment, for example, subject to LMPC and Insurance Committee approval. The LMPCs were also asked to advise on how the total capitation fees for patients who had not registered with a GP were to be distributed among the panel doctors at the year end. Insurance Committees and LMPCs were in regular correspondence about the distribution of these 'unallotted funds' in 1914, particularly in London, where GPs in the inner-city areas with small lists but high workload objected to dividing the surplus strictly according to panel list size. The matter was eventually resolved by a compromise whereby the number of patients for which the sum was apportioned was capped at 2,000 per GP.[82] The Lancashire LMPC, by contrast, wrote to its members in February 1914 that 'the division of the surplus at the end of the first year would be pro rata to the number of county members on the list of each Doctor on the county panel, excluding those associated with approved institutions'. This may be a reference to Medical Aid Institutes and demonstrates the GPs' continuing antipathy towards them.[83] These examples demonstrate that the advice given by LMPCs was guided by individualistic and sometimes idiosyncratic notions of what was in the profession's, and sometimes the public's, best interests.

Another of the more important matters falling within the remit of LMPCs was the investigation of 'excessive' or 'extravagant' prescribing. Discussion centred around the cost of individual items and whether they were necessary and effective. There was, theoretically, no financial limit on what panel GPs could prescribe for patients. The only limit on the practitioner, as the chairman of the IAC explained in 1930, was that of satisfying 'not the officers of the Ministry, but his own colleagues, that what he has ordered was reasonably necessary for the treatment of his patients'.[84] The cost of what the GPs prescribed impacted on the amount of profit the pharmacists made in dispensing items and the amount the Insurance Committee spent on drugs, but also, in terms of items dispensed by GPs themselves, on the amount left in the GPs' (pooled) drugs fund. Initially, the Insurance Committees' drug budget comprised 2s per patient, including a 'floating sixpence' for contingencies, the residue of which was available to be distributed to local GPs (and until 1916, pharmacists) on a per capita basis if there were unspent funds remaining at the financial year end.[85] The prospect of extra pay for their constituents gave LMPCs an incentive to investigate and discourage overprescribing. Practitioners found guilty of excessive prescribing could be surcharged, that is made to replace the 'excess'. In June 1920, the Staffordshire LMPC conducted one such investigation, finding that the practitioner 'had been careless in prescribing and caused an excessive charge on the drug fund'. It recommended that he be surcharged the sum of £5.[86] In Kent, an investigation into an allegation of excessive prescribing in December 1921 found that 'Dr L was in the habit of ordering tinctures where infusions would do equally well and ordering acqua chloroform as a vehicle'. The GP promised to comply with the LMPC's advice, and no further action was deemed necessary.[87] LMPCs were also required to advise on 'whether a substance prescribed was a drug within the meaning of the pharmaceutical regulations'. Thus, in 1928, the Manchester Panel Committee opined that 'Roboleine' should be classed as a food and could not therefore be prescribed as a drug.[88] In 1936, the North Riding of Yorkshire Panel Committee agreed that Myocrisin be added to the drug formulary, recognising its use in the 'modern treatment' of Rheumatoid Arthritis, TB, and Lupus.[89]

One area in which LMPCs were strenuous in asserting their expertise was in determining whether a particular service rendered by a panel doctor fell within the scope of insurance practice. If outside it, the practitioner might be able to claim (on form GP11) an item of service fee or be permitted to charge the patient as a private service. The 1913 Regulations spoke of 'service of a kind which can, consistently with the best interests of the patient, be properly undertaken by a general practitioner of ordinary professional competence and skill'.[90] LMPCs considered this to be a matter which they alone could decide.[91] In May 1915, the Kent committee ruled that treatment of a 'smashed finger joint' was within the scope of medical benefits, but in 1916 ruled syringing of ears and operative treatment of haemorrhoids 'out of scope'.[92] When considering questions involving the scope of practice, LMPCs were often wary of setting any kind of precedent. In November 1920, for example, the Staffordshire LMPC's executive subcommittee supported a practitioner's claim for an item of service fee with the caveat that 'no general definitions are possible or expedient and each case must be decided on its merits'.[93] However, not all LMPCs supported this lack of definition. Many committees, including that of Lancashire in July 1913, lobbied the IAC to specify the procedures lying within the scope of the practitioner's responsibilities under the Act to prevent GPs being overloaded with additional duties.[94] Some who favoured definition did so in the belief that it would support the profession's claim for increased remuneration. It was for this reason that in 1919, the IAC Chairman, Henry Brackenbury, advocated inclusion, within the scope of services, of the administration of Salvarsan, a drug used in the treatment of venereal disease.[95] This suggestion was highly contentious. In May 1914, the Lancashire LMPC advised that Salvarsan should not be included in the drug tariff 'because of its cost and questionable value and because administration has serious results…sometimes fatal, and the technique of its administration is complicated and can only be acquired by considerable practice'.[96] By contrast, the neighbouring County Palatine of Chester LMPC proposed that Salvarsan should be available for use by GPs, informing its County Council that 'the only way of seriously combating venereal disease was through the General Medical Practitioners'.[97] The LMPCs Conference rejected the IAC's proposal, concluding that most GPs preferred to leave the administration of such a dangerous drug to specialists employed in local authority clinics.[98]

Where Insurance Committees disagreed with LMPCs, they sought advice from advisory committees set up, after 1919, by the Ministry of Health. Such enquiries most frequently concerned anaesthetics, vaccination, venereal disease, contraceptive advice, and minor surgery.[99] Norman Eder lists 13 examples of what were typically considered within the scope of medical benefit, including things that would be considered quite hazardous to perform today outside hospitals, such as curetting of the uterus and chest drains.[100] While exercising the rights accorded to them to determine the scope of service, the judgement of LMPCs was almost always conservative: they sought to discourage GPs from undertaking innovative treatments until such times as they had become commonplace and relatively free of risk. Consequently, the nature of GPs' practice changed very little during this period, in contrast to the significant advancements made in treatment in hospitals.[101] However, the Ministry of Health's rulings prove that LMPCs did not always succeed in frustrating attempts to broaden the scope of service. Among items regularly declared by Insurance Committees, on the advice of Panel Committees, to be outside the scope of medical benefit was 'removal of varicose veins'.[102] This ruling was subsequently challenged and offers a perfect illustration of the controversy often accompanying changes in medical practice. In January 1929, the Ministry appointed referees to consider a case involving a Manchester practitioner who considered that he possessed the necessary skill to undertake the treatment of varicose veins via 'injection of a sclerosing solution', a procedure first tried and shown to be effective in 1925. Their consideration took note of similar cases which had occurred in Sussex and Leicester.[103] Kent LMPC subsequently wrote to the Ministry objecting that such injections should not be carried out by GPs 'as they were still in an experimental stage and no uniformity has yet been arrived at as to the best type of injection to be used'.[104] A motion to that effect was submitted to the LMPCs Conference in 1930 by Inverness LMPC.[105] The referees nevertheless found in favour of the practitioner, a decision which, in a memorandum on the subject, IAC member E. Rowland Fothergill described as 'almost unintelligible'. He noted that several LMPCs were refusing to accept the ruling which, he said, represented 'an illegal attempt to lay down a general rule'.[106] The Ministry subsequently appointed a committee of inquiry which in August 1931 ruled that although the treatment was novel, it was now widespread, with very few cases of complications, and was not therefore beyond the skill of GPs.[107] A critic of the London Panel Committee and its LMC was clear where he stood on the matter when, after a lengthy explanation of the controversy, he stated, 'Every right-minded practitioner will agree with the decision of the referees'.[108] He later qualifies this statement by stating, 'Can one expect such doctors as those who serve on Panel Committees to add new treatments for panel patients to their already overworked practices?'[109] When the IAC questioned LMPCs about remuneration and workload the following year, several, including the London Panel Committee, agreed that workload had increased due to 'the popularity of sclerosing methods of tackling varicose veins' and it was subsequently listed in an IAC memorandum in support of increased remuneration as one of the factors contributing to the increase in 'timeage (sic) rendered per insured patient'.[110]

There were, moreover, other matters affecting panel practice in which the GPs' determination to 'have the final say' did not go unchallenged. The rules covering certification of sickness benefits were a constant source of dispute between medical practitioners, LMPCs, and the Approved Societies, in which the Insurance Committees were often reluctant arbitrators. The doctors resisted the Societies' efforts to make it compulsory to state the nature of patient's illness on the certificate on the grounds that it would breach doctor/patient confidentiality and felt that the doctor's professional opinion that the patient was unfit for work should be sufficient. At its first meeting in May 1913, the Lancashire Panel Committee objected to the wording of a proposed standard certificate stating its opinion that 'it would be seriously detrimental to the interests of the public to place upon certificates the nature of the disease'.[111] At a subsequent meeting with the Insurance Committee, the LMPC stated that what they wanted was a form stating simply, 'I certify that the patient from (start date) to (end date) is unable to perform his or her duties'.[112]

Insurance Committees often looked to the Insurance Commissioners, and later the Ministry of Health, and the IAC, to help resolve these disputes. In July 1914, the Insurance Commissioners invited chairs and secretaries of Panel Committees to a conference to 'discuss difficulties...experienced by approved societies in dealing with sickness benefit and...giving of medical certificates for that purpose'.[113] It failed to resolve the issue and subsequent discussions proved equally fruitless. In December 1914, the London Insurance Committee dismissed as 'frivolous' complaints by two Approved Society secretaries that panel doctors had failed to state the nature of the disease 'on a form of certificate not modelled on that issued by the Commissioners'.[114] Insurance Committees were sometimes content, moreover, to let LMPCs deal with breaches of certification rules, as in Lancashire in July 1915 when the LMPC summoned three practitioners to explain why they had, contrary to the rules, ante-dated and post-dated certificates. The Committee concluded that the GPs had not breached the rules 'wilfully', that is to save themselves work, but 'through ignorance' and, perhaps because no harm was suffered by the patients, the trio were let off with a warning.[115] Beginning in 1920, the Ministry of Health appointed Regional Medical Officers (RMOs) to support panel GPs with second opinions, rule on disputed cases of malingering and inappropriate certification and carry out inspections of medical records.[116] The profession itself had long campaigned for the appointment of what they described as 'medical referees' to prevent the inevitable clashes between GPs and Approved Societies over certification but LMPCs not infrequently took issue with RMOs' decisions.[117] Among other duties, the RMOs were also meant to collect statistical information about disease prevalence by random examination of GPs records. This was abandoned in 1926 due to the lack of uniformity and general illegibility of the records![118] However, as explained in a later chapter, the profession's leaders eventually found it expedient to cooperate with the Approved Societies and the Ministry on ways to tackle perceived abuses. Thus, in October 1932, Staffordshire LMPC wrote to GPs recommending that they should 'furnish information in confidence as to the nature and duration of illness when requested to do so by Approved Societies in cases of difficulty'. The LMPC suggested that GPs carry out the recommendations 'as far as possible' but added that 'it is not compulsory for you to do so'.[119] LMPCs were thus prepared to advise constituents to act in ways that to them seemed reasonable while always acknowledging GPs' rights, as independent contractors, to determine their own course of action.

The range of matters relating to the administration of medical benefit on which the LMPCs were invited to advise the Insurance Committees was increasingly broad. In 1920, the Kent Insurance Committee asked the Panel Committee's opinion of 'irregularities' in one GP's accounts. The committee informed the Insurance Committee that the accounts submitted by a Dr Swindale 'show evidence of grave irregularity and warrant the further action applicable in such cases'.[120] The claiming of anaesthetic fees also proved the subject of a long-running correspondence between the Kent LMPC, its Insurance Committee, and the Ministry of Health in the early 1920s. Initially, the LMPC decided to allow claims for anaesthetics for operations considered within the scope of the Act even if carried out in a hospital.[121] However, they later ruled that no fee should be paid to 'a man who administers and anaesthetic himself for an operation which he also performed'.[122] A claim disallowed on these grounds led to an appeal to the Ministry by the practitioner concerned, Dr J.H. Bennett, on which the Ministry ruled that the LMPC had erroneously interpreted earlier advice and a number of disallowed claims had to be reconsidered.[123] The Committee was still free to determine what was within the scope of benefit, however, as when it disallowed claims for anaesthetics accompanying extraction of teeth, removal of tonsils and adenoids, curetting of uterus, and intravenous injection of Salvarsan.[124] Claims approved included removal or drainage of cysts, abscesses, carbuncles, whitlows, and cellulitis and 'stretching of anal sphincter'.[125] Fees for emergency treatment of other practitioners' patients were another area of the LMPCs' responsibility. When allowing a claim in 1923 for the treatment of a scalp wound following a bicycle accident, the Kent LMPC opined that such fees should be paid from ' the practitioners' fund' and not, as the regulations required, deducted from the remuneration of the patient's usual doctor.[126] In September 1928, the Manchester LMPC circulated an admonitory letter stating that 'the business of the panel committee is being increasingly devoted to consideration of (emergency treatment) claims, and in a large number of cases, the patient is on the list of a neighbour of the doctor who makes the claim'. It went on (in underlined capital letters to add emphasis): 'Your committee feels very strongly that most of these claims should not be made but that neighbours should more often act for one another in a friendly way'. It continued, 'In future the panel committee will be inclined to CONSIDER ADVERSELY claims for emergency treatment where both doctors concerned practice in the same district'.[127]

Mileage grants constituted a substantial addition to the income of rural practitioners.[128] In the North Riding of Yorkshire, a total of £7,539 was paid out to panel doctors in 1934.[129] The 1913 Benefit regulations also allowed practitioners to make claims for sundry items from the 'reserve portion' of the central mileage funds subject to approval by Insurance Committee subcommittees containing LMPC nominees.[130] In Lancashire in December 1914, the LMPC approved payment from this source for 'tolls over the ship canal'.[131] Claims could also be made for emergency dressings. In the North Riding of Yorkshire, claims for emergency dressings in the years 1930–1933 were £333, £222, £113, and £122, respectively.[132] From 1928, claims for postgraduate courses were included in what the reserve portion could be spent on. Eder notes that in that first year nationally, only 86 GPs took advantage of that provision.[133] In 1938, however, the Ministry reported that it had received 2,500 separate applications.[134] In 1933, 85 GPs in the North Riding of Yorkshire received between them a total of £165 for attending such courses.[135] At a meeting of the LMPC in that year, the RMO, Dr A.E. Huxtable, explained why one claim had been rejected. He said that payment from the special expenses part of the central mileage fund was meant to provide locum cover for GPs in isolated rural areas who could not otherwise afford to attend courses without assistance. The applicant in this case was in the habit of attending courses at his own expense and his intention to attend was not dependent on being given the grant. Moreover, he had declined to divulge his net professional income.[136] A report to the North Riding of Yorkshire LMPC in 1936 categorised claims totalling £2,202 made from the reserved portion under schedule 2. These covered, *inter alia*, grants for postgraduate study, holiday and sickness locums, and exceptional motor car and telephone expenses.[137]

Another of the LMPCs' duties involved assisting the Insurance Committees with inspections of GPs' premises to ensure that they were in a fit and proper condition. In 1921, Surrey LMPC objected when its Insurance Committee sought to make approval of a GP taking on 'a substantial number of new patients' conditional on his having 'satisfactory' premises.[138] However in Kent in 1923, the LMPC chairman visited the premises of a Dr Edmanston of Greenhithe, reporting that he found the accommodation to be 'grossly inadequate' and the LMPC consequently supported a decision that permission for the doctor to appoint an assistant be withheld pending improvement in the accommodation.[139] In Staffordshire in 1925, the Insurance Committee wrote to the LMPC that a practitioner who had been requested to improve the conditions of his waiting room had so far taken no action. The LMPC secretary subsequently wrote to the practitioner pointing out that 'the matter must be remedied forthwith'.[140] In the 1930s in the North Riding of Yorkshire, general inspections of GPs' surgeries took place every five years conducted by teams involving LMPC-nominated GPs and the LMPC shared the cost on a 50/50 basis.[141] However, the approach was less systematic in Staffordshire, where the LMPC participated in a general survey of waiting room accommodation in 1936 'on the same lines as that carried out in 1924' and subject to the LMPC warning practitioners that it was taking place.[142] In Cheshire the same year, the LMPC objected when the Insurance Committee sought information about GPs' surgery premises via a questionnaire. They informed their constituents that they were under no obligation to complete this and were supported by the BMA's Deputy Secretary, Charles Hill, who described the Insurance Committee's actions as 'unusual, undesirable and vexatious'.[143] In 1931, *Medical World* commended one Insurance Committee and its LMPC for sidestepping the contentious issue of whether every GP's consulting room should contain an examination couch by stating that it was 'more a matter of equipment than "accommodation"'.[144] Other functions fell to the LMPCs by default. Some Insurance Committees felt it necessary to set local limits on the number of patients GPs could have on their lists and were obliged to seek the LMPCs' approval.[145] But some LMPCs took a more active role in policing their constituents' behaviour. In 1925, the Kent LMPC recommended that the Insurance Committee impose a limit on the patient list of a Dr Jefferis following the upholding of a complaint about failure to visit a patient, and in 1934 the North Riding of Yorkshire LMPC objected to a GP living too far from his patients and in a separate case to the 'illegal retention' of an excess of patients following the departure of his assistant.[146]

Mediation and self-government: the management of complaints and discipline

A responsibility which LMPCs took very seriously was the adjudication of patient complaints. The LMPCs were allowed to nominate three of the seven members of the medical service subcommittees which oversaw this function. The very first hearing of the Nottinghamshire Insurance Committee's medical service subcommittee took place in June 1913 when they heard a complaint from a Mrs Burton about the treatment she had received from a Dr Park. The accusation of a poor standard of treatment was found to be 'unsubstantiated' but the committee concluded that 'the words and manner of Dr Park were wanting in sympathy and showed an unjustifiable loss of temper'.[147] This echoes a case cited by R.W. Harris in the appendix to his book on National Insurance in which the London medical service subcommittee 'deprecated very strongly' the conduct of a practitioner who thought it 'a confounded impertinence to ring up a doctor at 8.30am about a panel call'.[148] In such cases, the practitioner was invariably advised 'to adhere more closely in future to the terms of his agreement with the Insurance Committee'. Sanctions were only employed where there was evidence of a breach of the terms of contract or a failure to perform one or more of the required services, such as a failure to visit or examine a patient or inappropriate charging, in which case the practitioner might suffer a 'withholding' (of part of their contractual remuneration). In rare cases, a practitioner might be removed from the panel. In December 1916, Nottinghamshire GPs Coughlan, Hine, Hawson, and Simpson were all subjected to withholding for failure to properly complete patient record cards.[149]

The necessity to keep medical records was resented by many GPs as the records were, initially at least, simply an aid to the administration of medical benefit rather than any useful source of clinical information. When, following changes in 1921, they became more comprehensive, Kent LMPC drew up a memorandum listing criticisms of the new regulations which it sent to the Ministry of Health and the IAC.[150] This was little comfort to their constituent who refused to keep *any* records and in 1922 was accordingly fined £25 and told that repetition would result in his removal from the panel.[151] Anne Digby contends that complaints to service subcommittees of poor treatment or negligence were usually rejected but less serious complaints upheld.[152] Eder says that charges of negligence were uncommon but not as rare as accusations of incompetence.[153] Further examples given by Harris based on his experience as a Medical Service Subcommittee chair in London give a flavour of what the subcommittees considered. These included a failure to visit or facilitate the admission to hospital of a patient who was severely burned – the GP was censured and subjected to a withholding of £20, a case in which a GP had provided backdated sickness certificates to a patient whose absence from work turned out to be due to him being in prison – the practitioner received a warning and a withholding of £10, a blatant case of inappropriate charging in which two GPs charged patients wanting speedier access a shilling to be admitted to their consulting rooms via a separate waiting room – the GPs were 'severely censured' and subjected to a withholding of £150. In the final case described by Harris, an exasperated GP recommended that a patient suffering from a psychosomatic illness attend his surgery rather than expect him to visit as he had done unnecessarily several times previously. The patient called in another GP and sent the first GP their bill. The subcommittee's sympathies are obvious from its laconic finding that, 'There was no failure on the part of the (accused) practitioner to comply with the terms of service'.[154]

An interesting reflection on the insurance complaints procedures can be found in the novel *The Old Doctor* by the panel GP, Frank Layton, published in 1923.[155] Layton is scathing about fellow doctors who are neglectful of their professional responsibilities. His hero, the 'old doctor', Luke Dennison, is pleased that the new insurance panel system provides a means to hold such doctors to account and subject their conduct to peer review and sanction. To Dennison's obvious delight, one of the characters typifying these attitudes, McFadd, quickly finds himself subject to a complaint which, the author says, was 'thoroughly well-founded'. He was charged with 'refusing to visit a patient who had sent for him one evening; with writing for the patient, whom he had not seen, a prescription for a disorder which he had not investigated'.[156] At the hearing, McFadd is forced to admit to his negligent practice under interrogation by the medical members. For Layton, peer review is what made a difference. He states: 'McFadd seemed uncomfortable. He was rather afraid of the Doctor members of committee. He had no delusions as to how he stood with his professional brethren. They knew all about him and his ways. He knew that he might bluff the lay people, but he could never bluff the doctors'.[157]

In Layton's book, the accused GP is 'severely admonished and heavily fined'. His portrayal of service subcommittees may, however, represent wishful thinking. Critics suspected that the medical members were inclined to be lenient towards accused doctors and, as the lay members did not know what constituted ordinary competence and skill, they generally bowed to their expertise.[158] Anne

Digby illustrates this with the case of Retford GP, Dr H.R. Chibber-Want, who was censured numerous times for failure to visit, irregular prescriptions and certification, and wrongly charging patients for private treatment. His deficiencies prompted the Ministry of Health to question in 1923 if his continuance of the Panel would be 'injurious to the service'. He remained on the panel list, according to Digby, because local doctors on the Medical Services Subcommittee excused his failings, ascribing them to his youth and inexperience.[159] Contributors to *Medical World* took an altogether different view of the service committee process. An article in July 1915 claimed the fact that of 100 cases investigated between July 1914 and June 1915, 42 were unsubstantiated, was an indictment of the system. It criticised the conduct of the medical members of the subcommittees, stating provocatively that 'it is often to the laymen on the subcommittee that the doctor has to look for fair play'.[160] It is perhaps ironic that *Medical World's bête noire*, the BMA's secretary Alfred Cox, appears to have agreed with them on this point. In his memoirs, he states that, 'Many a man who has been hauled over the coals for extravagance or neglect has told me that he would have got off more easily had he been dealt with by a body of laymen'.[161] *Medical World* did not view this as a good thing. In a comment on the case of 'a Croydon practitioner' who in 1922 won his case against the Insurance Committee on appeal, its editor stated, 'We repeat that we protest against a system which compels medical men to prosecute and fine a brother practitioner in cases of which they can have only imperfect knowledge'.[162] Cox, however, commented later: 'I do not hesitate to say that it was this increased reliance on the doctors to "police" their own service that made it the smoothly running service it was eventually to become'.[163]

While its nominees served on the medical service subcommittees, LMPCs often expressed concern about the sanctions imposed by Insurance Committees and sought modifications to their rules. In February 1919, the London Panel Committee suggested that a time limit of three months after the event giving rise to the complaint be established. However, the Insurance Committee rejected the idea.[164] In Kent in 1922, the LMPC compiled a comprehensive list of issues justifying changes to the service committee procedure. These were members having no legal training; inclusion within complaints of prejudicial statements; admission of hearsay evidence; failure to formulate definite charges and cite regulations breached; inclusion of supplementary charges for which the accused was unprepared; leading questions; self-incrimination; awarding of costs to the unsuccessful party if the complainant but not the defendant; increasing of penalties by the Ministry; no right of appeal to the courts; and the waste of public money investigating trivial complaints.[165] The Insurance Committee set up a special subcommittee to consider these criticisms and, after acknowledging their validity, drew up new rules of procedure which were circulated to Panel Committees across the country.[166] They were welcomed by LMPCs in Stockport, Nottingham, and Birmingham but rejected by the West Riding of Yorkshire

LMPC, and by Staffordshire LMPC with the pointed reply that 'so far as this area is concerned there is no need of any alteration'.[167] LMPCs sometimes considered the punishment meted out for contractual failings disproportionate, as in a celebrated case in Lancashire in which two GPs accused of inappropriate charging were subjected to a fine of £1,000.[168] However, they sometimes took the opposite view. GPs removed from the panel could appeal to be readmitted, as appears to be the case in Lancashire in 1928 when, on learning that a Dr Godfrey had been reinstated following an appeal to the Minister, the LMPC expressed its disapprobation by informing the Insurance Committee that it 'would accept no responsibility for Medical Services as far as Dr Godfrey is concerned'.[169]

Despite the concerns of some LMPCs about procedures, very few complaints resulted in a fine or withholding. This is not surprising, given the relatively low number of patient complaints. The highest number recorded, 520, in 1922, represented a ratio of one to every 24,000 patients.[170] In 1924, only four of 404 complaints resulted in a practitioner being removed from the panel. The same year, the Court of Inquiry into GPs' remuneration heard that there had been only 324 withholdings in the previous four years.[171] However, some authorities questioned the weight that should be attached to such statistics. In evidence to the Royal Commission on National Insurance in 1925, an Approved Society representative, Mr E.E. England, alleged that for every complaint brought before the Insurance Committees, there were 99 that were not, 'merely because the insured person is either afraid of the doctor or is loth to lodge a complaint, or is too lazy to do it'.[172] Although the friendly societies frequently criticised panel doctors in the press, it was mostly about lax certification. Patient dissatisfaction with the standard of care given by panel doctors was only occasionally reflected in the press and then only in terms of reporting of medical service subcommittee decisions.[173] When, in a rare example, the *Daily Sketch* voiced a concern about 'collusion' during a Medical Service Committee hearing, in London, it was forced to issue a retraction and an apology to the medical members.[174]

Practitioners subject to hearings were entitled to be accompanied by a medical colleague who, though not permitted to act as an advocate and address the subcommittee, could offer the individual advice on how to respond. The Staffordshire LMPC justified this by stating that the accused practitioner 'is liable to prejudice his case in his reply to the accusations made against him' and thus advised any practitioner who may have a charge against them 'to obtain expert medical advice before making any reply to the charge'.[175] Concerns about conflict of interest were compounded when the individual entrusted with accompanying the accused was the Secretary or Chairman of the LMC or Panel Committee. An unnamed LMPC explained in *Medical World* in February 1922 that the Panel Committee chairman was accepted by the Insurance Committee as the defendant's representative and 'is always present at hearings'.[176] Kent LMPC noted in July 1922 that the Insurance Committee had confirmed its agreement that one of the Panel Committee members should accompany an accused practitioner to medical service subcommittee hearings.[177] LMPC representatives also accompanied practitioners at interviews with RMOs investigating inappropriate certification, a practice recognised and endorsed by the Ministry in a communication to Panel Committees noted by the North Riding of Yorkshire LMPC in June 1933.[178]

LMCs (and, where recognised as LMCs, Panel Committees) were also given responsibility to investigate and decide on complaints by GPs about other GPs.[179] This was an essential part of self-government and reflected the profession's long-cherished desire for 'courts of honour'.[180] It is also consistent with what recent European researchers have referred to as 'regulated self-regulation'.[181] Allegations of 'serious professional misconduct' were the preserve of the General Medical Council (GMC) which had statutory authority to strike off doctors' names from the medical register. But canvassing patients, the most common cause of friction between GPs, although considered unethical, being a serious breach of professional etiquette, was seldom deemed serious enough to warrant GMC involvement and became the concern of LMCs and LMPCs. In January 1913, for example, Kent LMC were asked to investigate an allegation that a Dr Morris had registered patients 'touted' for him by a Prudential insurance agent.[182] Comyns Carr et al. state that on the subject of malingering and GPs wrongly issuing certificates to gain patients, 'it will be to the personal interest of other members of the panel and to the Local Medical Committee to keep a sharp watch on any practitioner who is seen to be attracting an unusual number of patients'.[183] One exception to this was Manchester where there was an established medical ethical committee.[184] In October 1928, the Lancashire LMPC referred to it a case of alleged canvassing after the accused doctor could not be found to explain himself.[185] In another case, the same LMPC pursued its own investigations more assiduously. In January 1929, they noted an alleged incident in which, on investigation, 200 patient registrations were found to have been completed the same day, mostly in the same handwriting. Summoned before the LMPC in April 1929, the two accused GPs admitted that they had filled in registration forms 'for patients' convenience' seeing that they expected to receive a large number of registration requests after being appointed the colliery medical institute doctors. The Committee initially decided to refer the matter to the medical service subcommittee as a 'flagrant breach of insurance practice procedures' but subsequently made do with a letter of admonishment.[186] In 1921, the London LMPC conducted a lengthy hearing of a case under article 36 of the medical benefit regulations in which both parties were legally represented, the committee being assisted by its own 'legal assessor', and evidence was taken from 17 witnesses.[187]

There were several problems, however, with this exercise in professional self-government. Firstly, having no funds to draw on, LMCs found it difficult to recoup costs incurred in conducting investigations. Salford LMPC, for example, had requested reimbursement of funds but found that these costs were 'taxed' and they were left with a shortfall.[188] Secondly, statutory recognition notwith-standing, LMCs had no legal protection if those they investigated or sanctioned claimed that they had been unjustly injured by the Committee's actions. In 1926, the IAC established an 'Emergency subcommittee' to draw up guidance for LMCs and LMPCs on how to avoid accusations of bias. They asserted that 'until tested in court it cannot be assumed that any privilege attaches to any of the proceedings of the LMC or its officers'. They suggested that the LMC could only warn or advise the practitioner found in default, their only real sanction be-ing, in extreme cases, to advise the Minister to remove the defaulting GP from the panel list on the grounds that their continuation would be 'detrimental to the good of the service'.[189] Eventually, amendments were made in 1928 permitting investigations under Regulation 39 by Panel Committees, in recognition of the LMCs' absence of funds.[190] The issue of touting continued to trouble LMPCs. In June 1934, the Manchester LMPC felt it necessary to issue a circular letter to its constituents stating that touting and other 'illegitimate means of acquiring pa-tients' were 'on the increase in Manchester particularly in some of the new hous-ing estates'. The letter stated that 'several districts are being carefully watched' with a view to obtaining evidence and that 'the committee will not hesitate to take appropriate action'.[191]

What do this, and other interventions described in this chapter, tell us about how LMPCs viewed themselves and their role? Clearly, they believed that ad-monishment by locally elected peers was an effective check on poor practice or questionable behaviour and that LMPCs were the most appropriate judges of such matters. Comyns Carr et al. appear to have agreed, stating that the LMCs intervention 'may prove to be of the greatest value in what will always be a most difficult and odious business'.[192] LMPCs acknowledged the existence of mini-mum standards but, fearing lay attempts to enforce them, were as anxious to pre-serve local discretion over conduct and discipline as they were over determining the extent and quality of treatment offered to patients. Were LMPCs in any other ways proactive in how they led and policed the profession? Critics of panel prac-tice like W.A. Brend lamented the fact that the 'public health' role of insurance practitioners in prevention of ill health, which Addison and others had hoped to see, had not materialised.[193] Hermann Levy noted that 'Doctors have other more pressing duties to perform than to elaborate schemes of health improvement'.[194] In the 1920s and 1930s, however, some LMPCs assisted Insurance Committees' 'Health Propaganda Committees', nominating GPs willing to give public lec-tures on hygiene and ill-health prevention.[195] In Cheshire, the LMPC addressed the issue of preventing ill health in a singularly eccentric fashion. At the prompt-ing of its colourful secretary, Dr Lionel J. Picton, who had written a book on nutrition and health, a meeting of Cheshire doctors and local farmers in 1939 signed a 'Medical testament on nutrition and its relation to Agriculture'. This championed the belief, with which the *BMJ* was in sympathy, that poor nutrition lay at the heart of most preventable illness and that the adoption of what would now be called 'organic' methods of agriculture would result in immediate health benefits.[196] In a move which seems less eccentric in the context of the war years, the LMPC devoted considerable energy to encouraging householders to grow their own food by organising gardening competitions (!)[197]

The same LMPC had long argued against allowing the growth of specialisation to reduce the role of GPs and, unusually, actively encouraged its constituents to undertake antenatal examinations of pregnant women who were not covered by NHI. Lengthy negotiations with the County Council resulted in a scheme whereby the latter paid GPs 10s 6d for each of two examinations.[198] Many LMPCs were involved from their earliest beginnings in drawing up local drug formularies, which they had printed and distributed at their own expense, as the Report of the Committee of Inquiry into GPs' Remuneration noted in 1924.[199] Others took the time to draft useful guidance for their constituents which served to benefit both practitioners and their patients. An example can be found in Manchester where in 1931 the LMPC produced at their own expense a 'Handbook of hospital and general information' listing specialists' locations, clinics, and appointment times. In 1933, this was expanded to include contacts for district nursing institutions, ophthalmic practitioners, and lists of notifiable diseases, and in 1934 they added details of vaccines, child welfare services, and pre-maternity centres.[200] This serves to qualify slightly Levy's statement that the LMPCs 'offered little or no encouragement to the dynamic and progressive improvement of the medical services rendered under national health insurance'.[201] That they were also proactive in seeking to address their constituents' personal needs was demonstrated by the West Riding of Yorkshire LMPC which devised a superannuation scheme for practitioners which was adopted as the model for a national scheme endorsed by the Conference of LMPCs in October 1932.[202]

LMPCs were also active in another aspect of health service delivery which has been largely overlooked by historians. This is the establishment of Public Medical Service (PMS) schemes in which GPs collaborated in organising GP services for dependants of NHI subscribers who were excluded from the state scheme. The BMA had provided a model scheme in 1911, the year which saw the establishment of the longest-lived and most successful of these, in Leicester. It was built around an existing hospital provident dispensary which in 1911 had 90,000 subscribers, and before long its membership comprised over 90% of the medical practitioners in the city and county utilising a network of branch dispensaries.[203] The scheme was run by the self-styled Union of Medical Practitioners but the membership of its Leicester subdivision was identical to the local Panel Committee and LMC which consequently held their meetings sequentially.[204] LMPCs were clearly the driving force behind PMS in other areas such as Kent, where the first draft scheme was considered in October 1924 and an East Kent branch was launched in Bromley in September 1925 to 'face down a threat from a public dispensary with imported full-time salaried doctors'.[205] The Kent LMPC agreed to provide the scheme with £100 from its voluntary levy to pay for 'the necessary stamps and cards'. In April 1926, the LMPC resolved that the committee 'transform itself' into the governing body of the Kent County PMS and recorded in September 1926 that governing body meetings would now routinely follow meetings of the LMPC.[206]

The same was true of the London PMS which began in 1927.[207] In 1932, as will be described later, the Conference of LMPCs actively encouraged the setting up of PMS schemes across the country and resolved that the National Insurance Defence Trust be required to collaborate with the BMA 'in assisting the effective development of Public Medical Services'.[208] This meant permitting the Trust to provide loans for groups of GPs, often led by their LMPCs, to set up new PMS schemes. There was already a precedent for this. In January 1924, the Essex PMS set up by IAC member C.H. Panting had requested a temporary loan which the IAC thought deserving of consideration by the Trust.[209] The *National Insurance Gazette* noted, in March 1924, that the Essex PMS 'had already made a promising start'.[210] A Dr Eldred informed the Defence Trust that it comprised 170 doctors, including some non-panel GPs and in Colchester it ensured 'all club arrangements had been wiped out of existence'.[211] The stimulus given to PMS schemes by the BMA and LMPCs in the 1930s saw a significant expansion in the number of such schemes, such that at the first national conference of PMS schemes in 1935, representatives of 43 areas attended. In the development of PMS, as in all matters affecting the interests of GPs when NHI was in operation, LMPCs played a pivotal but not always obvious part in bringing doctors together in a common cause.

Conclusion

Referring to the LMPCs, the Royal Commission on National Insurance 1926 (majority report) stated that 'to secure the full cooperation of the Medical Profession so necessary to the scheme of medical benefit, the independent position given by the two statutory and purely professional committees was essential'.[212] According to Eder, direct contact between GPs and Insurance Committees was minimal and sporadic – 'Quarterly checks (sic), occasional information circulars, and the filling up of sickness and prescription forms were usually the only reminders of panel service'.[213] In evidence to the Royal Commission, the chairman of the Middlesex Insurance Committee, Sir William Glyn-Jones, stated: 'the average practitioner – I say it with great respect…does not worry himself very much about the machinery (of insurance committees) provided the terms and conditions are alright for him personally'.[214] As this chapter has demonstrated, this laissez-faire approach may be explained by the fact that LMPCs were involved in regular communication with the Insurance Committees on GPs' behalf on a wide range of issues and mediated between them on matters requiring a collective response. They were also able to articulate local GPs' concerns and present them when necessary to the Insurance Committees, the NHI Commissioners, the Ministry of Health, and the IAC, and give vent to concerns at the Annual LMPCs' Conference. LMPCs were not without their critics. In its weekly journal, *Medical World*, the PMPU frequently attacked the representative credentials of individual LMPCs in its desire to demonstrate the need for a proper trade union to represent panel practitioners.[215] While stating that the LMPCs were a 'useless expense and have not justified their existence', it went on to urge panel doctors to take 'a more lively interest in the personnel of these committees'.[216] However, the Union did, unwittingly, identify the LMPCs' chief virtue, that is their mediatory role, when its editorial opined that they were 'in an equivocal position', and 'have confused in some measure the position of public and medical representative' conceding that 'the task of an intermediary is never an easy one'.[217] A more sardonic commentary in the same journal in June 1915 describes LMPC members as 'men who are willing to devote their time and money to a thankless task', and comments: 'Should however any financial crisis arise, or should there be any addition to the clerical work, the profession momentarily awakes, curses its representatives on the Panel Committee and goes to sleep again'.[218] The anonymous author of *This Panel Business*, a severe critic of LMPCs, or at least the London Panel Committee due to its apparent failure to weed out incompetent GPs, stated, 'Panel Committees have again and again shown themselves to be incompetent' but admitted that, because insurance doctors 'do not exhibit much enthusiasm to serve on panel committees…a certain amount of credit is due to those who undertake to give their time to this work'.[219] By 1926, however, the *Medical World* columnist, 'Hereward', acknowledged that 'the newer Panel Committees represent more and more the rallying point of the best brains and the most important business in each district'.[220]

Whatever their critics within the profession may have sometimes felt about them, the LMPCs were clearly a functional necessity for NHI, offering the authorities a pool of expertise and advice, a professional 'temperature gauge' offering early warning of problems, and a means of managing professional discipline more acceptable than the alternative of bureaucratic diktat. In that sense, they were effectively part of the state apparatus and essential to the smooth running of NHI. However, it is unlikely that the members of any LMPC would have seen themselves as agents of the state. Despite the criticisms of the PMPU and its successor organisations, many members of LMPCs saw their role as fighting the profession's corner and preserving at all costs their independent contractor status and right to professional self-determination. They were therefore perfectly well prepared, as will be seen in the following chapters, to abandon their partnership with the state when it failed to accommodate their needs or acted against what they saw as GPs' professional interests.

Notes

1 *The New Statesman*, 21 April 1917, vol. IX, issue 211, 'Special Supplement on Professional Associations.' p. 9.
2 *Report of the Royal Commission on National Health Insurance*, cmd. 2596 (1926). p. 61.
3 R.W. (Robert William) Harris, *National Health Insurance in Great Britain, 1911–1946* (2nd edn, London, 1946). p. 143.

4 Anne Digby, *The Evolution of British General Practice, 1850–1948* (Oxford, 1999); Peter Bartrip, *Themselves Writ Large: The British Medical Association, 1832–1966* (London, 1996); Frank Honigsbaum, *The Division in British Medicine: A History of the Separation of General Practice from Hospital Care, 1911–1968* (London, 1979). p. 60, footnote.

5 Norman Eder, *National Health Insurance and the Medical Profession in Britain, 1913–1939* (New York, 1982). p. 194, note 72. John Marks, *The History and Development of Local Medical Committees, their Conference and its Executive,* 1974 Edinburgh University MD Thesis.

6 John Turner, 'Experts' and Interests: David Lloyd George and the Dilemmas of the Expanding State, 1906–1919', in Roy MacLeod (ed) *Government and Expertise: Specialists, Administrators and Professionals, 1860–1919* (Cambridge, 1988). p. 204. See also Nikolas Rose, 'Government, Authority and Expertise in Advanced Liberalism.' *Economy and Society*, 22 (3) (1993). p. 285.

7 James Vernon, *Cambridge History of Britain: 1750 to the Present* (Cambridge, 2017). pp. 114–115.

8 Tom Crook, *Governing Systems: Modernity and the Making of Public Health in England 1830–1910* (Berkeley, CA, 2016). p. 11.

9 Harold Perkin, *The Rise of Professional Society: England since 1880* (London, 1989). p. 288.

10 'Regulated self-regulation from a legal historical perspective': www.rg.mpg.de/1921124/regulated-self-regulation-from-a-legal-historians-perspective?c=2019245 Last accessed November 2020. Project completed 2020.

11 Michel Foucault 'The Subject and Power.' *Critical Inquiry*, 8 (4) (1982). p. 790.

12 Marc Stears, Progressives, *Pluralists and the Problems of the State: Ideologies of Reform in the United States and Britain, 1909–1926* (Oxford, 2002). pp. 105, 108–115.

13 *Medical World*, 30 May 1919 'The National Insurance Defence Fund', pp. 454–455.

14 Alfred Cox, *Among the Doctors*, (London, c.1949). pp. 98–99.

15 Jane Morgan and Kenneth O Morgan, *Portrait of a Progressive: The Political Career of Christopher, Viscount Addison* (Oxford, 1980). p. 14.

16 *Ibid.*

17 John Turner, "Experts' and Interests', pp. 204 and 211.

18 Brian Abel-Smith, *The Hospitals 1800–1948: A Study in Social Administration in England and Wales* (London, 1964). p. 33.

19 Charles Hill, *Both Sides of the Hill: The Memoirs of Charles Hill (Lord Hill of Luton)* (London, 1964). p. 77.

20 Honigsbaum, *The Division in British Medicine*, p. 13.

21 *Manchester University Medical Collections,* MMC/7/4/3/4, Official Report of the Conference on Medical Organisation 1900, p. 51.

22 Bartrip, *Themselves Writ Large*, pp. 145–146.

23 Cox, *Among the Doctors*, p. 99.

24 *National Insurance Act 1913*, 3 & 4 Geo V. Ch. 37, s. 32.

25 Marks, *The History and Development of Local Medical Committees*, p. 32.

26 *BMA Archive*, B/203/1/1, Insurance Acts Committee, minutes of meeting on 19 March 1914. Correspondence between Alfred Cox, BMA and S.P. Vivian, National Insurance Commissioners.

27 *Medical World*, 8 July 1915, 'The Surcharge Problem – Who Is Responsible?' p. 52.

28 C.V.J. Griffiths (September 2004). "Bentham, Ethel (1861–1931)". *Oxford Dictionary of National Biography*. Oxford University Press.

29 Mabel Ramsay, *The Doctor's Zig-Zag Road*, Unpublished memoir, 1953, Royal College of Physicians Archive, p. 116.

30 *Ibid.*, p. 120.
31 *BMA Archive*, B/203/1/2, minutes of IAC meeting on 19 October 1914.
32 *Ibid.*, LMC/1/1, minutes of London Panel Committee meeting on 26 May 1914, min 6.
33 *Ibid.*, LMC/1/2, minutes of London Panel Committee meeting on 18 July 1916.
34 *North Staffordshire LMC Archive*, agenda for Staffordshire LMPC meeting on 21 April 1914.
35 *Ibid.*, Staffordshire LMPC minutes of meeting on 5 May 1914.
36 *Kent LMC Archive*, KCMC minutes of meetings on 9 October 1913, and 14 July 1914. They eventually merged in 1921.
37 *NI Amendment Act 1913*, Section 59 (3) a) to e).
38 Hermann Levy, *National Health Insurance: A Critical Study* (Cambridge, 1944). p. 19.
39 *Report of Royal Commission on National Health Insurance*, Cmd. 2596, (1926). p. 167, para 379.
40 *Nottinghamshire County Archives*, SO NHI/ 1–3; NHI Committee minutes 1913–48, vol. 1.
41 *Lancashire and Cumbria LMCs Archive*, minutes of LMPC meeting on 11 September 1929.
42 Eder, *National Health Insurance and the Medical Profession*, p. 270.
43 *BMA Archive*, minutes of London Panel Committee meeting on 17 February 1914.
44 *YORLMC Archive*, Appendix to minutes of a meeting of North Riding of Yorkshire LMPC on 19 March 1936.
45 *Ibid.*, minutes of meeting on 1 December 1932, min 7.
46 *Kent LMC Archive*, minutes of LMPC meeting on 26 May 1920.
47 *Ibid.*, minutes of meeting on 7 December 1921.
48 Marks, *The History and Development of Local Medical Committees*, p. 26.
49 *BMA Archive*, B/203/1//12, Minutes of IAC meeting on 27 January 1921 'Expenses of LMCs', min. 36.
50 *Lancashire & Cumbria LMCs Archive*, minutes of Lancashire LMPC meeting on 18 March 1914.
51 *BMA Archive*, LMC/1/1, minutes of London Panel Committee meeting on 15 December 1914.
52 *Lancashire & Cumbria LMCs Archive*, levy consent form enclosed with LMPC minutes 1914.
53 *Kent LMC Archive*, minutes of KCMC meeting on 12 June 1913.
54 *Lancashire & Cumbria LMCs Archive*, minutes of LMPC meeting on 8 July 1914.
55 *North Staffordshire LMC Archive*, minutes of LMPC meeting on 29 August 1914.
56 *Medical World*, 11 March 1915, Alfred Salter, 'The Panel Practitioner and his interests', pp. 298–304; and response by C.W. Hogarth, 18 March 1915, pp. 333–334.
57 *Kent LMC Archive*, minutes of LMPC meeting on 18 October 1921.
58 *North Staffordshire LMC Archive*, Statement of Committee accounts enclosed with minutes of LMPC meeting on 29 September 1921.
59 *YORLMC archive*, minutes of North Riding of Yorkshire LMPC meeting on 13 July 1933, min 4.
60 *Kent LMC Archive*, minutes of LMPC meeting on 21 October 1920.
61 *Ibid.*, minutes of meeting on 7 February 1924.
62 *Lancashire & Cumbria LMCs Archive*, minutes of Lancashire LMPC meeting on 27 May 1913.
63 *North Staffordshire LMC Archive*, minutes of LMPC meeting on 14 January 1915. The Staffordshire accounts show total committee expenditure to be only £300, 1s. 8d, and separate receipts for 'the medical defence trust' totalling £405,11s.7d.

64 *BMA Archive*, B/203/1/2/, minutes of IAC meeting on 9 October 1914.
65 *Kent LMC Archive*, minutes of LMPC meeting on 13 January 1921.
66 *Ibid.*, minutes of meeting on 11 May 1922.
67 *Ibid.*, minutes of LMPC meeting on 21 March 1923.
68 *Ibid.*, minutes of LMPC meeting on 28 April 1925.
69 *BMJ* 12 April 1913, Dr A.E. Larking, Supplement, p. 325.
70 Eder, *National Health Insurance and the Medical Profession*, p. 166.
71 *Medical World*, 22 April 1915, p. 500 and 29 April 1915, 'Great Protest Meeting in London', p. 530.
72 *Ibid.*, p. 533.
73 *Medical World*, 21 January 1916, pp. 81–82.
74 *Ibid.*, 4 February 1916, p. 148.
75 *Kent LMC Archive*, minutes of LMPC meeting on 17 November 1915.
76 *Cheshire County PRO*, NHL 7135/ 1, minutes of meetings of the County Palatine of Chester LMPC on 3 September and 24 September 1915.
77 *BMA Archive*, B/203/1/19, minutes of the IAC meeting of 20 January 1928, 'Report of Inquiry into Dorset Case', Doc. 16. See also Eder, *National Health Insurance and the Medical Profession*, pp. 163–166.
78 *Kent LMC Archive*, minutes of LMPC meeting on 28 April 1925. *North Staffordshire LMC Archive*, minutes of LMPC meeting on 5 April 1933.
79 *YORLMC Archive*, North Riding of Yorkshire LMPC accounts enclosed with minutes of meeting on 13 July 1933.
80 *Manchester University Medical Collections*, MMC 11/2/1/1, Manchester LMPC 'Information to every member of the Medical Profession in Manchester 1913'.
81 Eder, *National Health Insurance and the Medical Profession*, pp. 316–351. Lancashire and Kent had also briefly considered attendance rather than capitation payments.
82 *Ibid.*, pp. 69–70.
83 *Lancashire & Cumbria LMCs Archive*, Letter from Dr Thomas Campbell, Hon Secretary, dated 4 February 1914.
84 Quoted in Harris, *National Health Insurance in Great Britain*, p. 159.
85 The 'floating sixpence' was abolished in 1920, becoming part of the local drugs fund. Eder, *National Health Insurance and the Medical Profession*, pp. 42, and 129. *The National Archive/Public Record Office Kew*, MH 62/119, Memorandum by J.S. Whitaker, 20 September 1919.
86 *Staffordshire LMC Archive*, minutes of LMPC meeting on 16 June 1920.
87 *Kent LMPC Archive*, minutes of Kent LMPC meeting on 7 December 1921.
88 *Manchester University Medical Collections*, MMC/11/2/2/3. Manchester Panel Committee circular to panel practitioners dated 7 March 1928.
89 *YORLMC Archive*, minutes of meetings of North Riding of Yorkshire LMPC on 14 June 1934, min. 2, and 19 March 1936, min. 7.
90 *NHI (Administration of Medical Benefit) Regulations 1913*; Part V, Reg. 50 and First schedule, part 1 (Conditions of service for practitioners) 2 (i).
91 This was, technically, one of the functions reserved to LMCs and exercised by them on referral by Panel Committees other than where the LMC and Panel Committees were combined.
92 *Kent LMC Archive*, minutes of Kent Panel Committee meetings on 11 May 1915, 3 February 1916, and 3 May 1916.
93 *North Staffordshire LMC Archive*, minutes of LMPC meeting on 9 November 1920.
94 *Lancashire & Cumbria LMCs Archive*, minutes of Lancashire LMPC meeting on 3 July 1913.
95 Honigsbaum, *The Division in British Medicine*, p. 131.

96 *Lancashire & Cumbria LMCs Archive*, minutes of Lancashire LMPC meeting on 20 May 1914.

97 *Cheshire County PRO*, NHL 7135/1, Minutes of a meeting of the County Palatine of Chester LMPC on 16 June 1917, point 4.

98 Honigsbaum, *The Division in British Medicine*, p. 131.

99 Eder, *National Health Insurance and the Medical Profession*, p. 168.

100 *Ibid.*, pp. 168–169.

101 Digby, *The Evolution of British General Practice*, pp. 220–223.

102 Eder, *National Health Insurance and the Medical Profession in Britain*, pp. 168–170.

103 *BMA Archive*, B/203/1/23, minutes of IAC meeting of 2 July 1931, Memorandum by E. Rowland Fothergill, Doc. 58 p. 4, point 30, and correspondence with LMPCs in Sussex, Caernarvonshire and Kent, Doc.64.

104 Kent Local Medical Committee, *The History of Kent Local Medical Committee, 1912–2012* (2nd edn., Harrietsham, Kent, 2012). p. 21.

105 *BMA Archive*, B/203/1/22, minutes of IAC meeting of 20 November 1930, 'Minutes of the Annual Conference of LMPCs on 23 October 1930' min. 49.

106 *Ibid.*, B/203/1/ 23, minutes of IAC meeting of 2 July 1931, Doc 58, p. 4, point 30.

107 *BMJ* 8 August 1931, Supplement pp. 126–127.

108 'AGP', *This Panel Business* (London, 1933). p. 219.

109 *Ibid.*, p. 270.

110 *BMA Archive*, B/203/1/24, minutes of IAC meeting on 12 May 1932, Doc 54. Min. 35; B/203/1/25, minutes of IAC meeting on 2 May 1933, Doc. 80, point c).

111 *Lancashire & Cumbria LMCs Archive*, minutes of Lancashire LMPC meeting on 27 May 1913.

112 *Ibid.*, minutes of meeting on 23 June 1913.

113 *BMA Archive*, LMC/1/1, minutes of meeting London Panel Committee on 7 April 1914, min 4.

114 *Medical World*, 3 December 1914, 'Complaints against Panel Practitioners', p. 638.

115 *Lancashire & Cumbria LMCs Archive*, minutes of Lancashire LMPC meeting on July 1915.

116 Eder, *National Health Insurance and the Medical Profession*, p. 177. See below, p.198.

117 *Ibid.*, p. 178.

118 *Ibid.*

119 *North Staffordshire LMC Archive*, Letter to Panel Doctors from Dr A.V. Campbell, Hon. Secretary dated 1 October 1932.

120 *Kent LMC Archive*, minutes of Kent Panel Committee meeting on 21 July 1920.

121 *Ibid.*, minutes of meeting on 8 September 1920.

122 *Ibid.*, minutes of meeting on 21 October 1920.

123 *Ibid.*, minutes of meeting on 19 January 1922.

124 *Ibid.*, minutes of meeting on 13 July 1922.

125 *Ibid.*, minutes of meeting on 13 July 1922 and 18 January 1923.

126 *Ibid.*, minutes of meeting on 21 March 1923.

127 *Manchester University medical collections*, MMC/11/2/2/7, Letter from Manchester Panel Committee dated 28 September 1928.

128 Levy, *National Health Insurance*, p. 123.

129 *YORLMC Archive*, minutes of North Riding of Yorkshire LMPC meeting on 14 June 1934, min 4.

130 *Kent LMC Archive*, minutes of Kent Panel Committee meeting on 2 March 1921.

131 *Lancashire & Cumbria LMCs Archive*, minutes of Lancashire LMPC meeting on 23 December 1914.
132 *YORLMC Archive*, minutes of North Riding of Yorkshire LMPC meeting on 14 June 1934, appendix to schedule 2 of report on mileage fund.
133 Eder, *National Health Insurance and the Medical Profession*, p. 194, note 59.
134 *BMA Archive*, B/203/ 1/30, minutes of IAC Remuneration Subcommittee meeting on 4 April 1938 para. 19.
135 *YORLMC Archive*, minutes of North Riding of Yorkshire LMPC meeting on 13 June 1933.
136 *Ibid.*, minute 2.
137 *Ibid.*, minutes of meeting on 19 March 1936.
138 *BMA Archive*, B/203/1/13, minutes of IAC meeting on 17 November 1921.
139 *Kent LMC Archive*, minutes of LMPC meeting on 20 December 1923.
140 *Staffordshire LMC Archive*, minutes of LMPC meeting on 8 October 1925.
141 *YORLMC Archive*, accounts attached to minutes of North Riding of Yorkshire LMPC meeting on 13 July 1933.
142 *North Staffordshire LMC Archive*, minutes of LMPC meeting on 19 September 1936.
143 *Cheshire County PRO*, NHL 7135, 7, Minutes of a meeting of the County Palatine of Chester LMPC on 12 August 1930, p. 6.
144 *Medical World*, 18 September 1931,'National Health Insurance', p. 61.
145 Anne Digby, 'The Economic and Medical Significance of the British National Insurance Act 1911,' in Martin Gorsky and Sally Sheard (eds) *Financing Medicine: The British Experience since 1750* (Abingdon, 2006). ch.11, p. 186.
146 *Kent LMC Archive*, minutes of meeting of Kent LMPC on 29 October 1925. *YORLMC Archive*, minutes of North Riding of Yorkshire LMPC meetings on 5 April 1934 and 10 November 1934.
147 *Nottinghamshire RO Archives*, SO NHI/ 1–3; NHI Committee minutes 1913–48, Vol.1, meeting in June 1913.
148 Harris, *National Health Insurance in Great Britain*, Appendix 7, Case A, p. 206.
149 *Nottinghamshire RO Archives*, SO NHI/ 1–3, NHI Committee minutes 1913–1948, vol. 1, meetings in December 1916 and March 1917.
150 *Kent LMC Archive*, minutes of LMPC meeting on 19 May 1921.
151 *Ibid.*, minutes of meeting on 13 July 1922.
152 Digby, *The Evolution of British General Practice*, p. 311.
153 Eder, *National Health Insurance and the Medical Profession*, p. 174.
154 Harris, *National Health Insurance in Great Britain*, Appendix 7, pp. 206–211.
155 Frank G. Layton, *The Old Doctor* (Birmingham, 1923). pp. 165–166.
156 *Ibid.*, p. 162.
157 *Ibid.*, p. 166.
158 Eder, *National Health Insurance and the Medical Profession*, p. 170.
159 Digby, 'The Economic and Medical Significance of the National Health Insurance Act 1911,' p. 185.
160 *Medical World*, 24 July 1015, 'Complaints Against Practitioners – the Medical Service Subcommittees'.
161 Cox, *Among the Doctors*, p. 124.
162 *Medical World*, 13 January 1922, 'Comment on "Letter from Croydon practitioner"'.
163 Cox, *Among the Doctors*, p. 124.
164 *BMA Archive*, LMC/1/3, minutes of the London Panel Committee meeting on 25 February 1919, min 6.
165 *Kent LMC Archive*, minutes of LMPC meeting on 20 December 1922.

166 *Ibid.,* minutes of LMPC meeting on 18 January 1923.
167 *Ibid.,* minutes of meeting on 10 May 1923; *North Staffordshire LMC Archive,* minutes of LMPC meeting on 6 April 1923.
168 *BMJ,* 22 December 1923, Supplement, pp. 277–278. It was subsequently reduced to £600.
169 *Lancashire & Cumbria LMCs Archive,* minutes of Lancashire LMPC meeting on 19 September 1928.
170 Honigsbaum, *The Division in British Medicine,* p. 208.
171 Marks, *The History and Development of Local Medical Committees,* p. 118.
172 Quoted by Levy, *National Health Insurance,* p. 116.
173 For example: *Daily Mail,* 29 June 1923, 'Panel Doctors fined' and 9 October 1929, 'Panel Doctor and a patient.'
174 *Daily Sketch,* 10 March 1923 reprinted in *Medical World* 16 March 1923, p. 47.
175 *North Staffordshire LMC Archive,* minutes of meeting of LMPC Executive Subcommittee on 29 September 1914.
176 *Medical World,* 3 February 1922, pp. 534–535.
177 *Kent LMC Archive,* minutes of LMPC meeting on 13 July 1922.
178 *YORLMC Archive,* minutes of North Riding of Yorkshire LMPC meeting on 15 June 1933 referring to Ministry circular ICL 808.
179 *The National Insurance (Provision of Medical Benefit) Regulations* 1912, Reg. 49 and *National Insurance Amendment Act Regulations* 1913, Reg. 53.
180 See Chapter 2.
181 Peter Collin, Sabine Rudischhauser, and Pascale Gonod (eds), "Autorégulation régulée. Analyses historiques de structures de régulation hybrides = Regulierte Selbstregulierung. Historische Analysen hybrider Regelungsstrukturen", in *Trivium. Revue franco-allemande de sciences humaines et sociales,* (2016), vol. 21, available at http//journals.openedition.org/trivium/5245.
182 *Kent LMC Archive,* minutes of KCMC meeting on 29 January 1913.
183 A.S. (Arthur Strettel) Comyns Carr, W.H. (William Hubert) Stuart-Garnett, and J.H.(James Henry) Taylor, *National Insurance* (London, 1912). p. 71.
184 See David B. Green, *Working-Class Patients and the Medical Establishment: Self-help in Britain from the Mid-Nineteenth Century to 1948* (Aldershot, 1985). p. 132.
185 *Lancashire & Cumbria LMCs Archive,* minutes of Lancashire LMPC meeting on 2 October 1928.
186 *Ibid.,* minutes of Lancashire LMPC meetings on 3 April and 15 May 1929.
187 *Medical World,* 6 January 1922, Report of meeting of London Panel Committee, LMC section, p. 443.
188 *BMA Archive,* B/203/1/17, minutes of the IAC meeting on 19 November 1925, Doc 17.
189 *Ibid.,* B/203/1/19, minutes of IAC Emergency Subcommittee on 28 January 1928, Doc.38, 1–4.
190 *Ibid.,* B/203/ 1/20, minutes of IAC meeting of 25 June 1928, Report of LMPCs' Conference, p. 6.
191 *Manchester University Medical Collections,* MMC/11/2/2/14, Letter from Manchester Medical and Panel Committee dated 26 June 1934.
192 Comyns Carr et al, *National Insurance,* p. 71.
193 William A. Brend, *Health and the State* (London, 1917). pp. 222–223.
194 Levy, *National Health Insurance,* p. 271.
195 *North Staffordshire LMC Archive,* Minutes of LMPC meeting on 17 February 1927.
196 *BMJ,* 15 April 1939, 'Annotations', 'Nutrition, Agriculture and the Family Doctor', pp. 783–784.

197 *Ibid.,* 27 November 1948, Picton Obituary, p. 960.
198 *Cheshire County PRO,* NHL 7135/8, Minutes of a meeting of the County Palatine of Chester LMPC on 13 September 1934, Appendix, 'LMPC Antenatal Scheme.'
199 *BMJ,* 5 January 1924, Supplement 'Report of Court of Inquiry into GPs' Remuneration', para 25, p. 8.
200 *Manchester University Medical Collections,* MMC/11/2/2 'Practitioner handbooks'.
201 Levy, *National Health Insurance,* p. 271.
202 *BMA Archive,* B/203/1/24, minutes of IAC Pensions Subcommittee meeting on 30 November 1932.
203 *University of Leicester, David Wilson Library medical archive,* E1/1/3, 1960, F.A. Alexander 'Leicester Royal Infirmary Maternity Hospital'.
204 *Ibid.*
205 *Kent LMC Archive,* minutes of Kent County LMPC meetings on 25 September 1924 and 24 September 1925.
206 *Ibid.,* 24 June 1926 and 23 September 1926. Plans to extend the service were considered in June 1936.
207 *Medical World,* 4 February 1927, 'London Panel Committee', p. 494.
208 *BMA Archive,* B/203/3/21, minutes of Annual Conference of Representatives of LMPCs, 20 October 1932, minute 51.
209 *Ibid.,* minutes of IAC meeting on 17 January 1924, min 242.
210 *National Insurance Gazette,* 8 March 1924, p. 93.
211 *Wellcome Collection* (BMA archive), SA BMA/H.10 Box 258, extract from report of Conference of LMPCs October 1924.
212 *Report of the Royal Commission on National Health Insurance,* 1926, HMSO, cmd. 2596 p. 61.
213 Eder, *National Health Insurance and the Medical Profession,* p. 176.
214 Quoted in Levy, *National Health Insurance,* p. 271.
215 *Medical World,* 8 July 1915, 'The surcharge problem -who is responsible?' (Alfred Salter). p. 52.
216 *Ibid.,* 15 April 1915, Editorial.
217 *Ibid.,* 25 March 1915, 'The Panel Committees and their relation to the PMPU', p. 370.
218 *Ibid.,* '24 June 1915, Apathy - The Curse of the Profession', p. 786.
219 'AGP', *This Panel Business,* pp. 269–270.
220 *Medical World,* 22 October 1926, 'On financing the Panel Profession' (Hereward). p. 126.

7 'Black-coated Bolshevists'

The Ministry of Health, political brinkmanship, and the 'ideologies of class', 1919–1926

During the First World War, the BMA had laid the foundations of 'bargained corporatism' by forging a constructive relationship with government officials and through their largely successful efforts to manage the supply of medical personnel to the armed services. When the Ministry of Health was created in 1919, the profession's leaders expected to extend their working relationship with civil servants and hoped for more success in collective bargaining on the panel GPs' behalf. However, their efforts in this regard generally fell short of their expectations. The Insurance Acts Committee (IAC) was convinced that if they could only provide sufficient and convincing evidence to back their claims for an increase in the insurance doctors' remuneration, Ministry officials would advocate their cause to ministers and to His Majesty's Treasury. This negotiating strategy was undermined, however, by changes of government and in civil service personnel. Moreover, the policy of retrenchment which successive governments felt obliged to adopt in the early 1920s in response to the post-war depression put the continued existence of NHI in jeopardy. The consequent need to square up to their old adversaries, the Approved Societies, brought the insurance doctors together as never before in preparing in 1923 for one brief but effective attempt to challenge government authority. When their leaders' negotiating prowess fell short of expectations, militant action was an inevitable default for the panel GPs. This action was fuelled not only by a justified set of grievances on the GPs' part, but also by a fear, common to the professional middle class during this period, that their status and economic power were being eroded relative to their working-class clientele. While two-thirds of GPs in the early 1920s maintained panel lists and devoted a considerable proportion of their time to the care of working-class patients, their aspirations to be family doctors still relied on the custom of the fee-paying middle class.

However, the middle class, of whom the GPs counted themselves members, believed themselves to be suffering at that time a significant decline in living standards. The post-war squeeze on middle-class incomes made GPs more anxious than ever to obtain an adequate financial return from their exacting panel work. They were also fearful that their hard-won autonomy might be wrested

DOI: 10.4324/9781003438274-7

from them by a newly assertive Approved Society lobby demanding increased influence as a quid pro quo for increased financial support for the NHI scheme. The insurance doctors looked to their representatives for resolution of these concerns, but their limited success exposed the IAC to trenchant criticism from the trade union lobby. Historians of this period largely agree that the economic recession which followed the end of the First World War enabled opponents of state expansion to force the coalition government and its successors to return to budgetary orthodoxy and cut back on commitments to widen the scope of welfare provision.[1] Their efforts therefore punctured hopes of expanding NHI. This, as will be seen, made it difficult for the doctors' leaders to reconcile their desire to expand and develop the scheme with the need to meet their constituents' overarching need for remuneration sufficient to maintain their status as middle-class professionals. It also led, inexorably, to a questioning of the benefits of partnership between GPs and the state and a further political showdown between the Government and the profession.

The Ministry, the IAC, and the 'cantankerous minority'

As the survey conducted by the IAC in 1917 had demonstrated, the medical profession was broadly supportive of the idea of a Ministry of Health.[2] The process by which the Ministry came into being was tortuous and punctuated by attempts to reconcile the very different objectives of reformers within central government, the profession, and the Local Government Board (LGB). The latter, according to Kenneth Morgan, had 'provided a steady, depressing resistance to change, especially to the proposed formation of the new Ministry'.[3] The fusion of the NHI Commission and the Board was precipitated by Addison's appointment as the Board's president in 1918. For the profession at this time, a satisfactory conclusion to the negotiations over their remuneration was paramount. Dr H.J. Oldham informed the Local Medical and Panel Committees (LMPCs) Conference that year that GPs' work deserved recognition as marked as that given to other workers but added that 'they were not going to be paid the wages of scavengers for doing it'.[4] Addison's eyes were firmly fixed, however, on a different objective, that is realising his ambitions for an integrated model of health and social services, extending coverage to include, at one end, preventative public health measures, and, at the other, a range of secondary care services not confined to hospital settings. He had set out proposals to achieve this in a memorandum written in 1914 to LGB president Lord Rhondda with the help of Morant and Sir George Newman.[5] He was also preoccupied with the task of building hundreds of thousands of new houses, something added to his ministerial brief as a consequence of Lloyd George's pledge to create 'homes fit for heroes'.[6] Addison was in no hurry to forgive the personal attacks on him by diehards within the BMA even if its GP leaders' views of NHI were now more closely aligned with his. However, the BMA were anxious that in his zeal for consolidating health services, Addison did not sacrifice what the profession had gained in the way of autonomy by making GPs salaried and subordinating them to local authority control.[7]

When a BMA delegation met with Addison and the chairman of the NHI Joint Commission Waldorf Astor in April 1919, Addison deflected discussions of their concerns by suggesting that they would be addressed in the recommendations of the new medical consultative council he had established which he had tasked with drawing up plans for the development of NHI and its integration with other health services.[8] The Council, chaired by the respected physician, Sir Bertrand Dawson, comprised a number of medical luminaries though initially only one GP, Dr Adam Fulton of Nottingham, who was described as being 'a GP of special experience'.[9] The membership of the Council proved to be the subject of debate and argument in the medical journals. An article in *Medical World* in October 1919 alleged that it was full of BMA 'bigwigs' and 'controlled by a body of middle-class nobodies inexperienced in affairs'.[10] However, some of the BMA's own nominations, including that of Brackenbury, had also been ignored, though the Council eventually comprised additional GPs, including IAC members H. Guy Dain and J.A. Macdonald.[11] Always keen to impugn its rivals, the MPU alleged that Morant and the NHI commissioners were involved with the BMA in a conspiracy to keep their nominees out of the inner circles of power.[12] The truth, however, was more mundane. Addison was clearly irritated by the political infighting among the medical representative bodies and soon made it clear that while they could put forward names, he alone would decide who was to be on the Council and what its remit was. He informed those appointed that, 'they did not sit upon the council in a representative capacity, and he hoped that he might rely upon receiving the best advice they could furnish as independent individuals'.[13]

Addison had supported the establishment of the Panel Medico-Political Union (PMPU) in 1914 when it seemed like a logical extension of State Medical Services Association (SMSA), but he was now beginning to find his erstwhile friends a handful. The PMPU had changed its name to the Medico-Political Union (MPU) in 1918. In April 1919, its secretary, Alfred Welply, circulated MPU members about its stance on remuneration and insurance practitioners' terms and conditions stating that the Union 'has interviewed Dr Addison and the commissioners' [sic], and 'the promise of amendment has been made'. In June, an irritated Morant wrote to Astor that if a substantially increased war bonus was to be given to the doctors, it should be given without delay lest it seem 'due to pressure from the PMPU *which is not the case*' (added emphasis).[14] In reference to the upcoming discussions with the IAC, an undated civil service memorandum from around the same time refers to 'a certain small but noisy section of insurance doctors who have been increasingly cantankerous and difficult throughout the five years and have been combined in a rival organisation' which had been 'carping' at the IAC for being 'inexcusably supine'.[15] The Ministry was clearly unwilling to entertain the arguments of this cantankerous minority. A

Commission document entitled 'Memorandum of agreement for medical services under the Insurance Act' described the LMPCs as the principal means by which the profession was consulted and concludes with a statement that the IAC is 'the executive body of the successive conferences of the Local Medical and Panel Committees of Great Britain'.[16]

The strident demands of the MPU with regard to the level of GPs' capitation fee had the effect of making the IAC's proposals seem reasonable by comparison. The civil servant R.W. Harris wrote in a memorandum of September 1919 that:

> It is difficult to know what figure is intended...The wild men are talking about £1 or even more; in other areas opinion is hardening in favour of 15s while it appears likely that the moderate elements in the profession would concentrate on some figure between 12s and 13s.[17]

The IAC finally settled on a requested capitation fee of 13s 6d per annum but the Ministry were only prepared to offer 10s. However, the Treasury's unwillingness to support an award of this size concerned James Smith Whitaker who opined that the resultant average GP income 'can hardly be maintained to be high'.[18] He repeated his concern that if remuneration was 'not sufficiently high to attract the best men in the profession to insurance work (we) should at least aim at retaining the best men who are present on the panel'. In a subsequent memorandum, Whittaker said that 'a strike, that is a general withdrawal from service, is not much to be feared' but he suggested that there should be a further test by which the profession's claim should be judged, that is: 'whether it will secure a service of the quality that any reasonable insured person would expect to be delivered if he were paying for it as a private patient'.[19]

Although his officials were happy to accept that the BMA had the authority to represent the profession in negotiations with the Ministry, Addison briefly pinned hopes on an alternative means of developing professional consensus. This was an independent body established in 1918 to support the campaign for the Ministry of Health called the Medical Parliamentary Committee.[20] It was originally chaired by Sir Henry Morris and was given strong support by the *Lancet*.[21] In February 1919, a meeting of GPs was held at Wigmore Hall, London to discuss the need for more effective representation. At the meeting, the IAC chairman, Brackenbury, wearily pointed to the futility of trying to reach a medico-political consensus. Citing the diametrically opposed views of the National Medical Union (NMU) and the MPU, respectively, he said that 'they always would have in medical politics...views that would never meet' and which were 'were absolutely antagonistic'.[22] The editor of the *Lancet*, Sir Samuel Squire Sprigge, therefore moved that, as an ostensibly non-partisan body, the Medical Parliamentary Committee be empowered to speak for the profession but, crucially, he failed to win sufficient support.[23] The meeting ended inconclusively and, despite Addison's encouragement, the Medical Parliamentary Committee ceased to have any influence in debates about the profession's future. In May 1919, it changed its name, at his suggestion, to the British Federation of Medical and Allied Services.[24] However, Sprigge later regretted that 'the BMA saw no reason to revise its opinion that the Federation has no reason for its existence'.[25] The Medical Women's Federation (MWF) maintained its membership of the new body but, given its close working relationship with the BMA, 'found this gradually becoming a source of embarrassment'.[26]

Concerned that the constant anti-BMA refrain voiced by *Medical World* and a minority of representatives at the Annual LMPCs Conference undermined the IAC's authority and threatened to impede its negotiating prowess, Alfred Cox responded with an article in the *BMJ* in March 1919 explaining why it was unnecessary for the BMA to become a trade union. Taking account of the Association's conclusions about the Coventry case, the article cited advice from the 'foremost experts on trade union law', F. Gore Brown K.C. and H.H. Slesser, 'author of the most recent book on the legal position of trade unions and standing council of the Labour party'. These experts had said that the benefits of being a trade union were doubtful in the BMA's situation, as a loophole in the Trades Disputes Act could still leave the Association vulnerable.[27] The article prompted a letter to *Medical World* from the York GP Dr J.C. Lyth who described advice given to the MPU by one of the same experts stating that in respect of the Coventry case, the MPU as a trade union would be protected from accusations of restraint of trade, whereas the BMA would not.[28] Cox took great pleasure in describing in his article the successes the BMA had enjoyed in supporting doctors engaged in industrial disputes, citing opponents' begrudging acknowledgement of their power and influence. These included an MP who in 1916 described them as 'the most powerful syndicalist trade union in the kingdom', miners' leaders praising the Association's robust defence of its members' interests, and a *Daily Express* editorial in 1918 which described them as 'the strongest trade union in the world'(!) He might have added the admiration of Beatrice Webb, the assumed author of an article in the New Statesman in 1917 which described the BMA as 'one of the most highly developed and most efficient of all British Professional Organisations' which had 'adopted some of the most efficient methods of warfare of the manual-working Trade Unions'.[29]

Cox's article also served to advertise the introduction of the new National Insurance Defence Trust which was formally established by the BMA in March 1919. Its objects were, firstly, to help meet expenses incurred in organising or taking any action to protect the profession in connection with NHI; secondly, to provide financial support for medical practitioners disadvantaged by participating in such action. The trust was to be entirely separate from the BMA, but the IAC would constitute the trustees.[30] The memorandum establishing the trust recommended the LMPCs ask their constituents to contribute ½d per patient per annum, but it was a voluntary contribution separate from any statutory levy supporting LMPCs. The issue of whether individual LMPCs would support the trust was complicated by the attacks which the MPU levelled against the BMA, the IAC, and its motives during increasingly rancorous exchanges throughout 1919 and the advice given to LMPCs by the Union to decline the BMA's request and pay instead into the MPU's political objects fund.[31] One MPU supporter reported in *Medical World* that Middlesex LMPC, which was chaired by Brackenbury, had voted 11 to 3 in favour of supporting the BMA. He advised his colleagues to ignore this and pay it to the MPU, claiming that he would 'rather feed a live dog than a dead lion'.[32] In June 1919, the Kent County Panel Committee pointedly rejected the BMA's request and decided to pay £100 from voluntary contributions to the MPU and the following month wrote to its constituents seeking permission to donate to the Union the accumulated fund of £2,000.[33]

Why was it that certain LMPCs at this time were so critical of the IAC and anxious to promote the MPU in its place? A careful reading of extant LMPC minutes suggests opinions regarding support for the IAC and for the MPU, respectively, fluctuated depending on the presence or absence of key personalities, and on internal politics. The London Panel Committee had been firmly supportive of the PMPU/MPU, and the latter was, as has been seen, largely London-centric. The combative MPU Secretary Alfred Welply was absent from the committee between July 1918, when he was called up for military service, and September 1920, when he was finally re-elected, and during that period, a significant change of attitude is detectable. In June 1919, for example, two London Panel Committee representatives, B.A. Richmond and H.G. Cowie, withdrew from a conference called by the Union after refusing to condemn the BMA's report of its negotiations over amendments to terms and conditions.[34] In July, moreover, the committee instructed its representatives to the LMPCs' Conference to support the aforementioned report (M25) and recognise the IAC as the Conference's executive, mandated to negotiate on their behalf.[35] The same month, after learning that the Association of Panel Committees (APC) had not come to a decision about which defence fund to support, it decided to support the BMA defence trust and in September, when invited to send to representatives to the MPU's annual conference, resolved that 'no action be taken on the matter'.[36] Following Welply's return to the London Panel Committee in 1920, however, the committee resumed its previously hostile stance towards the IAC/BMA.

In Cheshire, the LMPC minutes reveal a growing dissatisfaction with the efforts of the IAC during the First World War and in 1917 they considered correspondence from York LMPC urging them to join the PMPU alongside a competing entreaty from Gloucestershire LMPC stating that this would weaken the national negotiating position.[37] The committee angered the IAC by continuing to collect 'contingent' resignations from their constituent GPs in a unilateral attempt to force the local Insurance Committee to concede an increase in their capitation fee.[38] When reporting on the LMPCs Conference in 1918, the Cheshire representative, Dr Hodgson, complained that provincial LMPCs 'do not get a chance to get our wishes ventilated'.[39] He urged his committee to join the APC but this prompted the LMPC's secretary, Dr Lionel Picton, to tender his resignation.[40] Due to his frequent and voluminous correspondence with the IAC, the eccentric Picton may have been thought of as a nuisance by Cox and his colleagues at BMA House but he was at heart a solid 'BMA man' and a firm believer in professional unity. Although disapproving of his committee's actions, he was persuaded to remain as its secretary and promulgated their wishes, even when disagreeing with them. Under the influence of Hodgson and the chairman, Dr Marsh, the Cheshire LMPC not only joined the APC but later urged its members to join the MPU, Picton being one of three dissentients.[41] Hodgson was elected to the IAC in 1919 but found that he was a lone voice opposing its corporatist policies, complaining that 'the central influence of the Association was too closely connected with governmental circles for independent action in the interests of the profession'.[42]

Many within the profession were dismayed by the spectacle of the MPU and BMA trading insults and calls were repeatedly made in letters to the respective journals for the two organisations to set aside their differences. One of the peacemakers was E. Rowland Fothergill, who chaired the BMA's Ministry of Health subcommittee. At its first meeting in February 1919, the subcommittee sought to co-opt members of the MPU 'if they will act' and committed itself to organising a conference involving the MPU, and other organisations to 'define obstacles to cordial relations'.[43] He was subsequently persuaded to withdraw his suggestion but the joint conference he campaigned for went ahead in May 1919. It was attended by representatives of the APC, the MPU, the Medical Parliamentary Committee, the MWF, and the BMA. The NMU and SMSA were invited but failed to field any representatives. The meeting quickly ran into difficulties when E.H. Stanscombe vainly called on BMA representatives to recognise the MPU as the only body capable of conducting collective bargaining in negotiations with government.[44] The Conference established a liaison committee, however, which met ten days later. At this meeting, the APC chairman Peter Macdonald pointed out that if the IAC consisted solely of insurance practitioners, a 'modus vivendi' could be established between the BMA and MPU and then 'his association would be quite satisfied and would probably cease to exist'.[45] As a compromise, Brackenbury proposed that MPU representatives to be invited to 'accompany IAC representatives in meetings with the NHI commissioners and officials of the new Ministry'. However, at a second meeting, Welply dismissed this proposal and the APC's suggestion of a permanent liaison committee, and further dialogue was abruptly curtailed.[46]

The extent of the animosity between the IAC and MPU over the issue of defence funds can be gauged from an unpublished draft circular to insurance practitioners and LMPCs considered by the IAC in July 1919 which the committee decided not to approve, fearing that its intemperate language would only inflame the situation. It seems likely to have been written by Cox who, despite his experience, was more thin-skinned and less statesmanlike than Brackenbury.[47] The document states that the MPU's recent circulars were 'grossly mendacious in character and...vulgarly offensive in language' and that insurance practitioners deserved to know the facts of the matters referred to.[48] The document describes the MPU's circular on the IAC's memorandum of changes to conditions of service, M25, as 'one colossal lie', rejecting among other claims their allegations that the insurance commissioners wrote it as well as agreeing to pay for its distribution.[49] The document claimed that these attacks showed how 'hopelessly ignorant' the council of the MPU were about matters of administration, ridiculing their instruction to panel doctors to leave representation of GPs' interests in their hands.[50] The circular reveals why attempts to establish a professional consensus at this time were doomed to failure.

Arbitration, retrenchment, and the renewed threat of the Approved Societies

The ongoing conflict with the MPU was in any case an unwelcome distraction for the BMA from the difficult business of securing improvements in the panel GPs' pay. In September 1919, the IAC reported a wide range of responses to its survey of LMPCs about the appropriate amount by which the capitation fee should be increased. These ranged from 10s to £1, 3s, 6d.[51] At the Annual LMPCs Conference in November, the York representative, Peter Macdonald, congratulated the IAC on 'the strong fighting lead which had been given' but proposed a rider to a debated motion calling on the IAC to refuse to accept anything less than 13s 6d.[52] Brackenbury opposed this on the grounds that it would tie the hands of the negotiators and the amendment was lost, prompting E.H. Stanscombe to wonder if the LMPCs 'had sent up men or rabbits'.[53] However, the LMPCs accepted the non-financial provisions of the proposed amendment regulations contingent on there being a sufficient increase in remuneration. Morant clearly sympathised with the doctors, opining that 'the moderates in the profession had succeeded in keeping the extremists at bay and 13s 6d was not an unreasonable figure'.[54] Due to pressure from the Treasury, however, Addison had little room for manoeuvre and was unmoved even by the IAC's agreement to broaden the range of services to the insured, something which Brackenbury had only with difficulty persuaded conference to accept.[55] In January 1920, Addison informed the IAC that he was prepared to offer them 11s in spite of Treasury opposition.[56]

Despite having won the vote at Conference, Brackenbury insisted that the LMPCs would not permit the IAC to accept anything less than 13s 6d and proposed the matter be settled by arbitration. After further correspondence, Addison reluctantly agreed and the IAC accepted 11s as an interim award.[57] A board of arbitration was hastily convened and considered the evidence presented to it, including the IAC's data which Ministry officials had previously deemed insufficient and unconvincing. The Arbitration Board noted that 'there was unfortunately a surprising absence of evidence from the doctors' side' before concluding that the 11s offered by the government was a fair and reasonable settlement.[58] The IAC was left to shamefacedly report its failure to the profession. A *BMJ* editorial initially praised Brackenbury's performance in the negotiations which it said were 'wisely handled' by the IAC.[59] In an article in the *Lancet* in March 1920, Brackenbury said that, given the pressure on the Ministry, 'the extraction of the offer of 11s...appears something of an achievement'.[60] He admitted, however, that the absence of data was 'our chief weakness before the arbitrators'. This was not, he said, the fault of the IAC 'who have appealed over and over again to the profession to produce such statistics'.[61] Reinforcing his confidence in the process, he added that, 'The machinery of negotiation was not at fault' and in an indirect reference to the lack of unity, and arguments over the defence fund, he said that negotiations could not succeed 'without the entire support, both moral and financial, of the whole profession'. The LMPCs seem to have appreciated Brackenbury's candour, and during the course of 1920, a large number wrote expressing their gratitude for the IAC's efforts.[62] *Medical World*, however, condemned his 'apologia' as 'a whitewash'.[63]

Following the arbitration award, the IAC committed itself to gathering the most persuasive data it could find to support its case for an increase in the capitation fee. In March 1920, however, Morant died unexpectedly, and his place as Permanent Secretary was taken by the altogether less sympathetic Sir Arthur Robinson. By the following year, Addison too was gone, shortly to be cast into the political wilderness as a matter of expediency by his once great friend Lloyd George.[64] In September 1920, the London Panel Committee, following Welply's return to it, once again expressed its opinion that the interests of panel GPs could only be served by an independent body devoted to them alone. It politely declined to nominate candidates for seats on the IAC and invited other LMPCs to support the APC instead.[65] The IAC once again found itself having to face down militants questioning its right to represent the insurance GPs, although over the ensuing months, most LMPCs responded with expressions of support.[66] In September 1921, Robinson wrote to Cox on behalf of the new Minister, Sir Alfred Mond, conveying the devastating news that, rather than increase the capitation fee, the government proposed to reduce it to 9s 6d.[67] Cox replied that the IAC 'were at a loss to understand why the minister has decided to set aside the decision of the arbitrators'.[68] A subsequent meeting with the minister took place on the eve of the annual LMPCs Conference. Mond explained that he was responding to the Geddes committee's call for the complete abolition of the government's supplemental payments into the National Insurance Fund, amounting at that time to £1.7 million annually.[69]

Appointed in August 1921, the Committee on National Expenditure chaired by the businessman Eric Geddes was seen by many as a response to the Anti-Waste campaign supported by the Rothermere and Northcliffe press. It was very much attuned to the views of Treasury hawks who urged a return to budgetary orthodoxy and the abandonment of further government investment in social welfare.[70]

A dismayed and angry Conference of LMPCs debated whether to accept the proposed reduction or to continue to press for a higher fee than that awarded by arbitration, and what to do in the event of a continued refusal of their reasonable claim.[71] The Conference decided to nominate its own delegation to join the IAC negotiators in the reconvened meeting with the Minister and his officials on the evening of the first day of the Conference. One of those chosen was Henry Cardale, chair of the London Panel Committee, who had earlier withdrawn a motion critical of the IAC and urged Conference to rally behind them. The meeting showed how determined Mond was and revealed his implied threat that if that GPs did not accede to his proposed reduction 'on grounds of citizenship', the Government might abandon NHI altogether. Mond said that 'There is a question on a paper in the House of Commons tomorrow asking whether in view of general dissatisfaction, I should not be well advised to scrap the whole thing'.[72]

The GPs were clearly taken aback by this announcement, which was all the more surprising, given the cavalier manner in which it appeared to contemplate the destruction of a key part of the serving Prime Minister's legislative legacy. Even Mond's Conservative successors proved to be more circumspect in that regard. Brackenbury proposed a face-saving compromise by describing the reduction as a temporary 'rebate' but Mond dismissed this as 'mere camouflaging'.[73] When the deputation reported back the following day, the representatives were in a sombre mood when debating what to do next. A crestfallen Cardale said that he got the impression that the insurance system was 'in a bad state' and that the government thought they were being generous in offering 9s 6d.[74] In the debates which followed, several LMPC representatives confessed that their constituents had no stomach for a fight. A Scottish representative said that GPs in Scotland would accept the offer and E.A. Gregg had to admit that even in London 'men would not refuse service for 9s 6d'.[75] The Conference acknowledged the necessity to capitulate but ended defiantly with an unprecedented show of unity and promises from erstwhile dissenters to contribute to the defence fund.[76]

The IAC subsequently informed Mond that the profession reluctantly accepted his proposals while maintaining that they did not believe 'that anything less than 11s was sufficient to maintain an adequate service for the public'.[77] The IAC also made it clear to the Minister that to maintain the panel GPs' remuneration at the level recommended in the 1920 arbitration award if not to increase it, the Approved Societies should be compelled to meet the shortfall from their accumulated reserves. In 1922, these amounted to about £42 million.[78] The Societies made it clear, however, that if they were required to contribute more, they would expect to be a party to the negotiations over the GPs' remuneration and enjoy a greater share in the administration of medical benefit.[79] The MPU and the London Panel Committee were greatly alarmed at this prospect, but Cox and Brackenbury were less fearful.[80] Robinson had assured him, Cox informed the IAC, that the Ministry had no intention of giving the Societies any more say in the administration of NHI but could not say so publicly. Cox admitted to fuelling the London Panel Committee's fears by telling them that 'there may shortly be a time when it is necessary for London doctors to join a national fight'.[81] Welply echoed this when urging Union members to prepare for 'the biggest fight the profession has ever had to wage'. To support this concern, he circulated an article from *The Star* newspaper of 8 March 1922 by Mr Percy Rockliffe of the New Tabernacle Friendly Society, one of the Approved Societies' most uncompromising and unrepentant critics of the panel GPs.[82] In order to disprove the MPU's accusations of inertia on their part, the IAC published a timetable of its discussions with the Ministry, exchanges of letters and memoranda, and press briefings.[83] They further demonstrated their resolve when in March 1922 they informed Robinson that 'under no circumstances would they tolerate interference by the approved societies in negotiations with the profession as to the regulations or the capitation fee'.[84] Fear of the Societies' resurgence was sufficient to compel the MPU towards rapprochement with the IAC and in April 1922 they set aside their differences, stating that they would 'be pleased to afford every possible assistance to the Insurance Acts Committee to prevent Approved Society control'.[85] Before considering the profession's preparation for this new conflict, it is important to understand the root causes of the panel GPs' discontents at this time.

The 'ideologies of class' and renewed attempts at professional consensus

In their discussions with both government and the Approved Societies in the early 1920s, the IAC vented their constituents' growing sense of anger at what they saw as a refusal to accord a proper value to their services. This reflected a common feeling among the professional and managerial classes that they had lost out during the war and its aftermath to the working class which had grown in relative prosperity and influence. The wages of unskilled workers doubled between 1917 and 1924, whereas the cost of living rose by only 70%.[86] As Kenneth O. Morgan states, 'the middle class…felt themselves to be, in major respects, a casualty of the war and suffering a real cut in its living standards'.[87] In October 1921, an editorial in *Medical World* stated:

> There have been sad stories of late of the passing of the family doctor. We are told that the one-time friend of the household has gone for ever…The root cause is financial exiguity. The middle class, at one time the doctor's mainstay, is now the new poor.[88]

The description of the middle class as 'the new poor' was popularised by newspapers like the *Daily Mail*.[89] In his book, *The Ideologies of Class*, Ross McKibbin states that the problems faced by many middle-class households 'were seen as directly proportional to the gains made (as they supposed) by the working classes'.[90] The Middle Classes Union founded in 1919 and the Anti-Waste

League founded in 1921 were manifestations of this feeling.[91] Other 'bourgeois demons', as McKibbin describes them, included 'profiteers, the Lloyd George government, and capital'.[92] For the militant columnists of *Medical World,* the latter two were personified in the new Minister of Health, Sir Alfred Mond, whom Gordon Ward, under his nom de plume 'Hereward', pointedly described as 'a Hebrew financier'.[93] Ardent supporters of the MPU saw the Union as the modern inheritor of the medical guild traditions which had become resurgent in the 1890s. Some, including the GP and later Labour MP Alfred Salter, were clearly attracted to ideas of guild socialism. While he was one of the leading lights of the Socialist Medical Association founded in 1930, he had earlier been in favour of the idea of a 'health guild' of doctors, dentists, midwives, and nurses to replace both the panel and voluntary system.[94] By the 1920s, guild socialism had become, in Morgan's words, 'an idea of the past'.[95] It was being supplanted by a socialist pluralist movement which championed the concept of 'associational independence', emphasising the capacity of groups to protect the individual from the growing influence of the central state. Modifying and indeed rejecting some of the guild socialist ideas of F.N. Figgis, the leaders of this movement, principally G.D.H. Cole, Harold Laski, and R.H. Tawney, believed that 'democratic mechanisms were essential to any and every form of association'.[96] It is ironic that the MPU, and Salter in particular, did not recognise that LMPCs, despite their proximity to the state apparatus, could arguably be viewed as a reification of these ideas. The socialist pluralists were also responsible for popularising the 'functional theory of social justice' and principles of 'economic reciprocity' which would certainly have resonated with the panel GPs. As individuals who made a productive contribution to the community, many GPs subscribed to the view that, to borrow Ben Jackson's words, 'as a matter of right the community owed them a fair share of the social product'.[97] This view, combined with notions of the 'professional social ideal', added to the GPs' sense of injustice, and underlined the government's failure to properly value or reward their services.

GPs also feared that their declining economic status was leaving them vulnerable to renewed attack by some of those who had sought dominion over them before the advent of NHI. The 1920s saw a resurgence of the conflicts which had characterised relationships between GPs and the miners' Medical Aid Societies in South Wales before and during the First World War. A dispute in Abertridwr in 1920 saw GPs dismissed by the workmen's committee from their contracts to treat dependants and replaced by salaried doctors and led to a rival scheme being set up by the GPs.[98] A disagreement between the miners and the doctors in Llanelli was settled by an agreement in 1921, only to resurface in a dispute in 1934 which saw the creation of rival schemes and vehement recriminations.[99] In all these disputes, class consciousness played a prominent part as the GPs found themselves the unwitting target of an assault by working-class activists on the political establishment and the liberal bourgeoisie. According to Steven

Thompson, the workmen's committees saw themselves as 'the disinterested protectors of "the public good" against the selfish, egotistical interests of the medical profession'. He speaks admiringly of the determination of the mining communities to create a proletarian 'public sphere', to use the phrase coined by Jurgen Habermas, based on a collectivised mutuality in which the sick and old were made a charge on the whole community.[100] Thompson admits, however, that these 'subscriber democracies' should not be idealised. The doctrinaire views of a dominant few left little room for dissenting views and entirely excluded those of women who were equally if not more reliant on the services under discussion.[101] The committees spoke of 'justice', 'liberty', 'freedom', and 'equality' in asserting working-class rights, but their medical opponents could use equally emotive language in defending their professional independence and voicing their opposition to this subscriber tyranny.[102] Alfred Cox used the words 'wage slaves' to describe the condition in which he felt that the miners' societies desired to leave the doctors. He overstated his case somewhat, however, when he said that doctors had no problem in accepting service under town councils, Insurance Committees, or poor law Guardians because these were 'public bodies' subject to public, government, or judicial scrutiny, whereas workmen's committees were not.[103] As subsequent events were to show, the panel GPs were equally resistant to the efforts of these and indeed any lay institutions which sought to exercise control over their activities.

The MPU was especially vocal in encouraging panel GPs to fear state interference in their 'craft'. They shared with their conservative rivals a contempt for state bureaucracy, Alfred Salter famously informing the London Insurance Committee on one occasion that 'I am a doctor not a clerk'.[104] In common with many LMPC members and their IAC representatives, they viewed independent contractor status as central to their understanding of what a GP was and aspired to be.[105] This view was shared by others, including, surprisingly, many Approved Society representatives. When the Societies met with the IAC in January 1923, Sir Thomas Neal, chair of the Executive Committee of the National Association of Approved Societies, acknowledged the benefits of GPs working in private practice and hospitals saying that 'he did not want an insurance practitioner who was *only* an insurance practitioner'.[106] In contrast to the small minority of socialist doctors who made up the SMSA, the MPU's leaders were not, at this stage, wedded to the idea of becoming state employees and were increasingly protectionist, and suspicious of attempts by either the BMA or the government to alter the nature of GPs' professional responsibilities.[107] The Kent GP Gordon Ward was the only prominent MPU member to advocate a contrary view. He had advocated salaried service in 1917 and continued to argue that better working conditions, sick pay, and pensions were a price worth paying for the loss of autonomy.[108] Though not without progressive ideas, the MPU became increasingly fixated on the material well-being of their GP members at the expense of all other considerations. For example, their commentary on the IAC's report of its negotiations with government in 1919 stated that, 'The amount of remuneration is the most important matter affecting medical men' and that it is 'not the business of a defensive medical association to help towards securing a really satisfactory service for insured persons'. This prompted Cox to ask moralistically: 'Could the objects of the Union be put on a lower plane?'[109] While Brackenbury and his successors sought to promote a more expansive vision of the family doctor service, the MPU pursued a defensive policy focused on maintenance of the status quo and the submission of unrealistic demands for increased remuneration while refusing to accept any corresponding increase in public scrutiny or accountability. Their focus was directed more towards the pragmatic concerns of panel GPs struggling to maintain their economic and social status than on lofty ideals of public service.

In May 1922, following the unsatisfactory outcome of the latest meeting with Robinson, a special Conference of LMPCs was convened. It passed a resolution insisting on the continuance of the existing system of direct negotiations between the profession and government without the interference of any third party. But, in an attempt to make the GPs appear reasonable to public opinion, Brackenbury secured the addition of the rider 'but will continue to welcome cooperation of all those interested in the best possible medical service for insured persons'.[110] In the debates which followed about the use of the defence fund to support political action, a number of LMPC representatives attacked the London Panel Committee for not contributing. This prompted E.A. Gregg to respond by way of explanation that 'a big whacking fund was needed, and such a fund could not be left unprotected'.[111] Believing a fight with government over the capitation fee and increased powers for the Approved Societies to be ever more likely, the IAC instructed its general purposes subcommittee to consider 'steps to be taken to organise the profession including the provision of a Public Medical Service (PMS), in case of suspension of medical benefit'.[112] In the resulting document, called 'Organisation of insurance practitioners in the event of a struggle with government', the subcommittee outlined various scenarios, including the Government abandoning the scheme and handing subscriptions to the insured themselves to spend on schemes of their choosing, or handing complete control to the Approved Societies.[113] The subcommittee admitted to a reluctance to develop PMS proposals fearing that organising contract medical practice as a substitute for the panel system 'would be bad policy'. But a newly revised version of the Association's original 'Public Medical Services scheme' was presented to and approved by the Annual Conference of LMPCs in October. This stated that 'in some circumstances it will be necessary for Public Medical Services to be worked not by a division of the Association but by the personnel of the Local Medical and Panel Committee'.[114] This was a significant acknowledgement by the BMA of the central importance of LMPCs.

Meanwhile, attempts to establish a professional consensus continued. Following a meeting in June 1922 chaired by Guy Dain between representatives of the

IAC and the MPU, the IAC considered a proposal that MPU representatives be co-opted onto the IAC.[115] In September, the IAC considered a paper by Brackenbury in which he underlined the threat of always having the MPU on the sidelines, noting that a small number of LMPCs had declined invitations to attend the Annual Conferences, preferring to attend MPU conferences instead. These were infrequent and not very important, he said, but if a significant number were to repudiate the LMPC Conference, 'its representative character and consequently its authority would be seriously undermined'.[116] The IAC accordingly invited the MPU to nominate two representatives to attend IAC meetings 'for the purpose of assisting in its deliberations during the remainder of the present session' and established a special subcommittee to look at cooperation between the two bodies. When the Annual Conference of LMPCs convened in October 1922, the representatives were fully expecting a fight with government and Brackenbury, knowing that ministerial observers were present to gauge the mood of the profession, made no attempt to dissuade them. A paper on the organisation of the profession in the event of the dispute with government explicitly referring to mass resignation, and another containing the model PMS scheme, was approved for circulation to all panel doctors to view and comment on, the IAC being anxious to ensure that panel GPs knew what was in store before any call for mass resignation was made.[117]

Efforts to cement better relations between the IAC and the MPU continued with the latter eventually offering in December 1922 to allow the merging of the two defence funds on the condition that three seats were reserved for them on the IAC.[118] Unfortunately, this proved too much for BMA loyalists. The aforementioned special subcommittee concluded that the MPU was not as great a threat to the BMA as many believed and advised the IAC at its meeting in November that direct representation of the MPU on the committee would 'be widely objected to and so would be impracticable to obtain'.[119] To undermine the MPU's support among LMPCs and increase links between the Conference and its executive, it suggested that the number of LMPC-nominated members of the IAC be increased. The subcommittee were influenced by a paper by BMA Council member, Dr Robert Bolam, which noted that of an estimated 12,000 panel doctors, 8,000 were BMA members and 3,000 MPU members. However, by the MPU's own admission, 75% of their members were also BMA members which meant that there were only 750 GPs who were MPU members only, and 3,250 panel doctors not belonging to either organisation.[120]

The IAC consequently declined to endorse the MPU's latest proposal. A document describing the attempts at reconciliation circulated to the profession by them in December 1922 explained that to reserve seats for the MPU on the IAC 'would provoke a division in the ranks of the profession' and would risk 'losing the support of many LMPCs who up to the present day have been absolutely loyal'.[121] *Medical World* denounced the decision which it said should be up to the LMPC Conference rather than the IAC to decide, stating that this was 'a good example of an executive committee which is responsible to two different bodies, the British Medical Association and the panel conference'.[122] The MPU had unwittingly provided its opponents with the means to counter such arguments, however, when, at some point in 1922, in an effort to broaden its membership to explicitly include Consultants and non-panel GPs, it restructured itself and consigned the representation of panel GPs to its National Health Insurance 'section'. The status of the latter within the MPU, its opponents gleefully pointed out, was exactly equivalent to that of the IAC within the BMA.[123] Ignoring such comparisons, *Medical World* subsequently branded Brackenbury 'a last ditcher' opposed to a closer bond between the two organisations and claimed: 'We are now condemned as heretics and if not yet consigned to the stake we are already excommunicated'.[124]

Believing that the Government would seek to exploit the animosity between the panel GPs and the Approved Societies, the LMPCs Conference supported a proposal in October 1922 that the IAC meet with representatives of the Societies in a public forum.[125] A conference between the two sides and representatives of the Insurance Committees took place in London in January 1923.[126] The discussions began respectfully though in Eder's words 'pleasant words could not hide the implacable hostility of the Societies towards the continued independence of the panel medical service'.[127] The meeting nevertheless gave rise to a series of recommendations aimed at reducing the causes of tension between panel GPs and the Societies, which subsequently featured in discussions between the IAC and the Ministry. These included certification arrangements, the work of RMOs, delays in payments of benefits to the insured, and possible extensions of the scope of service. Both sides agreed to continue to meet periodically to progress discussion of these matters.[128] While separate negotiations took place over remuneration, the IAC continued to discuss with the Ministry necessary changes to the benefit regulations, including clarification of the scope of service. Their suggestions for reducing the burden of paperwork on GPs were rejected by the Ministry which also decided, against the IAC's wishes, to reduce the recommended maximum list size from 3,000 to 2,500 patients. The IAC countered with a request for panel GPs to be able to employ more assistants but this was dismissed with the rather unassailable argument that it would restrict the insured patients' opportunities' to see their registered GP and therefore ran counter to the principle of 'free choice of doctor'.[129] Brackenbury and his colleagues eventually secured at least one thing from these negotiations: persuading the Ministry not to allow the Approved Societies to initiate complaints to Insurance Committees on their members' behalf.[130] This was something which the Societies were keen to do, arguing, as they maintained in evidence to the Royal Commission three years later, that their subscribers lacked the means to properly promulgate complaints themselves or feared antagonising their GPs by doing so.[131] The continuation of their negotiations with Ministry officials demonstrated the IAC's persistent confidence in the power of reasoned argument as a means of practising bargained corporatism. But on what was this confidence based?

The remuneration crisis and the threat of mass resignation

The public school-educated civil servants who ran the Ministry recognised the doctors' representatives as fellow technocrats with whom, though not quite their social equals, they shared a common set of values and cultural assumptions, and a common commitment to the ideals of public service.[132] Confirming Nikolas Rose's contention that 'Liberal government is inherently bound to the authority of expertise', these officials were thus content to countenance the doctors' leaders' suggestions when it served the broader interests of the state.[133] The IAC did not always succeed in convincing ministers or officials of the rightness of their arguments but were reassured that at least their representations would be received with equanimity rather than the hostility they might have expected from the Approved Societies. Brackenbury was convinced that, as educated and honourable men, ministry officials were open to reasoned argument. Cox subscribed to the same view, stating in a *BMJ* article in April 1923, 'Our Civil Service is incorruptible. It does not take sides. I would rather see the Government standing between the insured person and the medical profession than the approved societies'.[134] Eschewing the aggressive chest-beating of the MPU, Brackenbury explained to a meeting of GPs in Liverpool and Cheshire in April 1923 that 'It is no use going into negotiations with an ultimatum…in a bullying spirit'.[135] Contents of Ministerial memoranda show him to have been broadly correct in his assumptions. Those officials had little time for or sympathy with the MPU 'wild men' whose bellicose attitude Cox dismissed when stating that 'to be potentially pointing a pistol which will not go off or goes off at the wrong end is not the way to impress any one worth impressing'.[136] Morant's successors were not as well disposed to the doctors as he was, but Whitaker and Newman generally served to mitigate any antimedical bias, and in general the civil servants appreciated the IAC's restraint. Harry Eckstein describes the relationship which developed between the BMA and the Ministry of Health under the National Health Service after 1948 as a 'non-statutory partnership' whose origins he traced to the interwar period.[137] Reflecting on this relationship across the twentieth century, he concluded that the BMA had actually lost all the crucial public disputes over medical policy but conceded that 'behind the record of public failures is a much more impressive record of not so public successes, greatest of all on minor matters, points of detail, but impressive enough also in the case of principles'.[138]

In 1922, Brackenbury struggled to get this message across to those he represented. The 'minor matters' on which at that time the IAC could claim to have succeeded included securing a temporary reprieve for GPs from the burdens of completing medical records during wartime, negotiating the introduction of rural mileage allowances, and successfully campaigning for the establishment of a Regional Medical Referee service.[139] These successes failed to impress the IAC's critics, especially the MPU. Nevertheless, the IAC had succeeded in persuading government officials that they could be trusted to represent the true intentions of the majority, whatever their rivals or antagonists might say. In so doing, they achieved what Eckstein calls a 'clientele relationship' which gave them a privileged position.[140] This could also be viewed as a manifestation of what the philosopher Pierre Bourdieu refers to as 'the mystery of the ministry' whereby the spokesman or agent becomes the embodiment of the group it represents, and the agent's views are seen as normatively valid and authentic.[141] The fact that the showdown which occurred in 1923 and subsequent periodic contretemps were quickly followed by a return to 'business as usual' proves how mutually beneficial this relationship was both to the Association and to the Government.

In the early part of 1923, many LMPCs still hoped for a rapprochement between the IAC and the MPU. Some, like Sunderland, blamed the IAC for the breakdown in negotiations and henceforth refused to pay into the defence trust.[142] The IAC was in no mood to be distracted, however, from its primary goal of preparing the profession for a major showdown with government over remuneration. This was rendered even more likely when the coalition government was succeeded, following the 1923 general election, by a Conservative administration, led by Stanley Baldwin. The new administration was committed to a policy of even greater retrenchment, in compliance with the wishes of both the Treasury and the press-inspired Anti-Waste' campaign. The campaign found a willing supporter in the 'People's Union for Economy' founded by the Conservative MP Godfrey Locker-Lampson.[143] The new Minister of Health, William Joynson-Hicks, quickly signalled his intention to seek an even greater reduction in the capitation fee than his Liberal predecessor. The Minister was advised to offer to fix the capitation fee for five years, as a means to negate the efforts of the IAC whom, in a memorandum written in August 1923, Robinson described as 'incorrigible hagglers'.[144] At Robinson's suggestion, Joynson-Hicks decided to meet with representatives of the Approved Societies. His intention was to gather ammunition for his contest with the doctors but also to test the strength of the Societies' opposition to underwriting the cost of any increase in medical benefit from their reserves. Despite their recent polite discussions with the IAC, the Societies immediately sought to discredit the doctors' claims for increased remuneration, stating that the 7s 3d they had been awarded before the war was more than adequate.[145] Joynson-Hicks pointed out that the average number of patient attendances was now 3.25 per annum compared with the 1.25 which the Plender report had found to be the norm in 1912. Playing devil's advocate, the Minister said that 'that every working man earned more than he did before the war so why should doctors be treated any differently?'[146] In response, Alban Gordon, a Fabian society member who was later to become a firm advocate of a state medical service, opined that Lloyd George had been overly generous and that the pre-war figure now represented fair reward. The Minister made it clear that as regards the future funding of NHI, 'there was not the slightest chance of getting any more money out of the government' and that extra funding for the doctors would have to come from the societies' funds. Gordon then advised the Minister not to be intimidated by threats of industrial action, stating that 'Our friends, the black-coated Bolshevists of 429 Strand are past masters in the art of bluff'.[147]

The IAC were still hopeful that militant action would not be necessary. They believed in the strength of their case for increased remuneration and backed it with reasoned argument and statistics. The memorandum that formed the basis of their written submission in August 1923 acknowledged the need for economy in public services but stressed the importance of the remuneration being sufficient to attract the next generation of doctors.[148] It argued that remuneration of insurance practice must compare favourably with that of private practice and other branches of medical work. It supported this with statistical arguments about the cost of living, drawn from an attached memorandum on changes to the cost of living between 1914, 1920, and 1923 by the BMA's statistician, Professor A.L. Bowley. This concluded that the lowest fee the profession could accept was between 10s 4d and 10s 9d per head per annum.[149] In the Minister's meeting with the IAC, Brackenbury said that they were not concerned about remuneration per se but that a decision to reduce their income would curtail further development and lead 'to the service remaining at or sinking below a level we should not like'.[150] What GPs wanted he said was a service that would not only retain the best GPs but was capable of attracting in the one-third currently outside the service, thereby addressing the current shortage of GPs in some areas which led to unacceptably high patient lists and reduced choice of doctor. The meeting ended without agreement but when the Minister spoke of the Societies' contention that many of their members were dissatisfied with the quality of panel service, Brackenbury strongly disputed this and the extent to which the Societies understood or accurately represented their members' views, stating 'in no sense whatsoever did they really represent the insured person'.[151]

The Minister seems to have accepted this point, as he admitted in a subsequent meeting on 3 October with his key officials, Robinson, Whitaker, Sir George Newman, and Sir Walter Kinnear.[152] He was conscious, however, of the influence wielded by the Approved Societies in parliament. Robinson pointed out that the doctors had their allies in parliament too. He concluded that 8s 6d was the proper rate and would eventually be accepted by the GPs 'though not of course without alarums and excursions'.[153] As negotiating tactics, Robinson suggested offering the IAC the choice of 8s 6d per patient for three years or 8s for five years.[154] Whitaker felt that the GPs would not accept the lesser figure because they had been 'exasperated by the venomous attacks made upon them by the approved societies' which reinforced the risk of large-scale resignations, he said, especially by those doctors with small lists who, financially, had little to gain from remaining on the panel.[155] In conveying the Minister's offer in October 1923, Robinson argued that the 1920 arbitration 'took place at a period of optimism and inflation when increases of remuneration were being considered liberally on all hands' adding 'On economic grounds…medical incomes must be expected to fall' and the Ministry could not justify setting a higher rate than what it believed to be the norm in private practice.[156] The IAC declared the response 'very unsatisfactory', repeating the contention that any shortfall in funding could be met from the National Insurance Fund 'owing to windfalls of various sorts'.[157] The letter hinted that the IAC might accept the reduction if their case was referred to arbitration.[158] Robinson replied that the Minister did not propose to discuss it any further and would not go to arbitration since the results of the previous arbitration were fully taken into account in his decision.[159] As if to underline how far the moderate stance taken by the IAC was from that of the militants of the MPU, Alfred Welply wrote to the Minister submitting a memorandum in support of a claim for 10s 6d.[160] When the Annual Conference of LMPCs met in October 1923, they unanimously rejected the Minister's offer.[161] However, at a special meeting of the LMPC in Kent, the same month members acknowledged that most of their constituents would accept 8s 6d if it were 'stabilised' or guaranteed for an adequate period.[162]

The day following the Conference, Cox wrote to LMPCs and insurance practitioners advising them to prepare for resignations to become effective as from 1 January 1924.[163] He reminded them of the model scheme for PMS which the profession was now advised to adopt as an alternative to NHI, the significance of which was not lost on the press.[164] His missive included a letter for practitioners to use in giving notice to Insurance Committees.[165] The letter referred to the work of the propaganda committee which had been established to win public and parliamentary support for the GPs' cause. This Committee included the Walsall GP Frank Layton. The Defence Fund contributed £100 towards the publication of his novel *The Old Doctor* and, believing it to be a way of winning support for the GPs, encouraged LMPCs to purchase copies and send them to their MPs and other interested parties.[166] Fortunately for the panel GPs, support for their arguments came from an unexpected source. As reported in *The Times*, the Trades Union Congress (TUC) and Labour Party national executive had published a pamphlet setting out their views on NHI. It included things which needed addressing which the IAC itself had no real problem agreeing with, that is, a cap on list sizes, new rules on the use of assistants, and more effective means of securing removal of unsatisfactory doctors.[167] It stated that a Labour Government would be willing to guarantee a capitation fee of 9s 6d for five years on the grounds that 'we have satisfied ourselves that the National Insurance Fund in the aggregate contains sufficient money to meet the costs without lowering or endangering the revision of other benefits'. The pamphlet added that they considered it justifiable to lay claim to some of the societies' 'hidden reserves'. Although Robinson dismissed the document, Joynson-Hicks asked if he should invite to Labour leader Arthur Henderson to see him to ask if his party were supportive of giving more money to the doctors even if trade-union Approved Societies might not agree. In what seems like an overt breach of the civil service code of impartiality, Robinson replied that 'it would be sound tactics to spread confusion in the Labour ranks when the bill was introduced'.[168]

The Minister vented his concern that his policy of playing the doctors off against the Approved Societies might backfire when he said that 'he would not be made a cockshy by both the Approved Societies and the doctors'.[169] He was reported by the press as describing himself as like 'a buffer state' between them.[170] As a last resort, he admitted that he could ask the Commons to pass a suspensory Bill continuing the 9s 6d for two years and set up a Royal Commission to inquire into the operation of the scheme. Robinson still felt that the GPs would accept his offer and encouraged the Minister to call their bluff but that, as a contingency, the Government might consider arbitration 'objectionable as that might be'.[171] The Minister was clearly getting twitchy as reports of meetings of doctors around the country expressing support for the IAC and its call for mass resignations were sympathetically reported in *The Times*.[172] He dismissed talk of the Approved Societies' large surpluses saying that if the case was to go to arbitration, representations must be tripartite. His irritation was clear from his concluding remarks to the IAC that

> I am not enamoured of the panel system and if the doctors would prefer…a full enquiry into the best method of dealing with medical benefit…I am willing to submit a proposal for an early Royal Commission on the whole subject.[173]

To this, Cox responded bullishly, commenting that the profession hated 'this periodic dragging of its affairs before the public' and concluding that 'the profession is prepared for a full inquiry, either departmental committee or Royal Commission, at any point you like, provided it is a full inquiry'.[174]

Not all GPs were convinced, however, that arbitration would bring a satisfactory outcome. A meeting of Yorkshire and Middlesbrough LMPC representatives recorded that 'Some considered that arbitration was in a measure giving the position away'.[175] A final meeting took place shortly after between the Minister, his officials, and the IAC. Joynson-Hicks repeated that the Government actuary had confirmed that they could not afford to pay more than currently offered.[176] Brackenbury repeated that an adequate service could not be provided for that amount and said the fact that practically 95% of resignations had been sent showed how united and determined the profession was. Brackenbury advised the Minister that 'the desire to secure a worthwhile service and…the freedom of the doctors from approved society control' were the real issues on which the bulk of the profession were fighting. He continued that the IAC would welcome a full inquiry but as the process was likely to take some time wanted the existing capitation rate to continue pending its outcome.[177] Joynson-Hicks adjourned the meeting, stating testily that 'they had better send in their resignations because if no settlement could be reached there would be no alternative but to scrap the existing panel system'.[178] At a reconvened meeting on 31 October, the beleaguered Minister offered 8s 6d for five years, plus an additional £250,000 to the rural mileage fund and a Royal Commission to investigate all aspects of the scheme.[179]

The IAC rejected the offer and with 95% of panel doctors expected to resign (the figure was 100% in 59 areas), the Government found itself looking down the barrel of what Eder calls the 'gun with a single bullet' which the profession was now united in wanting to fire.[180] In a last ditch attempt to prevent this happening, the Ministry agreed to supplement the offer with a separate commission of inquiry into GPs' remuneration and guaranteed the rate offered, or a higher rate if recommended by the inquiry, for five years.[181] In light of this, a special LMPCs Conference was called in November 1923 at which Brackenbury declared the IAC finally willing to recommend that resignations be withdrawn.[182] The Conference recognised that the IAC's measured but determined approach had won significant concessions from a seemingly implacable opponent. More importantly, they were confident that the rightness of their cause would be self-evident to the independent inquiry and so, after a modicum of debate, the Conference voted to accept the Minister's offer by 141 votes to 29.[183] The Minister made it clear when setting up the inquiry that it was not to be a prolonged affair and indeed it was not, concluding its business and reporting its recommendations in less than a month. But it was to a different Government that the Court of Inquiry submitted its final report in March 1924 as in January, the Labour Party embraced for the first time the challenge of forming an administration following the inconclusive results of the general election in December 1923.[184]

When the Court of Inquiry met for the first time on 4 January 1924, the IAC put its case for the continuation of 9s 6d in a detailed memorandum supported by comparative data on incomes, expenses, and the cost of living by their retained expert, A.L. Bowley.[185] The Government presented its by now familiar case for 8s 6d and the Approved Societies argued that the doctors remuneration be reduced to the pre-war figure of 7s 3d.[186] On 23 January, the arbitrators announced their 'Solomon-like' decision, awarding the doctors 9s guaranteed until the end of 1927.[187] The IAC had no choice but to accept the result, which was arguably a victory of sorts but, to appease the many GPs who felt less than thrilled at the prospect of the modest reduction in their remuneration which this represented, responded that it was still unshaken in its opinion that 9s per capita per annum 'was not an adequate fee for services under the Act'.[188] The new Labour Government honoured the inquiry's recommendations and in March 1924 introduced a bill to enable it to be paid out of the insurance fund without the necessity to increase either employers' or employees' contributions, relying on 'previously unacknowledged funds from the sale of insurance stamps and interest since 1913'.[189] The Labour Party proved that the statement it had made in its joint leaflet with the TUC was correct and that Robinson and the previous Government actuary had not given an entirely accurate assessment of the situation. This must have dismayed the Approved Societies who saw a large part of their surpluses disappear, while their opponents, the panel doctors, exulted in the (partial) vindication of their claims.

Conclusion

The panel GPs' 'victory' in 1924 may seem a fairly hollow one, since it resulted in a reduction, though only by 6d per patient per annum, in the amount the panel doctors were up until then being paid. If Brackenbury and others were to be believed, moreover, it had left the service still unable to attract or retain the best doctors. But it was a victory nonetheless and represented a high watermark for unified professional action by GPs in support of political objectives. Proving that professional solidarity could be achieved and used effectively in the right circumstances, it set a precedent for future action because, as Eder puts it, 'the government and the approved societies recognised that the threat of a boycott of the panel system was no longer a fantasy'.[190] The reasons for the IAC's success in 1923 were twofold. Firstly, it had succeeded in obtaining the backing of an overwhelming majority of insurance practitioners. The figure of 94.6% of eligible doctors being ready to resign represented a degree of professional unity that was never equalled before or since. This was due at least in part to the fact that the IAC had acted reasonably and honourably in their pursuit of economic reciprocity and service improvements over a considerable time period and called for resignations only as a last resort once other avenues had been exhausted. The profession was thus able to enjoy a good deal of support from the public, if not from all sections of the press, and to take the moral high ground. This was due to its leaders having emphasised continually that the dispute was not purely about money but about the desire to provide a proper and sustainable medical service of which the profession could be proud and with which the public could be satisfied. An example of this can be found in Brackenbury's speech to the LMPCs Conference in 1921 when he said, 'The profession has a right... on public grounds, to say that the government must not go beyond the point at which the profession considered it possible to carry on a service satisfactory to the public'.[191]

The GPs' leaders' confidence was boosted by comments such as those made by *The Times* medical correspondent, McNair Wilson, who observed that the arbitrators' decision 'disposed at once of the idea that...the doctors were exhibiting a greedy spirit'. In an unconscious acknowledgement of the 'professional social ideal', he added, 'On the contrary, they were entering a protest against the scale of payment which rendered efficient service difficult or impossible. *That action was their clear duty to the public as well as themselves*' (added emphasis).[192] The second factor influencing the outcome was the fact that, if the Government had not backed down, the panel doctors were confident that they had a viable alternative. The panel service was still relatively new and underdeveloped and covered only part of the population. GPs provided medical care for dependants of the insured and the middle classes excluded from the scheme through fully private, or alternative insurance or provident-based, schemes which could, with some effort, have been extended to include panel patients if the NHI scheme was wound up. Historians seem to have ignored or underestimated the potential viability of PMS as professionally run alternatives to Approved Societies' schemes in the event that the National Insurance Acts were rescinded. The IAC, at the prompting of Conference, had updated its model PMS scheme and now had, in the LMPCs, democratically enfranchised bodies through which to implement such schemes across the country using the knowledge they had gained from a decade of involvement in the administration of NHI. While it would no doubt have proved difficult, particularly in rural areas, it was nevertheless feasible for LMPCs to set up their own services with financial help from the defence funds, as indeed a number were to do during the 1920s and 1930s. This became necessary, as will be explained in the next chapter, when the Government's continued need for economy ended hopes that NHI could be extended to include the dependants of the insured population, a situation which left the profession agonising once again over the necessity to challenge government authority.

Notes

1 See Kenneth O. Morgan, *Consensus and Disunity: The Lloyd George Coalition Government, 1918–1922* (Oxford, 1979). *passim*; Ross McKibbin, *The Ideologies of Class: Social Relations in Britain, 1880–1950* (Oxford, 1990). pp. 28–30 and 269–299; James E. Cronin, *The Politics of State Expansion: War, State and Society in Twentieth Century Britain* (London, 1991). ch.5–7. Peter Clarke, *Hope and Glory: Britain 1900–2000* (2nd edn, London, 2004). ch. 4–5.
2 *BMJ*, 23 June 1917, Supplement, p. 146.
3 Morgan, *Consensus and Disunity*, p. 81.
4 *BMJ*, 2 November 1918, 'Report of Conference of LMPCs 24 October 1918', Supplement, p. 66.
5 Kenneth O. Morgan and Jane Morgan, *Portrait of a Progressive: The Political Career of Christopher, Viscount Addison* (Oxford, 1980). p. 75.
6 Morgan, *Consensus and Disunity*, pp. 92–94.
7 Frank Honigsbaum, *The Division in British Medicine: A History of the Separation of General Practice from Hospital care 1911–1968* (London, 1979). p. 83 and pp. 86–87.
8 *National Archive/Public Records Office, Kew*, MH 62/117 Memorandum on meeting between Addison, Astor and IAC deputation 15 April 1919.
9 *Ibid.*, p. 3.
10 *Medical World*, 10 October 1919, 'Oestrus' comments on the Consultative Council, p. 351.
11 Peter Bartrip, *Themselves Writ Large: The British Medical Association, 1832–1966* (London, 1996). p. 211.
12 *Medical World*, 10 October 1919, p. 351.
13 Honigsbaum, *The Division in British Medicine*, p. 61.
14 *National Archive*, MH 62/124 Letter from Morant to Astor, 19 June 1919.
15 *Ibid.*, Unsigned undated memorandum, p. 2.
16 *Ibid.*, NHI Commissioners, Memorandum on 'Agreement for medical services under the Insurance Act.' p. 5.
17 *Ibid.*, MH 62/119, Memorandum to Commissioners from R.W. Harris 19 September 1919.

18 *Ibid.,* Undated Memorandum by J.S. Whitaker regarding Treasury response.
19 *Ibid.,* Undated memorandum by Whitaker.
20 *Lancet,* 23 November 1918, p. 712, 7 December 1918, p. 786, and 1 February 1919, p. 90.
21 *Ibid.,* Editorial 'Medicine and the State' p. 185.
22 *Medical World,* 7 February 1919 p. 90.
23 *Ibid.*
24 Honigsbaum, *The Division in British Medicine,* p. 60, note c. See also Roger Cooter 'The Rise and Decline of the Medical Member: Doctors in Parliament in Edwardian and Interwar Britain.' *Bulletin for the Society for the Social History of Medicine,* 78 (1) (2004). pp. 81–82.
25 *Lancet,* 2 August 1919, editorial, p. 207.
26 Joyce Cockram 'The Federation and the BMA.' *Journal of the Medical Women's Federation,* 49 (1967). p. 78.
27 *BMJ,* 22 March 1919, Supplement, 'Why should the medical profession be organised and how should it be done?' pp. 39–40.
28 *Medical World,* 28 March, p. 238.
29 *New Statesman,* 21 April 1917, vol. IX, issue 211, 'Special Supplement on Professional Associations', pp. 9–10.
30 *Wellcome Collection* (BMA Archive), National Insurance Defence Trust File, memorandum dated 20 March 1919.
31 *Medical World,* 27 June 1919, A. Welply, 'The snare of M.21', p. 539.
32 *Ibid.,* 13 June 1919, Letter from J.F. Holloway, p. 502.
33 *Kent LMC Archive,* minutes of Kent County LMPC meetings on 5 June 1919 and 15 July 1919.
34 *Medical World,* 4 July 1919 Report of Conference p. 13. and letter from Richmond and Cowie p. 24.
35 *BMA Archive,* LMC/1/3, minutes of the London Panel Committee meeting on 17 July 1919.
36 *Ibid.,* 23 September 1919.
37 *Cheshire County PRO,* NHL 7135, minutes of LMPC meeting on 17 November 1917, p. 23.
38 *Ibid.,* pp. 24–25, plus addendum enclosing list of 170 resignations set to take effect from 1 January 1918.
39 *BMA Archive,* minutes of LMPC meeting on 20 April 1918, p. 40.
40 *Ibid.,* pp. 40–41.
41 *Ibid.,* minutes of LMPC meeting on 17 March 1920, p. 195.
42 *Ibid.,* p. 193.
43 *BMA Archive,* minutes of Ministry of Health Committee meeting on 11 February 1919, min 34.
44 *Ibid.,* minutes of 'Conference of representatives of various medical bodies' on 6 May 1919.
45 *Ibid.,* minutes of meeting of Committee established by Conference of representatives of various medical bodies on 16 May 1919.
46 *Ibid.,* 16 July 1919.
47 *BMA Archive,* B/203/1/11, minutes of IAC meeting on 4 July 1919, Draft circular to Insurance practitioners and LMPCs.
48 *Ibid.,* point 1.
49 *Ibid.,* point 5.
50 *Ibid.,* point 9.

51 *BMA Archive*, B/203/1/11, minutes of the IAC meeting on 11 September 1919 (Doc IAC 4).

52 *BMJ*, 6 December 1919, 'Report of annual Conference of LMPCs 27 November 1919', Supplement p. 138.

53 *Medical World*, 12 December 1919, p. 604.

54 *National Archive*, MH 78/96, Memorandum from Morant dated 13 December 1919.

55 *BMJ*, 26 July 1919, 'Report of Special Conference of LMPCs on 17/18 July 1919', Supplement p. 29 (Range of Services).

56 Norman R. Eder, *National Health Insurance and the Medical Profession in Britain, 1913–1939* (New York, 1982). pp. 118–119.

57 *BMJ*, 24 January 1920, 'Insurance Remuneration', Supplement, p. 19.

58 *Ibid.*, 13 March 1920, 'Arbitration on rate of medical remuneration', Supplement, p. 74.

59 *Ibid.*, 6 December 1919, 'The Court's Award', p. 206.

60 *Lancet*, 13 March 1920, H.B. Brackenbury, 'Some thoughts on the arbitration', p. 621.

61 *Ibid.*

62 *BMA Archive*, B/203/1/12, minutes of IAC meetings on 22 July 1920 and 27 November 1920.

63 *Medical World*, 26 March 1920, 'Brackenbury's apologia', pp. 257–259.

64 Morgan, *Consensus and Disunity*, p. 81.

65 *BMA Archive*, B/203/1/12, minutes of IAC meeting on 23 September 1920, min. 53.

66 *Ibid.*, minutes of IAC meetings on 18 November 1920, min. 119, and B/203/1/13, minutes of meetings on 15 September 1921, min. 39, and 27 November 1921, min 135.

67 *Ibid.*, B/203/1/13, minutes of the IAC meeting on 11 October 1921, letter dated 27 September 1921.

68 *Ibid.*, letter from Cox dated 29 September 1921.

69 *BMJ*, 15 October 1921, Supplement, pp. 147–150.

70 Cronin, *The Politics of State Expansion*, pp. 89–91. Chris Renwick, *Bread for All: The Origins of the Welfare State* (2nd edn, London, 2018). pp. 146–147.

71 *BMJ*, 29 October 1921, Supplement, pp. 100–167.

72 *Ibid.*, p. 168.

73 *Ibid.*

74 *Ibid.*, p. 170.

75 *Ibid.*, p. 171.

76 *Ibid.*

77 *Ibid.*

78 *National Insurance Gazette*, 28 January 1933, H.A. Parker 'National Health Insurance', p. 46.

79 *Ibid.*, I July 1922, 'Doctors and Approved Societies', p. 307.

80 *BMA archive*, B/203/1/13, minutes of IAC, confidential letter from Cox to IAC members dated 29 March 1922.

81 *Ibid.*

82 *Ibid.*, minutes of IAC meeting on 30 March 1922, Appendix A. The IAC Appendix also includes a testy exchange of letters between Cox and Rockliffe.

83 *Ibid.*

84 *BMJ*, 8 April 1922, Supplement, p. 97.

85 *BMA Archive*, B/203/1/14, minutes of IAC meeting on 12 May 1922. Letter from MPU secretary Alfred Welply dated 13 April 1922.

86 Morgan, *Consensus and Disunity*, p. 295.

87 *Ibid.*, p. 299.

88 *Medical World,* 21 October 1921, p. 1921.
89 See Andrew McDonald 'The Geddes Committee and the Formulation of Public Expenditure Policy, 1921–1922.' *The Historical Journal,* 32 (1989). p. 645.
90 McKibbin, *The Ideologies of Class,* p. 298.
91 On the Union, later the Income Taxpayers Society, see Cronin, *The Politics of State Expansion,* pp. 74 and 79, and McKibbin, *The Ideologies of Class,* p. 299. On the Anti-Waste league see Cronin p. 89, Clarke, *Hope and Glory,* p. 108, and Renwick, *Bread for All,* pp. 144–146.
92 McKibbin, *The Ideologies of Class,* p. 299.
93 *Medical World,* 21 April 1922, (Hereward) 'The Great Betrayal.'
94 A. Fenner Brockway, *Bermondsey Story: The Life of Alfred J. Salter* (London, 1949). p. 149.
95 Kenneth O. Morgan, *Consensus and Disunity: The Lloyd George Coalition Government, 1918–1922* (Oxford, 1979). p. 93.
96 Marc Stears, *Progressives, Pluralists and the Problems of the State: Ideologies of Reform in the United States and Britain, 1909–1926* (Oxford, 2002). pp. 101–106.
97 Ben Jackson, *Equality and the British Left: A Study in Progressive Political Thought, 1900–1964* (Manchester, 2007). pp. 41–43.
98 Steven Thompson, 'A Proletarian Sphere: Working-Class Provision of Medical Services in South Wales, 1900–1948' in Anne Borsay (ed) *Medicine in Wales, 1800–2000: Public Services or Private Commodity* (Cardiff, 2003). p. 95.
99 *Ibid.,* pp. 95–98.
100 *Ibid.,* p. 89.
101 *Ibid.,* pp. 98–100.
102 *Ibid.,* p. 96.
103 *Ibid.,* p. 95.
104 Brockway, *Bermondsey Story,* p. 63.
105 See *Medical World,* 1 October 1926, 'Pharos' 'Improving the Medical Service', p. 37.
106 *BMJ,* 10 February 1923, 'Conference of parties interested in Insurance Act', Supplement, p. 35.
107 See *Medical World,* 30 June 1916, Editorial on 'State Medical Service', p. 825.
108 *BMJ,* 20 January 1917, 'The Future of Medical Service', pp. 86–88.
109 *BMA Archive,* B/203/1/11, minutes of IAC meeting on 4 July 1919, Confidential memorandum by Cox on MPU's response to M25, point 5.
110 *Medical World,* 26 May 1922 'Report of Special Conference of Local Medical and Panel Committees', p. 301.
111 *Ibid.*
112 *BMA Archive,* B/203/1/14, minutes of IAC's General Purposes Subcommittee meeting on 22 June 1922, min. 36.
113 *Ibid.,* Doc 83.
114 *Ibid., Report of Insurance Acts Committee 1921–22 to Annual Conference of Local Medical and Panel Committees,* 20 October 1922, item 23(c).
115 *BMA Archive,* B/203/1/14, minutes of IAC meeting on 6 July 1922, Doc 94, Report of meeting with MPU on 20 June 1922.
116 *Ibid.,* minutes of IAC, 5 October 1922, Memorandum by H.B. Brackenbury, item 7.
117 *Ibid.,* Document M 10 1922/23 circulated in January 1923.
118 *Ibid.,* minutes of IAC meeting on 22 December 1922, p. 387.
119 *Ibid.,* minutes of IAC's Special Subcommittee meeting on 16 November 1922.
120 *Ibid.,* minutes of IAC meeting on 5 October 1922.
121 *Ibid.,* minutes of IAC meeting on 30 November 1922 (Doc M31).
122 *Medical World,* 12 January 1923, pp. 441–442.

123 *Ibid.*, 2 February 1923, p. 47.
124 *Ibid.*, 10 August 1923, p. 595.
125 *Lancet,* 28 October 1922, p. 921.
126 *BMJ,* 10 February 1923, 'Conference of Interested parties on Insurance Medical Service on 30–31 January 1923', Supplement, pp. 31–38.
127 Eder, *National Health Insurance and the Medical Profession,* p. 209.
128 *Ibid.*
129 *BMJ, 16 June 1923,* Supplement, pp. 245–261.
130 *BMA Archive,* B/203/1/15, minutes of IAC meeting on 22 September 1923.
131 *Royal Commission on National Health Insurance,* Cmd. 2596, (1926). p. 188, para 440.
132 *Ibid.*, pp. 286–288.
133 Nikolas Rose, 'Government, Authority and Expertise in Advanced Liberalism.' *Economy and Society,* 22 (3) (1993). p. 285.
134 *BMJ,* 7 April 1923, Supplement, p. 106.
135 *Ibid.,* 28 April 1923, Supplement, p. 161.
136 *Ibid.,* 22 March 1919, Supplement, p. 40.
137 Harry Eckstein, *Pressure Group Politics: The Case of the British Medical Association* (London, 1960). p. 84.
138 *Ibid.,* p. 93 and p. 96.
139 *BMJ,* 10 February 1917, Supplement p. 23; *BMA Archive,* B/203/1/11, minutes of IAC meeting on 21 October 1919, Doc 24; *BMJ* 30 October 1920, Supplement, p. 116.
140 Eckstein, *Pressure Group Politics,* p. 38.
141 Pierre Bourdieu, 'The Social Space and the Genesis of Groups.' *Theory and Society,* 14 (1985). pp. 739–741.
142 *BMA Archive,* B/203/1/ 14, minutes of IAC meeting on 15 March 1923, doc. 64.
143 Honigsbaum, *The Division in British Medicine,* p. 76.
144 *National Archive,* MH 62/128, Memorandum from Robinson to Joynson-Hicks dated 1 August 1923.
145 *Ibid.,* Verbatim report of meeting between Minister of Health and Approved Societies dated 27 September 1923, p. 2.
146 *Ibid.,* p. 3.
147 *Ibid.* (429 Strand was the address of the BMA's Headquarters prior to its relocation to Tavistock Square, Bloomsbury in 1926).
148 *BMA Archive,* B/203/1/15, minutes of IAC meeting on 7 August 1923, Memorandum on Remuneration.
149 *Ibid.,* Bowley's memorandum dated 21 July 1923.
150 *National Archive,* MH 62/128, Undated verbatim report of meeting between Minister of Health and IAC, p. 6.
151 *Ibid.,* pp. 19–20. Brackenbury repeated this point in his speech to Conference reported in *The Times,* 19 October 1923, p. 9.
152 *National Archive,* MH 62/128, Memorandum of meeting on 3 October 1923.
153 *Ibid.,* pp. 1–2.
154 *Ibid.,* pp. 2–3.
155 *Ibid.,* p. 5.
156 *National Archive,* MH 62/128, Letter from Robinson of 3 October 1923, p. 3, item 6 and p. 15, item 9.
157 *Ibid.,* Letter from Cox of 8 October 1923, p. 1, item 1, and p. 7, item 17.
158 *Ibid.,* p. 8, item 18.
159 *Ibid.,* Letter from Robinson 15 October 1923.
160 *National Archive,* MH 62/128, letter dated 8 October 1923.

161 *BMJ*, 27 October 1923 Report of Annual Conference of LMPCs 18 October 1923, Supplement, p. 194.

162 *Kent LMC Archive*, minutes of Special LMPC meeting on 12 October 1923.

163 *BMA Archive*, B/203/1/15, Letter from Cox to LMPCs dated 18 October 1923 (M29) enclosing letter to insurance practitioners (M30) and notice of resignation to Insurance Committees (M 31).

164 *The Star*, 18 October 1923, p. 11.

165 *BMA Archive*, B/203/1/15, minutes of IAC meetings on 26 October 1923 and 7 November 1923.

166 *Ibid.*, Minutes of the London Panel Committee meeting on 23 October 1923, Finance & General Purposes subcommittee, min. 6.

167 *The Times*, 17 October 1923 'Panel Fees-Doctors to Decide Tomorrow-Labour Basis Proposed', p. 14.

168 *National Archive*, MH 62/128, Undated note of meeting between Joynson-Hicks, Robinson, Whitaker, Kinnear, Brock and Leishman, p. 2.

169 *Ibid.*, p. 3.

170 *The Manchester Guardian*, 24 October 1923, 'Minister's position', p. 5.

171 *National Archive, MH* 62/128, Undated note of meeting between Joynson-Hicks, Robinson, Whitaker, Kinnear, Brock and Leishman. p. 4.

172 See *The Times* articles of 13 October 1923, p. 12, and 15 October 1923, p. 12.

173 *National Archive*, MH 62/128, Letter to Cox from Joynson-Hicks dated 26 October 1923.

174 *Ibid.*, Letter from Cox to the Minister dated 27 October 1923.

175 *YORLMC Archive*, minutes of meeting of 'Group C' regional Committee of LMPCs on 10 October 1923.

176 *National Archive*, MH 62/128, Undated note of meeting between Joynson-Hicks, Robinson, Percy, Newman, Smith Whitaker, and IAC deputation, p. 2.

177 *Ibid.*, p. 3.

178 *Ibid.*, p. 4.

179 *Ibid.*, note of meeting between Minister of Health, officials, and IAC deputation, 31 October 1923.

180 Eder, *National Health Insurance and the Medical Profession*, p. 211.

181 *BMJ*, 3 November 1923, Supplement, p. 209.

182 *Ibid.*, 24 November 1923, Report of Special Conference of LMPCs, 14 November 1923, Supplement, pp. 238–239 and 243.

183 *Ibid.*, p. 243.

184 Clarke, *Hope and Glory*, pp. 124–126.

185 *BMJ*, 12 January 1924, 'Report of proceedings of Court of Inquiry and statements of evidence by interested parties', Supplement, pp. 30–53.

186 *Ibid.*

187 *BMJ*, 2 February 1924, Supplement, p. 205.

188 *BMA Archive*, B/203/1/15, minutes of IAC meeting on 20 March 1924, min 264.

189 Eder, *National Health Insurance and the Medical Profession*, p. 231.

190 *Ibid.*, p. 230.

191 *BMJ*, 29 October 1921, Supplement, p. 164.

192 *The Times*, 25 November 1924, 'Panel Doctors' Fees', p. 11.

8 The consolidation of National Health Insurance

Administration, 'red tape', and the economics of contract practice, 1926–1939

In the late 1920s and 1930s, the central role which GPs played in the administration of NHI, through the LMPCs, and the day-to-day interactions between the Insurance Acts Committee (IAC) and their civil service counterparts were severely affected by external factors. Government retrenchment led to increased scrutiny of the key system pressure points of alleged overprescribing and lax certification. This tested the extent to which the profession was prepared, and was enabled, to self-regulate, or acquiesce in the official policing of professional activity. It led inexorably to increased bureaucratisation which GPs of all political persuasions viewed with distaste if not alarm. In the face of continuing challenges for the wider economy, the failure to control the costs of NHI forced governments in the 1930s to take actions which were hugely unpopular with the panel GPs. The Government-imposed cuts in the panel GPs' remuneration in the early 1930s and the expanding remit of the Regional Medical Service convinced the insurance doctors that firstly, the Government could not be relied upon to treat them fairly and accord them a just reward for their labours; and secondly, that the state was impinging on their autonomy by interfering in their professional affairs and suffocating them in 'red tape'.

The effect of both these developments was to encourage many GPs to focus more attention on their private practice, while for the rest, the significant number of panel GPs for whom such opportunities were limited, they resulted in increased dissatisfaction with their professional leaders and a questioning of the benefits of the IAC's negotiating strategy. In his book on National Insurance published in 1946, the civil servant R.W. Harris contended that the share accorded to the medical profession in the administration on NHI was unique in comparison to European counterparts and helped explain why, he asserted, panel GPs in Britain were generally more content with their lot and gave better service.[1] An assessment of his assertion depends on two questions: firstly, whether GPs involved in panel practice experienced an improvement in their financial or social status during this period; and secondly, how much British GPs knew about their European counterparts and the extent to which they considered those counterparts' situation to be less favourable or secure than their own. As

DOI: 10.4324/9781003438274-8

will be shown, neither of these questions affords a completely clear-cut answer. However, it must be said that statements by some historians suggesting that the majority of British GPs were 'comfortably off' in this period are somewhat wide of the mark.

System pressure points: overprescribing and lax certification

According to Norman Eder, 'Overprescribing and lax certification drew more attention than any other issues associated with the National Insurance panel service'.[2] But the IAC were not, it seems, prepared to admit to the existence of these problems until after the report of the Royal Commission in 1926 when they no longer feared the influence of the Approved Societies. It was only then that the GPs' leaders were prepared to address these issues as a matter of self-regulation in the wider interests of the service and the profession's public image. Concerns about 'excessive prescribing' began soon after the panel service began. The GP's capitation fee included a nominal 2s per patient to cover the costs of medicines GPs dispensed themselves as 'stock mixtures'. Of this, 6d per patient was retained in a shared fund by the Insurance Committee to cover any excess in the costs of medicines prescribed by GPs and dispensed by pharmacists above the amount in the Committee's drugs budget. The residue of this 'floating sixpence' could be distributed to local GPs on a per capita basis if there were unspent funds remaining at the financial year end.[3] It thus served as an incentive for GPs to keep prescribing costs under control. However, although LMPCs were assiduous in their efforts to police 'excessive' prescribing, they were unable to prevent increasing overspends.

In 1914, an extensive investigation into the causes of prescribing overspends in London proved inconclusive. It cost £2,400, yet resulted in a net saving for the drugs fund of only £500.[4] The average cost of prescriptions continued to rise during the war, however, as the demand for medical care from women workers and those invalided out of the services increased and GPs were more inclined to prescribe named drugs rather than dole out stock mixtures of questionable efficacy.[5] It was a difficult problem to tackle, recognising that overprescribing was 'less a matter of fact and more one of opinion' about the needs of the individual patient and the doctor's management of them.[6] The difficulty for many GP is summed up in a letter which the County Palatine of Chester LMPC considered in 1915 from one of its constituents, a Dr W. White of Hadfield, Manchester. He opined that it was useless to issue circulars encouraging economy in prescribing without any means of enforcement, stating: 'Only tonight I have been asked for a bottle of formamint tablets, and when I refused them I was told that a competitor of mine prescribed them regularly and that a friend of my patient's had had four or five bottles at different times'. He concluded that to avoid losing patients to competitors, 'One's only defence is to join the lavish prescribers'.[7] The 'floating sixpence' was abolished in 1920, and the amount assimilated into the local drugs fund. A Ministry of Health memorandum noted that one reason for abolishing it was a concern that it afforded 'an inducement to unscrupulous doctors to economise unduly in the ordering of drugs'.[8] However, the same officials subsequently realised that LMPCs now lacked an incentive to properly investigate allegations of excessive prescribing.[9] The Ministry therefore created pricing bureaux to collect comparative data on individual GPs' prescribing habits and asked Regional Medical Officers (RMOs) to target for investigation areas with exceptionally high costs.[10] Insurance Committees likewise appointed drug advisory committees and drew up local formularies to try to iron out variations in prescribing habits.[11] From 1927, chemists were instructed to institute generic substitution of named drugs in accordance with local formularies and from 1929 a national formulary was drawn up in agreement with the IAC.[12]

Rising drug expenditure from the mid-1920s onwards was attributed to a variety of causes. These included patients exceeding the recommended dosage or becoming addicted to medicines, patients demanding that medicines be flavoured to make them palatable and thereby more expensive, and doctors prescribing large quantities of Cod liver oil and other food substitutes to compensate for the effects of malnourishment.[13] Harry Roberts became something of a national celebrity when he and his partners were fined £100 for prescribing 'excessive' quantities of Cod liver oil and malt. The press took up the case with the headline 'Doctors fined for idealism'.[14] Francis Maylett Smith was another GP criticised by his local Panel Committee for overprescribing Cod liver oil.[15] A comparative study of prescribing costs in Leeds and Bradford revealed inexplicable differences and prompted the Ministry to establish a more effective disciplinary process.[16] Individuals whose prescribing costs were abnormally high were visited by an RMO and if no explanation was offered or the explanation was inadequate, the RMO could request a formal hearing of the case by the Panel Committee. The IAC were by this time happy to participate in a propaganda campaign to advise panel GPs to be more careful about prescribing.[17] The number of GPs investigated for this problem rose from 1,369 in 1929 to 1,885 in 1930 but the number subject to a punitive deduction from remuneration, which in 1928 was 45, dropped to only 13 in 1930 and thereafter never exceeded 10 a year.[18] Prescription expenditure remained stable in the early 1930s but rose steadily between 1933 and 1937 when Health Minister Sir Kingsley Wood complained that it was out of all proportion to the increase in the insured population.[19] Critics noted that the cost in England was significantly higher than in Scotland prompting the Minister's Chief Medical Adviser, Sir George Newman, to describe the English as 'a nation of medicine drinkers'.[20] Beleaguered panel doctors often felt unfairly singled out for blame in this regard. The eponymous hero of Frank Layton's novel *The Little Doctor* sums up their feelings when complaining: 'So much unnecessary fuss, he knew, was made over the cost of prescriptions dealt out by him and his fellows. None at all was made concerning the silly unthinking habits of the Panel patients themselves'.[21]

Allegations of lax certification meanwhile lay at the centre of the political antagonism between the Approved Societies and the medical profession. In 1913,
the London Insurance Committee appointed six medical referees to investigate
the problem and of 471 cases of alleged malingering, 208 were declared capable
of work.[22] The referees' report did not, however, support the Approved Societies'
view that doctors were complicit. The problem was felt to be one of definition.
Often, the patient was not fit to return to their usual work but not incapable of
any work and attempts by Ministry officials to clarify this matter only served
to confuse the panel GPs further.[23] The government actuary, Sir Alfred Watson,
reported that sickness claims by males rose by 51% between 1921 and 1927 and
disablement claims by 85%. For unmarried women, the figure was 60% and 98%
and for married women 106% and 159%, respectively.[24] Jacqueline Jenkinson
notes that the Scottish Health Board generally regarded women's claims as more
suspicious than men's.[25] When the Ministry gave its RMOs the primary responsibility to investigate malingering and lax certification in 1920, the profession
accepted this as preferable to Approved Society involvement.[26] RMOs were
eventually swamped with referrals, however, the number rising from 69,544 in
1921 to 372,324 in 1928.[27] The *National Insurance Gazette* complained in 1928
that 'False certificates given by doctors to persons who are not ill are in fact robbing persons who are ill of services they need'.[28] The IAC strenuously denied that
GPs knowingly issued certificates to those who were not ill but acknowledged
their reluctance to police the benefits system, as was made clear by the chairman
of York LMPC, Dr J.C. Lyth, who said in 1928 that 'Medical practitioners as a
profession are not trained to regard the issuing of medical certificates as the main
object of life, nor even an important part of it'.[29] As the economic situation wors-
ened, the Treasury became increasingly suspicious that the sickness benefit fund
was being denuded by kind-hearted doctors certifying the unemployed as ill or
disabled. Levels of sick certification certainly rose significantly during strikes,
especially in coal mining areas.[30] The Scottish Board of Health were certainly
convinced that panel GPs were happily certifying the unemployed and strikers
as sick.[31] It is worth observing, however, that when workers were laid off, they
had time to go to see their GP about medical conditions that had often been unat-
tended to and which may have warranted treatment and certification.

The Approved Societies continued to regard malingering as a national scandal, viewing GPs as the primary contributors and were supported by their allies
in parliament and the press.[32] The complaints of some MPs, such as Sir Henry
Cautley, were criticised as being based on hearsay, ignorance, or out-of-date
information.[33] The Ministry therefore confined its efforts during the mid-1920s
to issuing advice rather than taking punitive action. What has been described
as 'bureaucratic pressure' was thus said to be the 'preferred official strategy
for reducing lax gatekeeping' and consequently only a small number of aber-
rant GPs were 'singled out for deterrent financial penalties'.[34] The majority of
referrals to RMOs resulted in the suspension of benefit but there were often

legitimate excuses. Many patients had either already returned to work or were waiting for the certificate to run out.[35] Or, as the anonymous author of *On the Panel: General Practice as a Career* stated, they were too intimidated to turn up for the RMO's examination.[36] GPs were also severely criticised for issuing sick certificates to pregnant women. By 1930, women made up a third of NHI contributors, half of claimants and two-thirds of cases referred to RMOs. Claims reflected an inability to claim extended unemployment benefits or for 'illness directly attributable to pregnancy'.[37] While it was accepted that pregnancy was not an illness, medical problems associated with pregnancy made it difficult for GPs to determine what was the exact cause of patients being unable to work in the later stages of pregnancy and this undoubtedly added to the number of supposedly questionable sick certificates.[38] However in 1927, one GP reported that a large manufacturing firm was actively advising its pregnant employees 'to go on the funds'.[39] Another GP, the anonymous author of *This Panel Business*, writing in 1933, declared, 'The pregnant woman is a great nuisance in pestering for certificates. She is always able to give examples of other pregnant women who had nothing wrong with them and who drew benefit throughout their period of pregnancy'.[40] But to counter the arguments of critics who alleged that GPs issued certificates to patients whom they feared would otherwise seek to change doctor, the IAC persuaded the LMPCs Conference in 1927 to agree to a change in the regulations introducing a time delay in registration.[41] A further change was made in March 1931 whereby patients could change doctor only once during each quarter after a month's notice was given.[42] There were clearly some GPs who issued certificates more freely and with less discrimination than others. The GP novelist Frank Layton was unrestrained in his condemnation of such individuals whom he characterises as 'easy-going men who'll give their patients…exactly what they want', concluding that, 'They are very expensive for the country'.[43]

In 1928, the IAC began a series of regular conferences with the Ministry regarding the causes of the rising sickness benefit rate.[44] The IAC representatives offered a series of reasons as to why the cost of benefits had increased. In addition to the increasing number of elderly insured and the increasing tendency of women to seek sick benefits before and after pregnancy, they suggested that it was due to:

- 'the undermining of individual self-reliance, i.e., an awakening by the public to their sense of their rights and a grasping of such rights';
- 'the inclusion of additional NHI benefits which encouraged an increase in claims because 'the more there was to get, the greater the desire to get it';
- 'the success of the profession's health propaganda which meant that patients were no longer ignoring trivial matters which would get worse and were seeking preventative treatment' (which the IAC acknowledged 'was possibly bad for the insurance funds').[45]

For the acerbic author of *This Panel Business*, the rising costs of drugs and benefits and patients' determination to get their maximum entitlement to both were a proof that NHI 'was a failure' and had led to a 'lowered morale', by which he meant a lack of scruples, among both patients and doctors.[46] In Scotland, the Health Board felt that the problem of lax certification warranted special measures. In 1929, they initiated a campaign of closer monitoring of data and follow-up inspections by RMOs, and in 1930 sponsored a pilot scheme in Dundee involving full-time sickness visitors employed by Approved Societies which they were subsequently keen to extend to other areas. This brought the Board into conflict with the Ministry of Health.[47] In 1928, the IAC had conceded changes to the disciplinary procedures governing certification, and in 1930, while never accepting that GPs were at fault, agreed a change to the Medical Benefit Regulations requiring LMPCs to investigate cases where there was 'a prima facie case for considering that the doctor had failed to exercise reasonable care in the issue of certificates'.[48] The IAC insisted that under no circumstances were the Approved Societies to be involved in any investigation, and therefore accepted that disciplinary action under the new procedure, usually involving a withholding from remuneration, was reserved to the Ministry itself.[49] The Scottish Health Department disagreed, preferring their own system which, since changes instituted in 1928 and agreed with Scottish BMA representatives, was overseen by the Insurance Committees. While anxious not to antagonise the IAC and to maintain the integrity of a nationally uniform system, the Ministry was forced to concede that different procedures would pertain in Scotland.[50] In 1931, the Ministry and the IAC agreed that Panel Committees be grouped together into larger districts for the purposes of enquiring into lax certification so as to remove the embarrassment of their members having to investigate close colleagues.[51] Despite all these efforts to address the problem, however, by August 1932, the Ministry was forced to acknowledge, in Eder's words, that 'all attempts at defining and reducing lax certification had proved to be cosmetic at best' and it continued to be a problem for all concerned.[52] It was to re-emerge in the 1940s in professional debates about GPs being forced to become salaried employees, something which Ministry officials like Sir John Maude, in company with Sir William Beveridge, privately advocated as a means of bringing the rampant costs of social insurance benefits under control.[53]

Norman Eder says that the joint efforts by the Ministry and the IAC to address the problems of overprescribing and lax certification in the interwar period strengthened their relationship to the point that 'the IAC became almost an arm of the Ministry of Health'. He says that, 'The doctors, observing the close working relationship between their leaders and the Ministry could feel fairly certain that profession's views were receiving a fair and usually friendly hearing'.[54] However, this conclusion has to be challenged on two fronts. Firstly, the IAC's efforts to work constructively with the Ministry were, as will be shown, dealt a severe blow when the panel GPs' pay was unilaterally cut in 1931 and the Ministry declined repeated requests to restore the shortfall until four years later. This created tension between the IAC and the Ministry and made it hard for many GPs to accept that the Government was sympathetically disposed towards them. Secondly, the increasing number and complexity of new regulations and the zeal with which some RMOs exercised their inquisitorial functions on behalf of the Ministry convinced many ordinary GPs that the state was increasingly intruding into areas touching their judgement and responsibility, thereby diminishing what many doctors held most dear, that is their professional autonomy.

The 'national emergency' and the widening remit of the Regional Medical Service

Remuneration became once again the principal point of contention between panel GPs and the Government in 1931 when the Economy Committee chaired by Sir George May recommended total cuts in public spending of £96 million. These were to be met in part by cuts in benefits and a significant reduction in the remuneration of public servants, including the panel GPs.[55] In September 1931, the Ministry informed the IAC that as part of their contribution to national recovery, panel GPs would be expected to face a cut of 1s in the annual capitation fee (almost 11%).[56] Compared with the 15–20% cuts which teachers, the police, and members of the armed forces were expected to suffer, the doctors felt that they had come off lightly and a motion that panel GPs accept 'the decision of HM government', as their share of the burden falling on the community was carried by the IAC with only one dissentient.[57] Sir Arthur Robinson responded, expressing warm appreciation of the IAC's decision by the Minister, Neville Chamberlain.[58] Their mutual respect quickly dissipated, however, when, in the aftermath of the Inver Gordon mutiny and a well-publicised campaign of opposition by the teaching profession, the Cabinet revised its proposals for variable cuts to public sector salaries and opted instead for a 10% cut across the board.[59] Dain, the IAC chairman, claimed that this was unfair and seriously compromised the IAC's position as negotiators.[60] His reasoning seems at first glance a little obtuse as the cut was slightly smaller than that previously proposed. However, the fact that the cut was from the gross remuneration of the panel doctors, whereas for public sector employees it was their net remuneration, meant that GPs were hit harder than other public servants because of the effect of practice expenses equating to between 25% and 35% of their income.[61] The MPU estimated the cut to be the equivalent of 16% and Dain, the IAC chairman admitted that it was around 15% rather than, as some were alleging, 20%.[62] The MPU was indignant that GPs were once again being called on to make sacrifices in the national interest. They objected that those criticising the IAC's 'ill-advised actions' were called 'carping and unpatriotic', and questioned why panel doctors had to 'help the bogged nation out of the morass', asking, 'Has not the profession done its bit already?'[63] *Medical World* printed letters from angry GPs, including one who advocated 'passive resistance' by refusing to complete certificates and forms and one from a GPs' wife showing, by means of a detailed breakdown of practice costs, how close to penury the cut would bring them.[64] The author of *This Panel Business* stated: 'Many medical men whose sole earnings are from an average-sized panel are just about managing to keep themselves from starvation'.[65]

Given the parlous state of the national economy, the IAC felt helpless to resist the Government's entreaty and were supported by the LMPCs Conference. An amendment by London to a motion supporting the IAC's actions protested 'against the inequality of the sacrifice as compared with other sections of the community' but was overwhelmingly lost.[66] The IAC decided to set up a remuneration subcommittee, once again drafting in the statistician A.L. Bowley, to help prepare the case for increased remuneration when circumstances were propitious.[67] The MPU, however, expressed a view felt by many GPs that the inquiry process seemed rigged in favour of the government and that the IAC negotiators were no match for wily government officials. They condemned the IAC's failure to challenge the May Committee's contention that the panel GP's fee was too high or to secure a definite date for the cut to be reviewed and for not calling a special LMPCs Conference before agreeing to it.[68] The following year, Dr Manson of Warrington expressed his LMPC's fears that the cut might be permanent and that civil servants could not be trusted when stating, 'Many practitioners had a lurking fear lest the clever officers of the Ministry, by their powers of persuasion, should prevail over the Insurance Acts Committee'.[69]

In 1933, the IAC's subcommittee listed a number of factors in support of their claim. These included an increase in the time and cost of medical education, and increases in the number of items rendered to, and in the average amount of time spent with, panel patients. They were forced to accept that the cost of living had decreased but were able to demonstrate an increase in practice expenses.[70] Being a veteran of previous battles with the Ministry, Brackenbury counselled the IAC against reliance on the increased number of attendances which he knew the Ministry would attempt to explain away. He advocated instead a greater reliance on the increased responsibilities of panel GPs following recent regulatory amendments. These included the keeping of statistics and compiling of many more medical reports for official purposes.[71] Fortunately for the country, the departure from the gold standard in September 1931 led to a gradual improvement in the economic situation over the next few years such that the Annual Conference of LMPCs resolved in November 1933 that 'the time has arrived when the 10% reduction…voluntarily accepted in the national emergency of 1931 is not now justified and should cease'.[72] The author of *This Panel Business* stated bluntly, 'There seems no doubt that panel practitioners as a body have had to pay more than their fair share of the national burden'.[73] Initially, their remonstrations fell on deaf ears but in July 1934, the government agreed to restore half of the reduction, still leaving the panel GPs 5% short of what they had earned in 1930 and the fee was not restored to its full amount until July 1935, some time after other public sector workers' pay cuts had been restored.[74]

After further pressure from the BMA and its allies in parliament, the Ministry eventually conceded another Court of Inquiry into panel GPs' remuneration. The Court, chaired by Lord Amulree, met in 1937 but the IAC were dismayed when, in its submission to the court, the Ministry sought to undermine the profession's case by attacking the general quality of the panel service.[75] The GPs were particularly incensed by the evidence of two 'junior' RMOs who opined that the majority of panel GPs' work was concerned with the alleviation of catarrhal or rheumatic conditions and that they referred anything more complicated to the hospitals. The IAC angrily described this as 'as astonishing as it was grotesque'.[76] For once the Approved Societies' representatives were less critical of the panel GPs, their representative, Mr Stanley Duff, stating that there was 'no general dissatisfaction with the service' on their part and that 'the service deserved more commendation than was occasionally awarded to it in ill-informed quarters'.[77] It is possible that the experience of the two RMOs whose evidence the IAC so decried was confined to investigations into GPs in conurbations where large teaching hospitals were contiguous, whereas panel GPs outside these areas undertook most investigations and treatment themselves. This is attested by the comments of the Cheshire GP Sir William Hodgson, who informed his LMPC colleagues in 1923, 'These men in London have nothing like the throb of professional work that the provinces have. If they have a whitlow to deal with, they send it to a large general hospital'.[78]

Refuting with detailed economic arguments the IAC's claim for a capitation fee of 12s 6d, the Ministry argued that only 8s would be appropriate. The IAC put forward what they felt was a strong case but once again their evidence failed to impress, largely because of faults in its methodology such as the obvious fact that its sample practices were self-selected. The Court consequently awarded them 9s per patient.[79] Predictably, the profession's initial response was one of anger and disappointment but there was this time also a sense of resignation and a greater determination to ensure that the evidence presented in future was truly incontrovertible. The IAC negotiators noted that the Court had cited the statistician Bradford Hill when impugning the validity of their evidence. The IAC therefore enlisted Hill's assistance in improving the quality of their data.[80] This resulted in the institution of an entirely new and more robust form of evidence-gathering and in 1938 the IAC was pleased to report that the data collected using these now impeccable methods, from 500 randomly selected practices, 'had placed beyond doubt the fact that the figures placed before the Court…were substantially accurate'.[81] Hill was subsequently to revise upwards his assessment of the average value of GPs' expenses at this time, concluding that the figure of 33% with which the IAC countered the Ministry's estimate of 25% was itself an underestimate. In 1945, he estimated the true figure to be between 35.5% and

43%.[82] The IAC was insistent that their case be reconsidered, but the outbreak of war in 1939 brought a temporary halt to such considerations and it was not until 1946 that the Spens Report offered some vindication of their claims.[83]

The panel GPs' relationship with the state was further complicated by the growth in power and responsibility of the Regional Medical Service. Initially, the panel GPs welcomed the establishment of a medical referee service to offer advice and second opinions on disputed certification cases and to work with panel committees in the problematic area of overprescribing. The GPs did not initially object when RMOs, who until 1929 were known in Scotland as District Medical Officers, were also given powers to inspect medical records, but opinions changed when the limitations of these records, and the GPs' lukewarm commitment to record-keeping in general which these investigations exposed, led to punitive withholdings. Geoffrey Barber describes the rather cavalier approach which his predecessor took when it came to the annual RMO inspection of his records, which were kept in a cardboard box under a sofa in the dining room! When given notice of the inspector's annual visit, these would be pulled out and Dr Tench would go through all 600 of them and dictate from memory, for his wife to write down in them in each case, the details of certification, treatment, 'and a brief diagnosis in the notes section'. This was evidently sufficient for the RMO who, Dr Tench informed his young protégé, usually complimented him for keeping any records at all![84] When GPs began to be fined also for overprescribing and lax certification, RMO inspection visits came to be resented and eventually feared, such that GPs asked for and were granted the right to have a panel committee representative present during such visits.[85] From working constructively with RMOs, many panel committees were now jealous and resentful of the latter's widening remit, especially when it was made clear that the RMOs would not be accountable to Insurance Committees but directly to Ministry officials. A letter to the *BMJ* in 1923 attacked these 'government limpets' decrying the 'needless bureaucracy' that 'keeps him in power with his salary'.[86] An editorial in *Medical World* in 1926 complained that RMOs were 'almost a service per se, a department within a department, an *imperium in imperio*'.[87] This was in keeping with public fears voiced by the Anti-Waste League and others about the growth of government bureaucracy, which they condemned as one of 'the most pernicious evils of the modern world'.[88] Many GPs objected to what they saw as arbitrary judgements based on putative norms. Dr G. Rome-Hall, writing in *Medical World* in 1926, complained that, 'The exigencies of medical practice and the daily life of the industrial nation are of necessity unknown to the civil servant who sits in an office and studies disease by returns, forms and written evidence'.[89] In the Walsall GP Frank Layton's novel, *The Little Doctor*, his hero Steel says, 'The panel doctor is in danger of being tripped up at any moment. If he gives too much Cod liver oil he's fined for extravagance; if he gives too little he's fined for neglect'.[90] Steele vents his anger at RMOs whom he disparages as 'ex GPs who have got sick of practice and hanker after a pension' and who 'have the nerve to pose as superior to us who have stuck to the firing line'.[91] This view was based on Layton's personal experience. In a letter to the *BMJ* in 1933, he described how his opinion in one case was overruled by an RMO who admitted that he had been out of practice since 1914![92] Francis Maylett Smith gives a detailed account of an RMO's visit in 1928 which led to him being fined for overprescribing Cod liver oil and malt. He was principally unhappy about having to explain himself to the Panel Committee which nevertheless did its best to reduce the amount suggested. He subsequently earned some notoriety for writing to the *BMJ* about 'bureaucratic lunacy' after the Minister of Health failed to respond to his enquiry as to exactly when he *was* permitted to prescribe food supplements to his patients.[93]

The columnists of *Medical World* frequently decried 'a tendency to subordinate professional opinion to the views of officials'.[94] They also railed against and the stereotypical 'regulation-monger of officialdom' whose actions threatened to 'ruin' NHI.[95] This view is echoed by, Dennison, another of Layton's characters, who complains that NHI 'has been ruined since the Ministry was established. When once a Ministry is given power to issue what it calls Regulations it becomes capable of spoiling anything and sometimes does'.[96] The MPU were keen to support individual panel GPs willing to offer themselves as a means of challenging the legality of the procedures they felt were being applied unfairly or inappropriately against them. One would-be martyr was a Cheshire GP, Dr Fox, who was found guilty of irregular certification in 1915 after a complaint from an Approved Society that he had issued a repeat certificate without re-examining the patient.[97] Outraged at being fined £15 and 'advised of the necessity of his more strictly adhering to the medical certification rules', Fox enlisted the support of the MPU. On their advice, he challenged the decision of the Insurance Committee on the basis that his agreement with the committee was not a contract.[98] The LMPC subsequently debated the counsel's opinion obtained by the Insurance Committee refuting Fox's contention, together with an opinion from the IAC's solicitor, W.E. Hempson, who concurred with that opinion.[99] Fox continued to be a thorn in the side of the Insurance Committee, however, informing them in 1917 of his refusal to accept invalided soldiers and sailors onto his list.[100] It is not clear how that dispute played out, but it seems that Fox may have overplayed his hand as he wrote to the LMPC in 1920 expressing indignation that GPs were denied the opportunity of challenging removal from the panel in the high court. He informed them that his MP was to raise the matter in parliament.[101]

However, the Ministry's efforts to enforce regulations were not always successful.[102] In a number of cases in which they sought to make an example of GPs alleged to be 'in breach' of their contractual obligations, the profession quickly closed ranks, objecting that the Ministry's actions impinged upon the principle of professional autonomy. A notable example included a homeopathic GP, Dr Harvey, who in 1925 was accused of negligence after the death of a patient and was successfully defended by the MPU.[103] In another case, a Welsh

GP, Dr McQuillian, fined for lax certification in 1934, was absolved of blame after independent investigation.[104] Bureaucracy was something to which most GPs at this time professed an aversion but according to Alfred Salter, the public too were 'thoroughly fed up with civil service red tape'.[105] *Medical World* complained that it greatly added to GPs' workload. An editorial in 1933 complained of 'the numerous reports called for by Regional M.O.s at short notice, entailing special consultations or visits' which 'demand further time and labour'.[106] However, the IAC saw regulations as a necessary trade-off for the preservation of professional freedom, as the chairman of the IAC, Guy Dain, explained in the Foreword to the 1929 edition of the panel doctors' handbook, *Insurance Medical Practice*. The need for such a 'complex mass of regulations' was needed, he said, when the service rendered by the doctor to the patient was paid for by a third party and in light of 'the insistence of the medical profession on the right of every registered medical practitioner to go on to the panel if he wish, and on the right to free choice of doctor by both doctor and patient.'[107] While Dain characterised the constraints of regulations as a justified quid pro quo for professional freedom, an increasing number of GPs were less accepting, and deemed the rewards of panel practice insufficient to compensate them for such annoyances.

GPs' economic and social status and the quality of panel practice

Reflecting on GPs' economic and social situation in the 1930s, Rosemary Stevens states that while most GPs were not 'well to do', they were 'comfortably situated' with an average net income in 1936–1938 of about £1,000 a year.[108] Supporting Stevens' view, Anne Digby and Nick Bosanquet maintain that during the interwar period, the medical profession enjoyed a substantial improvement in both absolute and relative incomes.[109] The report by Political and Economic Planning (PEP) in 1937 noted that British doctors were comparatively well-paid compared with doctors in other countries.[110] But this included Consultants who on average earned double what GPs earned.[111] The perception of improved financial status led, according to Digby and Bosanquet, to an increase in public esteem. Thus, it was stated in the *BMJ* in 1937 that 'Medicine gives to those who follow it an honourable position…the well-educated doctor stands high among his neighbours'.[112] Noel and Jose Parry assumed that it was the greater security and improved incomes from NHI that led to a contemporary feeling that 'a better class of men was attracted to general practice'.[113] Some medical Deans were apparently concerned that many new entrants were motivated by the prospect of an assured income rather than a 'call' to become a doctor.[114] These new entrants were said to be 'staunchly middle class' with 70% in 1938–1939 being self-financing.[115] However as early as 1914, Alfred Salter complained that the profession 'had been recruited almost entirely from the upper middle classes' which he attributed to the cost of medical education.[116]

All of this might suggest that by the late 1930s, popular acceptance of the profession's demands for adequate reward had at last been achieved. But such views should be treated with caution. Charles Webster says, 'the burgeoning of medical incomes should not be exaggerated', pointing out that 42% of net incomes were below £1,000 p.a. which in itself represented, in the words of Ross McKibbin, 'a good but not outstanding professional income' and among urban GPs, 55% earned below that limit.[117] The relative lack of prosperity experienced by a significant proportion of GPs helps explain the remarks of the BMA president Colin Lindsay who said in 1938, 'There is a tendency for this branch of the profession to sink lower and lower in the estimation of the public and of the student body from which the profession itself is recruited'.[118] While Digby and Bosanquet maintain that GPs in the 1930s enjoyed 'a handsome income' and an ample measure of respectability, the GPs' leaders continued to argue that the panel GPs' financial rewards and public respect were insufficient. How can these viewpoints be reconciled? As proof that GPs incomes had improved, Digby and Bosanquet cite the shortage of applicants for public health posts where salaries rarely exceeded £600 a year, an argument used by the Court of Inquiry into panel GPs' remuneration in 1937.[119] But these salaries were clearly below what the profession estimated them to be worth judging by the fact that the Society of Medical Officers of Health joined with the BMA in urging that no doctor applying for such posts, other than in training, should accept a salary below this amount.[120] It is also useful in this context to look at Guy Routh's analysis of how GPs' income compared with those with whom doctors most readily, and reasonably, compared themselves with, that is, the legal profession. In general, GPs earned less than members of the legal profession throughout the interwar period, though the differential narrowed somewhat in 1935–1937 when GPs' average professional earnings per annum (£1,094) momentarily exceeded those of barristers (£1,090) but were still much less than solicitors (£1,238).[121] The number of panel patients rose from 13.7 million in 1913 to 19.2 million in 1936. However, the number of panel GPs also rose, from 13,700 in 1920 to 19,060 in 1938.[122] This was not surprising as during this period, in the words of one contemporary, 'the Medical Schools were pouring out young doctors far in excess of available jobs'.[123] The vast majority of GPs were involved in panel practice at this time. Stevens claims that it was around 90%.[124] However, Bernard Harris offers a much more cautious estimate of between 66% and 75% of registered GPs.[125] The PEP report on the British Health Services (1937) noted 19,000 panel GPs out of total workforce of 29,000 registered doctors. Allowing for at least 5,000 non-GPs, this suggests that more than 75% were 'on the panel'. This explains why the average panel list fell from 1,000 in 1920 to 930 in 1930.[126] The percentage of GPs' total income from panel practice consequently declined, from 60% in 1913 to 50% in 1922 and to as little as 33% in 1936–1938.[127]

There seems little doubt that any increase in their average earnings was, therefore, as Digby and Bosanquet maintain, entirely due to their earnings from private practice. This conclusion is supported by a contemporary observer. In answer to the question, 'How can one account for the large numbers of apparently prosperous panel doctors?' 'AGP' replies, 'The solution lies in private practice'.[128] In the interwar period, GPs' total average net earnings increased by about a third, boosted by a 79% increase in earnings from private practice.[129] However, the GPs' situation is not as clear-cut as these figures or analyses suggest and disguise a significant disparity between the net incomes of the average and lowest-earning panel doctors. Digby and Bosanquet state that there were substantially two groups of 'losers': rural GPs, and those practising in industrial and mining districts which were worst hit by the depression.[130] Some 40% of GPs were rural and their expenses, largely due to travelling costs, were higher than for other doctors. In an article in the *BMJ* in 1923, Dr J.P. Williams-Freeman, Chairman of Hampshire LMPC, offered a detailed explanation of the increased costs of rural compared with urban panel practice.[131] This helps explain the strenuous efforts LMPCs like his went to when lobbying for increases in rural mileage allowances and dispensing fees. In answer to queries put by the board of arbitration in 1925, he admitted that rural GPs were also facing fierce competition for patients from GPs in neighbouring towns due to their increased use of motor cars.[132] Urban doctors, however, suffered higher levels of bad debts owed by poor families for treatment outside NHI, which could be as high as 20% compared with the professional average of 5%.[133]

But the real 'losers', overlooked in Digby and Bosanquet's analysis, were the GPs' salaried assistants, very few of whom, even when whole time, earned more than £500 per year. It is unclear exactly how many practices during this period employed salaried assistants which was a means by which GP principals were allowed to increase list sizes from 2,500 to 4,000 patients.[134] In Bradford Hill's sample, the figure was 18% of those studied though the PEP report noted that the figure in London was just over 7%.[135] The BMA acknowledged the fact that a number of GP principals exploited or 'sweated' their assistants. In 1924, the IAC's propaganda subcommittee under the heading 'Question of giving more help to assistants' noted a stinging rebuke from an exploited assistant who had resigned from the BMA stating, 'The Association spends all its energies on those medical men who have passed the troublesome stage of getting a practice...As regards an assistant who in perhaps 50% of cases does as much work if not more than the principal, very little is done'.[136] In 1925, the BMA's representative meeting passed a resolution supporting actions recommended by the Medico Political Committee aimed at preventing exploitation of assistants by specifying minimum salaries. These ranged from as little as £120–£400 a year. The resolution was prefaced, however, by the substantial caveat that this 'opinion' was issued as 'advice' only and could not be enforced as policy.[137] Attempts to discourage the *BMJ* from advertising assistantships offering less than the recommended salary levels therefore quickly foundered.[138] The Medico Political Committee also found it impossible to prevent women doctors who worked as assistants or locums being paid at lower rates than their male counterparts. Even though the BMA had adopted a policy of equal pay as early as 1907, letters to the *BMJ* in 1924 suggested that female doctors received only ¼ of the BMA's recommended rates.[139] The Medico Political Committee undertook an investigation into locum emoluments in June 1934 at the prompting of the Medical Women's Federation. Correspondence with the principal locum bureaux established that in only 19% of cases did women doctors earn close to the average rates paid to men (about £8, 8s a week).[140] The Spens Report in 1946 found that all but a very small percentage of women GPs earned well below the putative average of £1,000 per annum gross.[141] The position of salaried assistants did, however, improve as a result of medical workforce shortages during the Second World War. In 1945, the BMA's joint committee on remuneration reported finding that the range of 'salaries of assistants (indoor)' (sic) had increased from a pre-war average of £300–£450 to between £600 and £750.[142]

An altogether more important factor not taken account of by Digby and Bosanquet is the high level of debt which many GPs found themselves in. The returns mentioned earlier show income net of allowable expenses but, as the Joint Committee on GPs' remuneration noted in 1945, these did not necessarily include repayments of loans used to pay for education (amounting to £1,500 on average according to PEP) or the cost of buying a practice (which was equivalent to 1½–2 years income, that is £2,500–£3,000).[143] When offered a partnership at a practice in Somerset in 1929, Kenneth Lane was already having to pay off a loan from the Kent County Council's education committee for his medical education. He despaired of finding any way of providing the requisite capital with which to 'buy in' to the practice partnership until he learned that the Medical Sickness Society had started to offer loans for the purpose. The Society were very discriminating, however, and had to be satisfied both that the practice was a going concern and that it was underpinned by a watertight partnership agreement. Lane's partners agreed to commission a new agreement but insisted he paid for it! Three years into the partnership, Lane still owed the partners £150 and was overdrawn at the bank. Due to their appreciation of his work, Lane's partners took pity on him and waived his debt to the practice, but he was still saddled with loan repayments for many years to come.[144] Many young singlehanded GPs at this time were even less fortunate as they were effectively sharing their practice income with third parties. These were either retired GPs from whom they were in the process of purchasing the practice in instalments, or others who had seen an opportunity to make a financial killing by buying a practice and employing an impecunious GP to work it for them on the promise of a later opportunity to purchase it outright. There is conflicting evidence about the extent of this problem. Honigsbaum seems in no doubt that it was widespread, stating that in the 1930s around a third of panel practices were in the hands of 'insurance companies or moneylenders'.[145] This is consistent with evidence from Lancashire. In November 1934, IAC member S.A. Winstanley, chairman of the Lancashire LMPC, submitted a memorandum to the IAC regarding the mortgaging of practices, stating that there were 102 cases in Lancashire in which the panel fees had been assigned to a third party.[146] One practice he knew of had changed hands four times in seven years, the fees being assigned to the same third party on each occasion. Doctors who were heavily mortgaged and in financial distress were, however, often reticent or too embarrassed to disclose details, but the Lancashire Insurance Committee was sufficiently concerned to wonder if a change should be made in the regulations to prevent this happening.[147] Initially, the IAC contended that a change in regulations was not called for 'in as much as the abuse complained of arises upon very rare occasions'.[148] However, the Annual Conference of LMPCs in 1935 disagreed, stating that the Conference 'viewed with alarm the rapid increase…in the traffic of insurance practices by bodies of lay persons'.[149]

In his report of a debate on this subject at the previous year's Conference, a Cheshire LMPC representative noted that as a condition of the loan, the unfortunate doctor 'signed an undated resignation from the panel and placed it in the moneylender's hands, as well as assigning his panel pay to that individual (who presumably allowed him a pittance till repayment was complete)'.[150] The IAC's chairman, Guy Dain, certainly recognised the problem, stating, when interviewed by American observers, that speculative buying and selling of practices had resulted in young doctors being exploited by 'commercially minded men', and resulted in what he described as 'share cropping'.[151] Others referred to it as 'farming out'.[152] *Medical World* believed that GPs were being exploited more by financial institutions and moneylenders than fellow GPs. This is consistent with Digby's contention that entrepreneurialism was not widespread among GPs and that the disorganised approach taken by most GPs towards the running of their practice businesses meant that 'GPs continued to operate in a cottage industry environment'.[153] There were certainly a small number of GPs, however, who knew how to make the most of an opportunity to turn a profit. Kenneth Lane knew of one GP in the west country, for instance, 'who spent his time buying run down practices, building them up and selling them again making a useful capital gain each time'.[154] The author of *This Panel Business* was certainly familiar with this practice but opines that 'even the few doctors who are managing to run several practices are not as well off as they are made out to be'.[155] The LMPCs Conference was sufficiently concerned that it instructed the IAC to devise a scheme by which practitioners 'with limited means' could obtain loans with which to acquire practices 'on reasonable terms'.[156] The result was the British Medical Finance Company Ltd. established in 1936. Together with the Medical Insurance Agency, it made obtaining loans an easier and less punitive process for practitioners from then onwards, charging reasonable rates of interest.[157]

Another factor which is often overlooked when looking at the comparative affluence of certain GPs in the 1930s is the maldistribution of panel practitioners which, as Martin Powell demonstrates, was often a reflection of local levels of general prosperity.[158] There were generally fewer panel doctors serving the impoverished areas of London and other major cities than in wealthier suburbs and there were also fewer doctors serving coalfield communities than spas and seaside resorts favoured by middle-class retirees. Powell notes a six-fold variation between highest and lowest numbers of doctors in County Boroughs but as much as a 24-fold variation between wealthiest and poorest areas of London.[159] Charles Webster notes that, 'In seaside towns, where GPs were found in the greatest density, two-thirds of the patients would commonly be private'.[160] Historians who have studied the fortunes of the middle classes in this period such as W.D. Rubinstein and Richard Trainor have nevertheless shown that the provincial middle class was no longer as wealthy, numerous, or influential as they were before the First World War and that London and the home counties sustained a much greater proportion of white-collar workers who would have been obliged to pay for medical treatment then could be found elsewhere in the country.[161] While it is too simplistic to talk of a 'north-south divide', the decline of the country's industrial base led to greater levels of unemployment during this period among both the labouring classes and white-collar workers outside the southeast of England, as was noted by contemporary commentators such as J.B. Priestley.[162] Musing on this, Frank Layton's hero, Andrew Steele, describes this lyrically when he distinguishes between 'comfortable England' which he says mainly comprises London and the South East, and 'uncomfortable England', that is, the industrial towns and deprived agricultural areas, declaring that 'Uncomfortable England's the real England'.[163]

For GPs in 'the real England', and much of Scotland and Wales, the opportunity to garner fees from middle-class patients was accordingly limited. Moreover, the situation of the lower middle class remained perilous. According to Richard Trainor, 'in the interwar years ordinary doctors' bills threatened family solvency'.[164] Kenneth Lane testified to this from personal experience. His family was left with a 'crippling' bill for his mother's treatment by a GP which, due to his headmaster father's 'stupendous efforts' to pay off, the family were for several years denied luxuries of any sort. He concluded: 'I can honestly say that that debt to the Margate doctor dominated my boyhood'.[165] In some areas, however, this was academic as there were no middle-class patients to speak of. Thus, from evidence given to the Spens inquiry in 1946, Charles Webster notes, 'Dr Pierce in the mining valleys of South Wales could not anticipate any income from private practice'.[166] For GPs dependent more on panel practice than on private fees who may have been having to share their income with others, the Government's attempts to reduce panel fees in the late 1920s and again in the 1930s must have seemed injurious and unfair but even more so when considering just how hard they worked. As the IAC had said in 1923, the work of the panel practitioner was 'strenuous and unremitting'.[167] Webster agrees, asserting that 'NHI income was hard-earned'.[168] Twelve- to fourteen-hour working days were taken as normal according to one Welsh GP who reportedly undertook up to 50 domiciliary visits a day in winter months.[169] While income from panel work declined, the demand for GP services from panel patients continued to rise. In 1912, the Plender Report had estimated the average number of patient attendances per annum at 1.25. In 1924, it was 3.5 according to Ministry estimates and 3.8 according to the BMA. In 1931, the Ministry's estimate was 3.68 but the BMA's much higher estimate of 5.13 was closer to Bradford Hill's later and more authoritative estimate of 5.02.[170] Thus, while in the late 1930s panel practice made up only 30–40% of GPs' income on average, it actually took up more than 60% of the GP's time.[171] But, unlike solicitors, the professional group which GPs might reasonably expect to compare themselves to, GPs did not enjoy the luxury of a 9 to 5 existence and lived in perpetual fear of 'the night bell'.[172] It was not uncommon even during the 1940s for doctors who lived above their premises to have a speaking tube adjacent to the surgery entrance connected to the doctor's bedroom so that patients could rouse the doctor from his/her bed when needed out of hours.[173]

The increasing use of telephones by doctors and patients only increased the risks of disturbed sleep. In Brackenbury's summing up of the IAC's arguments to the Court of Inquiry into GPs' remuneration in 1924, he complained that 'one was listening for the telephone bell all the time'. This, he felt, justified the description of the panel GPs' obligations as 'oppressive' if not 'menacing'.[174] It was not uncommon for a GP to spend a whole night attending a difficult labour and then be obliged to attend a full surgery of panel patients the following morning without the benefit of sleep.[175] Being on call 24 hours a day 365 days a year meant that general practice, as Digby acknowledges, 'was not for the fainthearted or lazy'.[176] Mortality figures among GPs were correspondingly much higher than in other professional groups. A footnote to the Spens Report notes that, 'In 1931 the mortality among doctors between the ages of 20 and 65 was 54% above that of higher civil servants and 26% above that of professional engineers'.[177] For the kind of doctor whom Layton portrayed in his novels, it was hard to discern any of the improvement in the doctors' well-being which Digby and Bosanquet imply and even those whose income meant that they could afford the trappings of a comfortable middle-class existence seldom had the leisure time necessary to enjoy it. A Scottish survey revealed that few doctors took more than half-day breaks and many had virtually no leisure.[178] In 1933 in a memorandum on the increased workload of panel GPs, the London Panel Committee stated:

> Amongst insured persons, social and cultural improvement has been accompanied by reduction in hours of work, improved conditions of life and a substantial rise in the economic value of wages. There has on the other hand been little improvement in the conditions or standard of life for the insurance practitioner.[179]

In this light, the efforts made by the profession's representatives to challenge the government's persistent refusal to increase panel fees do not seem unreasonable.

In the decade that followed, however, there was little improvement. In 1945, while preparing evidence for the Spens inquiry, the Joint Committee on GPs' remuneration noted from 104 returns to a practitioner survey that 50% had had a total of two weeks holiday the previous year, but while 32 had managed three weeks or more, ten had had no holiday at all.[180]

It seems obvious that partnerships and group practice offered a potential solution to the problems of workload and professional isolation of which so many GPs complained. By the end of the 1930s, the number of partnerships was beginning to rise and the number of practices employing staff or working in some way with other professionals was increasing. At the beginning of the twentieth century, about 20% of practices were partnerships. This figure had risen to 25% by 1929 but it did not reach 50% until 1950.[181] Given that general practice was so individualistic, partnerships between GPs often proved difficult to sustain, given the inevitable personality clashes which occurred when strong-minded individuals disagreed. As the GP MP Sir Henry Morris-Jones observed in relationship to the dissolution of his own partnership, 'Partnership in medicine is more difficult than in any other profession…There are abundant opportunities for disagreement, discord and dissension. Temperamental variation and dissimilarities are emphasised and accentuated'.[182] The GP's practice was essentially a personal enterprise in which individual doctors invested much of their waking lives, but it bore the hallmarks of a 'cottage industry'.[183] This often led to a narrowness of vision when it came to thoughts about the future, as Charles Webster noted when stating of GPs, 'like shopkeepers, they looked for little beyond their list'.[184]

Before the Second World War, it was common for middle-class people to employ domestic servants. Many doctors employed a housekeeper or maid and some a dispenser and even a chauffeur. The fact that many less well-off GPs were able to run their practices without employing ancillary staff was due to the active support of family members. In the mid-nineteenth century, a contemporary commentator had opined that 'a wife was almost a necessary part of the physician's equipment' because women were reticent about seeking advice from a bachelor medical man.[185] Margaret Stacey observes that because there was no separation between home and workplace in general practice, doctors' wives were effectively 'married to the job'.[186] As an unpaid domestic, they often managed the practice as well as household finances, performed secretarial duties, and passed on messages from patients. Male doctors who were unmarried or widowed relied on other relatives who were remunerated with food and board. In *My Brother Jonathan*, Dr Hammond's daughter serves as his practice dispenser and factotum, while in *The Citadel*, Dr Page relies on his formidable sister and in his Black Country practice, Francis Maylett Smith relied on his Aunt Sophie.[187] In her early career, Mabel Ramsay counted on administrative support from her mother.[188] In his application for a partnership in the 1930s, Kenneth Lane discovered that his wife's affability and fashion sense proved to be decisive in his success, by winning the approval of the other doctor's wives![189] Lane, as has been noted, struggled financially and managed without domestics although the partnership employed its own staff. The relative affluence enjoyed by his contemporary Geoffrey Barber is demonstrated by the fact that he managed to employ several domestic servants. In the 1940s, his entourage comprised two maids, a nurse, a nurse maid, a gardener, and an 'occasional boy'.[190]

International comparisons

When it began, NHI was hailed as one of the most ambitious forms of state-coordinated medical care in Europe. But, with the failure to extend the scope of coverage and medical benefits in the 1920s, it was soon eclipsed by more progressive European schemes. According to Sir Arthur Newsholme, the Scandinavian countries in particular 'set an example to the world in efficiency and amplitude of provision'.[191] Fears of increasing bureaucratisation notwithstanding, British GPs consoled themselves with the belief that the machinery of NHI gave them more influence over administration and freedom from lay interference than their European counterparts. This belief was bolstered by published reports of meetings of the *Association Professionelle Internationale des Médecins* in which insurance doctors from across Europe complained of concerted attempts to diminish their pay and status.[192] A contemporary American investigation into health insurance found 'the Germans are the most loud in their complaints and the British are apparently the most satisfied'.[193]

Before the Second World War, British doctors took a keen interest in what was happening with insurance medical practice in Germany. The accord brokered in 1914 between the German medical profession and the government had broken down as a consequence of the post-war depression and in 1923 insurance doctors undertook a three-month strike. However, measures taken by the German government in 1931 actively favoured the profession at the insurance funds' expense and placed the mechanism for resolving their disputes 'totally in the physicians' hands'.[194] Once they had purged the profession of Jewish doctors, moreover, the Nazis strengthened the role of the profession, due in part to their ideological obsession with health and fitness. The Italian medical profession likewise benefitted from its corporatist support for Mussolini and his regime. In France meanwhile, the profession secured a major victory when a legislative Act of 1928 accorded state recognition to the principles of the doctors' 'Medical Charter', guaranteeing free choice of doctor, freedom to prescribe, and direct payment of doctor by patient according to an agreed tariff.[195] This prompted *Medical World* to state categorically that French doctors 'enjoy a superior social and legal status to ours'.[196] Alfred Cox considered their victory to be nominal, however, and elsewhere in Europe the situation of doctors was said to be less favourable and in many countries specialists were beginning to outnumber GPs. In the USA, as in Germany, there was at this time increasingly little distinction between GPs and specialists. By 1928, two-thirds of American physicians held hospital appointments but patients could access specialists without the need for GP referral. According to Paul Starr, 'In the long run, this failure to gain a mediatory role contributed to the breakdown of general practice'.[197] This helps explain why Alfred Cox felt moved to exclaim that 'Too strong an emphasis cannot be placed on the gravity of the position of the profession in many countries'.[198] British GPs noted with alarm the declining numbers of GPs in Europe and the USA where hospitals and clinics were becoming the predominant providers of healthcare and where the detrimental effects of over-hospitalisation were beginning to be felt.[199] To that extent, they might have agreed with R.W. Harris's comments noted earlier and this increased their leaders' determination to defend the British system and, as we shall see in the later chapters, to extol the, as yet unappreciated, benefits of the continuity of care which the British family doctor provided.

Conclusion

GPs were given an important role in administering medical benefits under NHI. However, in the late 1920s and 1930s, the rising costs of the scheme forced the Ministry of Health to look critically and in more depth at how individual doctors exercised their responsibilities. In 1930, the Ministry found it necessary to introduce new regulations boosting the role of RMOs, bypassing to some degree the LMPCs, whose judgements were felt to be suspect when it came to punishing those deemed guilty of failing to comply with professional norms. While not questioning the panel GPs' ability to do their best for their patients, the Ministry sought but ultimately failed to find a solution to the rising costs of medical benefit, even when the IAC was at its most compliant and supportive of their efforts. The IAC could hardly have been expected to do more in any case when the panel GPs' pay was cut, and the government pointedly ignored their request for restitution. This was where their policy of 'bargained corporatism' found its limits. Many rank and file GPs, particularly those who relied on panel work as their main source of income, were resentful of their leaders' willingness to accept changes which seemed to bring them little benefit. According to Charles Webster, 'the profession was never satisfied that the level for the capitation fee had been fixed correctly or upwardly adjusted sufficiently'.[200] As testament to this, the MPU claimed that replies to questionnaires it sent to panel GPs in 1931 suggested that, due to its handling of the cut in remuneration, the IAC had lost the confidence of two-thirds of panel GPs.[201] Dissatisfaction with the IAC's quiescence may have contributed to the MPU's increased membership which reached a peak of 5,857 in 1938 before declining thereafter.[202]

By the late 1930s, many established GPs were economically secure and had achieved the prosperous middle-class status they had collectively aspired to as a profession since the turn of the century. A significant proportion of GPs were less fortunate, however, finding themselves struggling with debt, beholden financially to other GPs, financial institutions, or money lenders, and completely overburdened with work. The situation of this exploited underclass of GPs was not far removed from that of the 'medical proletariat' Digby had identified in the 1890s.[203] In the 1930s, it is safe to say that the majority of GPs remained firmly wedded to independent contractor status, although the MPU was now openly questioning its supposed benefits. However, the symbiotic relationship between private and panel practices on which this 'article of faith' relied had unintended consequences. One effect of the free market in GP services was the obvious maldistribution of GPs which the Ministry and professional leaders were aware of but made no attempt to address in the interwar period. This compounded problems of inequality and resulted in limited choice of doctor in 'under-doctored' areas, a lower quality of service for those most needing it, and a lower standard of living for those delivering it. The NHI system had its advantages for those working in it, but it also had serious deficiencies, allowing payment of 'substantial prizes to the few, if necessary, at the cost of penury for a substantial residuum'.[204] During the interwar years, the profession's leaders put forward many suggestions for improvements which it seemed were doomed to failure without the government's support. But while they continued to argue the case for an extension of NHI, others asked if what was needed was not merely reform, but the substitution of an entirely different system.

Notes

1 R.W. (Robert William) Harris, *National Health Insurance in Great Britain, 1911–1946* (London, 1946). p. 143.

2 Norman R. Eder, *National Health Insurance and the Medical Profession in Britain, 1913–1939* (New York, 1982). p. 304.

3 *Ibid.*, p. 42.

4 *BMA Archive*, LMC/1/1, minutes of the London Panel Committee meeting on 28 April 1914.

5 *Ibid*, LMC1/2, minutes of meeting on 27 March 1917.

6 Eder, *National Health Insurance and the Medical Profession*, p. 268.

7 *Cheshire County PRO*, NHL 7135/1, minutes of the County Palatine of Chester LMPC meeting on 29 September 1915, minute 5.

8 *The National Archive/Public Record Office Kew*, MH 62/119, Memorandum by J. S. Whitaker, 20 September 1919.

9 *Ibid.*, MH 62/118, Memorandum from J.S. Whitaker to Morant dated 24 July 1919; MH 62/107, memorandum by Whitaker dated 19 June 1922.

10 *Ibid.*, MH 62/107, Undated 'Extract from the Instructions Issued to the Medical Staff, Investigation of Prescribing'.

11 Eder, *National Health Insurance and the Medical Profession*, p. 270.

12 *BMA Archive*, B/203/1/19, minutes of IAC meeting on 23 June 1927, Doc 68.

13 Hermann Levy, *National Health Insurance: A Critical Study* (Cambridge, 1944). pp. 188–195.

14 Winifred Stamp, *Doctor Himself: An Unorthodox Biography of Harry Roberts MD* (London, 1949). pp. 82–85.

15 Francis Maylett Smith, *A GP's Progress to the Black Country* (Hythe, Kent, 1984). pp. 140–142.

16 *National Archive*, MH 62/109, Unsigned memorandum dated 8 February 1926.

17 *BMA Archive*, B/203/1/19, minutes of IAC meeting on 30 November 1927, Doc 23.
18 Eder, *National Health Insurance and the Medical Profession*, pp. 275–276.
19 *BMJ*, 30 October 1937, Supplement, p. 275.
20 Quoted by Eder, *National Health Insurance and the Medical Profession*, p. 277.
21 Frank C. Layton, *The Little Doctor* (Edinburgh, 1933). p. 34.
22 *The New Statesman*, 6 December 1913, p. 263 and the *Lancet*, 3 January 1914, p. 77.
23 *National Archive*, MH 62/45, Letter (undated) from L.G. Brock to Cox.
24 Eder, *National Health Insurance and the Medical Profession*, p. 282.
25 Jacqueline Jenkinson, *Scotland's Health, 1919–1948* (Bern, 2002). pp. 354–355.
26 *YORLMC Archive*, minutes of meeting of Group C Regional Committee of LMPCs 9 October 1929.
27 *Ibid.*, p. 286.
28 *National Insurance Gazette*, 4 August 1928, p. 367.
29 *BMJ*, 12 May 1928 Supplement, p. 206.
30 *Ibid.*, 15 November 1927, Supplement, pp. 44–46. Anne Digby, 'The Economic and Medical Significance of the British National Health Insurance Act 1911,' in Martin Gorsky and Sally Sheard (eds) *Financing Medicine: The British Experience since 1750* (Abingdon, 2006). p. 184.
31 Jenkinson, *Scotland's Health*, p. 353.
32 *Daily Mail*, 7 April 1930, 'Health Insurance Inquiry Needed', by special correspondent, p. 9. *The Times*, 7 April 1930, 'Claims for Sick Benefit', p. 11.
33 'AGP', *This Panel Business* (London, 1933). pp. 111–115. See also Jenkinson, *Scotland's Health*, p. 370 and comments about this by Leith GP, Dr Gilruth.
34 Anne Digby, *The Evolution of British General Practice, 1848–1948* (Oxford, 1999) p. 253.
35 *BMJ*, 20 June 1931, pp. 1079. *BMA Archive*, minutes of the IAC meeting on 23 September 1932, Doc 1.
36 'A Panel Doctor', *On the Panel: General Practice as a Career* (London, c.1924). pp. 144–145.
37 Noel Whiteside 'Central Control and the Approved Societies: Access to Social Support under the Interwar Health Insurance Scheme.' *Bulletin of the Society for the Social History of Medicine*, 32 (1983). p. 16.
38 See debate at Annual LMPCs Conference 1930, *BMJ*, 11 November 1930, Supplement, pp. 189–190. 'AGP', *This Panel Business*, p. 146.
39 *Medical World*, 27 January 1927, 'Over certification- a cause?', p. 468.
40 'AGP', *This Panel Business*, p. 146.
41 *BMA Archive*, B/203/1/22, minutes of IAC meeting of 20 November 1930, Doc. 9, reference to Medical Benefit (Amendment) Regulations 1930.
42 Eder, *National Health Insurance and the Medical Profession*, p. 300.
43 Layton, *The Little Doctor*, p. 52.
44 *BMA Archive*, B/203/1/19, minutes of IAC meeting on 19 January 1928, Doc 39.
45 *Ibid.*, pp. 2–4.
46 'AGP', *This Panel Business*, pp. 36–7, 43–49, 71–72.
47 Jenkinson, *Scotland's Health*, pp. 375–376.
48 *BMA Archive*, B/203/1/22, minutes of IAC meeting of 20 November 1930, memorandum on Medical Benefit Amendment Regulations 1930, Doc.9, point 1.
49 *Ibid*, minutes of IAC meeting on 6 March 1930, Doc 27.
50 Jenkinson, *Scotland's Health*, p. 377.
51 *BMA Archive*, B/203/1/23, minutes of IAC meeting on 24 September 1931, Doc IA 5 referring to ICL 751 MoH.
52 Eder, *National Health Insurance and the Medical Profession*, p. 300.

53 Frank Honigsbaum, *Health, Happiness and Security: The Creation of the National Health Service* (London, 1989). p. 37.

54 *Ibid.*, p. 305.

55 *Report of Committee on National Expenditure* chaired by Sir George May, Cmd. 3920 (1931). See James E. Cronin, *The Politics of State Expansion: War, State and Society in Twentieth Century Britain* (London, 1991). p. 100 and Peter Clarke, *Hope and Glory: Britain 1900-2000* (3rd edn., London, 2004). p. 186.

56 *BMA Archive*, B/203/1/23, minutes of IAC meeting on 8 September 1931, min. 5, point 6 (letter from Robinson dated 5 September 1931).

57 *Ibid.* The dissentient was the London GP, E.A. Gregg.

58 *Ibid.*, minutes of IAC meeting on 24 September 1931, min 18 (letter from Robinson dated 10 September 1931).

59 *Ibid.* See also Clarke, *Hope and Glory*, p. 159.

60 *BMA Archive*, B/203/1/23, minutes of IAC meeting on 8 September 1931, min. 19.

61 Anne Digby and Nick Bosanquet, 'Doctors and Patients in an Era of National Health Insurance and Private Practice 1913–1938.' *Economic History Review*, 41 (1) (1988). p. 84.

62 *Medical World*, 2 October 1931 'Insurance notes' p. 110 and 30 October 1931, 'The Cut and the Conference', p. 199.

63 *Ibid.*, 25 September 1931, 'National Health Insurance', p. 85.

64 *Ibid.*, 25 September 1931, letter from Henry H. Haward, p. 94, and 9 October 1931 letter from 'Wife', p. 138.

65 'AGP', *This Panel Business*, p. 91.

66 *BMJ*, 31 October 1931, 'Report of Annual Panel Conference'. Compare this with *Medical World*, 6 November 1931, 'The mystery of the Conference', p. 221.

67 *BMA Archive*, B/203/1/25, minutes of IAC Remuneration Subcommittee meeting on 9 February 1933.

68 *Medical World*, 2 October 1931, p. 109.

69 *BMJ*, 29 October 1932 'Report of Annual Panel Conference', Supplement, p. 222.

70 *BMA Archive*, B/203/1/ 25, minutes of IAC meeting on 2 May 1933, Doc. 80.

71 *Ibid.*, Doc. 91.

72 *Ibid.*, minutes of IAC meeting on 16 November 1933, B/203/3/22, minutes of Annual Conference of LMPCs 19 October 1933, min. 25.

73 'AGP', *This Panel Business*, p. 204.

74 *BMJ*, 24 August 1935, Supplement, p. 109.

75 *Ibid.*, 29 May 1937, Supplement, p. 330.

76 *BMA Archive*, B/203/1/30, minutes of IAC Remuneration Subcommittee meeting on 3 November 1938, Doc 10. p. 4, point 5.

77 *BMJ*, 5 June 1937, Supplement, p. 356.

78 *Cheshire PRO*, NHL 7135 NHL/5, minutes of meeting of County Palatine of Chester LMPC on 21 November 1923, p. 39.

79 *Ibid.*, 12 June 1937, Supplement, p. 369.

80 *BMA Archive*, B/203/1/29, minutes of IAC meeting on 20 January 1938, Doc. 29.

81 *Ibid.*, B/203/1/30, minutes of IAC Remuneration Subcommittee meeting on 3 November 1938, Doc. 10, pp. 3–4.

82 *Ibid.*, B/203/1/37, minutes of the meeting of the Joint Committee on GPs' remuneration on 27 June 1945, Draft memorandum of evidence to the Spens Committee.

83 *Report of the Interdepartmental Committee on the Remuneration of General Practitioners, 1945–46*, Cmd. 6810 (1946).

84 Geoffrey Barber, *Country Doctor* (2nd edn., Woodbridge, Suffolk, 1975). p. 46.

85 *North Staffordshire LMPC Archive*, minutes of the LMPC meeting on 5 April 1934.

86 *BMJ*, 10 March 1923, Supplement, G.B. Sleigh 'Administrative Expenses', p. 82.
87 *Medical World,* 17 December 1926, 'Health Insurance in 1925', p. 317.
88 Andrew McDonald 'The Geddes Committee and the Formulation of Public Expenditure Policy 1921–1922.' *Historical Journal*, 32 (1989). p. 647.
89 *Medical World,* 24 December 1926, G. Rome Hall, 'Civil Service Control', pp. 348–349.
90 Layton, *The Little Doctor*, p. 109.
91 *Ibid.,* p. 191.
92 *BMJ,* 8 April 1933 'Incapable', Supplement, p. 131.
93 Francis Maylett Smith, *A G.P.'s Progress to the Black Country* (Hythe, Kent, 1984), pp. 140–142.
94 *Medical World,* 21 October 1927, 'As we see it' pp. 121–122 and 18 December 1931, 'Court Martial Procedure', p. 35.
95 *Ibid.,* 1 October 1926, (Pharos), 'Improving the Medical Service', p. 36.
96 Layton, *The Little Doctor,* pp. 110–111.
97 *Cheshire PRO*, NHL 7135 NHL/1, minutes of meeting of County Palatine of Chester LMPC dated 4 June 1915.
98 *Ibid.,* minutes of LMPC meeting dated 15 October 1916.
99 *Ibid.*
100 *Ibid.,* minutes of LMPC meeting dated 28 October 1917.
101 *Cheshire PRO*, NHL 7135 NHL/2, minutes of meeting of County Palatine of Chester LMPC dated 18 March 1920, p. 218.
102 *The Times*, 'Health Ministry Challenged', 5 April 1928, p. 17.
103 Frank Honigsbaum, *The Division in British Medicine: A History of the Separation of General Practice from Hospital Care 1911–1968* (London, 1979). pp. 165–167.
104 Eder, *National Health Insurance and the Medical Profession*, pp. 301–304.
105 (Archibald) Fenner Brockway, *Bermondsey Story: The Life of Alfred J. Salter* (London, 1949). p. 149.
106 *Medical World,* 28 April 1933, p. 177.
107 R.W. (Robert William) Harris and L.S. (Leonard Shoeten) Sack, *Medical Insurance Practice* (3rd edn., London, 1929). Foreword by H.G. Dain.
108 Rosemary Stevens, *Medical Practice in Modern England: The Impact of Specialization and State Medicine* (New Haven, CT, 1966). p. 57.
109 Anne Digby and Nick Bosanquet 'Doctors and Patients in an Era of National Health Insurance and Private Practice 1913–1938.' *Economic History Review*, 41 (1) (1988). p. 77.
110 *Ibid.,* pp. 9–10.
111 Anne Digby, *The Evolution of British General Practice, 1850–1948* (Oxford, 1999). p. 192.
112 *BMJ*, 'The Profession of Medicine', 4 September 1937, p. 445.
113 Noel and Jose Parry, *The Rise of the Medical Profession* (London, 1976). p. 198.
114 Digby and Bosanquet, 'Doctors and Patients in an Era of National Health Insurance', p. 80.
115 Stevens, *Medical Practice in Modern England*, p. 57.
116 Brockway, *Bermondsey Story,* p. 51.
117 Charles Webster 'Doctors, Public Service and Profit.' *Transactions of the Royal Historical Society*, 40 (1990). p. 200. Ross McKibbin 'Politics and the Medical Hero: A.J. Cronin's 'The Citadel.' *English Historical Review*, 123 (502) (2008). p. 663.
118 *BMJ, 23* July 1938. 'The Profession and the Public', pp. 163–164.

119 Digby and Bosanquet, 'Doctors and Patients in an Era of National Health Insurance', p. 86.

120 Political and Economic Planning, *Report on the British Health Services* (London, 1937). p. 157.

121 Guy Routh, *Occupation and Pay in Great Britain, 1906–1979* (2nd edn., London, 1980). p. 63.

122 Digby and Bosanquet, 'Doctors and Patients in an Era of National Health Insurance', pp. 74–75.

123 Mabel Rew 'Looking Back.' *Journal of the Medical Women's Federation,* 49 (1967). p. 85.

124 Stevens, *Medical Practice in Modern England,* p. 53.

125 Bernard Harris, *The Origins of the British Welfare State: Social Welfare in England and Wales, 1800–1945* (Basingstoke, 2004). p. 223.

126 Digby and Bosanquet, 'Doctors and Patients in an Era of National Health Insurance', p. 75.

127 *Ibid.,* p. 79.

128 'AGP', *This Panel Business* (London, 1933). p. 286.

129 Digby and Bosanquet, 'Doctors and Patients in an Era of National Health Insurance', p. 79.

130 *Ibid.,* p. 85.

131 *BMJ,* 21 April 1923, 'The Plight of the Country Practitioner' by Dr J.P. Williams-Freeman, Supplement, pp. 117–119.

132 *Ibid.,* 30 May 1925, Supplement, p. 241.

133 Digby and Bosanquet, 'Doctors and Patients in an Era of National Health Insurance', p. 85.

134 A. Bradford Hill 'The Doctor's Day and Pay.' *Journal of Royal Statistical Society,* Series A (Gen) 114 (1) (1951). p. 23.

135 *Ibid.,* p. 23, Table 14. PEP, *The British Health Services,* p. 143.

136 *Wellcome Collection* (BMA Archive), SA/BMA/C 522. Box 139. Minutes of meeting of Propaganda Committee on 11 March 1924.

137 *Ibid.,* Extract from minutes of BMA's ARM 1925, min 125, point f).

138 *Ibid.,* Extract from minutes of Medico-Political Committee meeting on 16 March 1927.

139 *BMJ,* 18 October 1924 p. 743. For a comprehensive analysis of the challenges facing women GPs in this period see Digby, *The Evolution of British General Practice,* ch. 7.

140 *Wellcome Collection* (BMA Archive), SA/BMA/C 522. Box 139. Extract from Minutes of Medico-Political Committee meeting of 3 January 1934, memorandum on 'Emoluments of Women Practitioners'.

141 *Report of the Inter-Departmental Committee on the Remuneration of General Practitioners, 1945–1946,* Cmd. 6810 1946, (the Spens Report) reproduced in *BMJ,* 18 May 1946, Supplement, pp. 149–150, tables 8 and 9.

142 *BMA Archive,* B/203/1/37, Agenda of Joint Committee of IAC and the BMA's General Practice Committee on GP Remuneration, meeting on 17 April 1945 (item 5).

143 PEP, *The British Health Services,* p. 9. *BMA Archive,* minutes of a meeting of the Joint Committee on GPs' remuneration on 27 June 1945, Draft memorandum of evidence to the Spens inquiry.

144 Kenneth Lane, *Diary of a Medical Nobody* (London, 1982). pp. 17 and 125–128.

145 Honigsbaum, *The Division in British Medicine,* p. 275.

146 *BMA Archive,* B/203/1/26, agenda of IAC meeting on 13 November 1934, Doc. 6. p. 1.

147 *Ibid.,* p. 2.

148 *Ibid.,* minutes of IAC meeting on 13 November 1934, min. 85.

149 *Ibid.,* B/203/3/24, Report of the Annual Conference of Representatives of LMPCs 1935, min. 19.
150 *Cheshire PRO*, NHL 7135 NHL/6, minutes of meeting of County Palatine of Chester LMPC dated 12 December 1934.
151 Douglass W. Orr and Jean Walker Orr, *Health Insurance with Medical Care: The British Experience* (New York, 1938). p. 147.
152 'AGP', *This Panel Business*, p. 191.
153 Digby, *The Evolution of British General Practice'*, pp. 125, 153.
154 Lane, *Diary of a Medical Nobody*, p. 24.
155 'AGP', *This Panel Business*, p. 169.
156 *Ibid.,* minutes of IAC meeting on 23 April 1936, Appointment of Subcommittee on Mortgages of Medical Practices.
157 *BMJ*, 9 June 1945, 'The Purchase of a Practice', Supplement, pp. 103–104.
158 Martin Powell 'Coasts and Coalfields: The Geographical Distribution of Doctors in England and Wales in the 1930s.' *Social History of Medicine*, 18 (2) (2005). pp. 245–263.
159 *Ibid.,* pp. 255–256.
160 Charles Webster 'General Practice under the Panel: The Last Phase.' *Bulletin of the Social History of Medicine*, 32 (1983). p. 21.
161 W.D. Rubinstein, 'Britain's Elites in the Interwar Period 1918–1939' and Richard Trainor 'Neither Metropolitan nor Provincial: The Interwar Middle Class' *passim* in Alan Kidd and David Nichols (eds) *The Making of the British Middle Class? Studies of Regional and Cultural Diversity Since the Eighteenth Century* (Stroud, Glos, 1998).
162 Trainor 'Neither Metropolitan nor Provincial' pp. 206–207. J.B. Priestley *English Journey: being a rambling but truthful account of what one man saw and heard and felt during a journey through England during the autumn of the year 1933* (London, 1934). *passim*.
163 Layton, *The Little Doctor*, p. 77.
164 'Richard Trainor, 'The Middle Class' in Martin Daunton (ed) *Cambridge Urban History of Britain, vol. 3 1840–1950* (Cambridge, 2001). p. 687.
165 Lane, *Diary of a Medical Nobody*, p. 158.
166 Webster, 'General Practice under the Panel', p. 21.
167 *BMA Archive*, B/203/1/15, minutes of IAC meeting on 7 August 1923,'Memorandum on Remuneration'.
168 Webster, 'Doctors, Public Service and Profit', p. 201.
169 Webster, 'General Practice under the Panel', p. 22.
170 Digby and Bosanquet, 'Doctors and Patients in an Era of National Health Insurance', pp. 86–87.
171 *Ibid*, p. 79; *Report of the Interdepartmental Committee 1945–46* (The Spens Report). p. 11.
172 For an illustration of this see Frank Layton, *The Little Doctor* (Edinburgh, 1933). p. 6.
173 Atholl MacLaren, 'Fifty Years On: How a fledgling Health Service Proved Its Worth,' in Chris Locke (ed.) *General Practitioners in Nottinghamshire, 1948–1998: A Health Service Record* (Nottingham, 1999). p. 16.
174 *BMJ*, 12 January 1924,'Insurance: The Court of Inquiry', Supplement, p. 49.
175 For an illustration of this occurrence see Frank Layton, *The Old Doctor* (Birmingham, 1923). pp. 18–21.
176 Digby, *The Evolution of British General Practice*, p. 149, based on the Spens report.
177 *BMJ*, 18 May 1946,' The Spens Report', Supplement, p. 143.
178 Webster, 'General Practice under the Panel', p. 22.

179 *BMA Archive*, B/203/1/ 25, Minutes of a meeting of the IAC's Remuneration Subcommittee on 9 February 1933. 'Memorandum by London Panel Committee's specially appointed section' Doc. 55 p. 3 point d.
180 *BMA Archive*, B/203/1/37, agenda for meeting of Joint Committee on GPs' remuneration, on 17 April 1945.
181 Digby, *The Evolution of British General Practice*, p. 131.
182 Sir Henry Morris-Jones, *Doctor in the Whipps' Room* (London, 1955). p. 80.
183 Digby, *The Evolution of British General Practice*, p. 136.
184 Webster, 'General Practice Under the Panel' p. 23.
185 M. Jeanne Peterson, *The Medical Profession in Mid-Victorian London* (London, 1978). p. 92.
186 Margaret Stacey, *The Sociology of Health and Healing* (London, 1988). p. 86.
187 Smith, *A G.P.'s Progress to the Black Country*, pp. 77–79.
188 Mabel Ramsay, *The Doctor's Zig Zag Road*, Unpublished autobiography, Royal College of Physicians, London, p. 62.
189 Lane, *Diary of a Medical Nobody*, p. 17.
190 Barber, *Country Doctor*, pp. 75–76.
191 Sir Arthur Newsholme, *Medicine and the State* (London, 1932). p. 76.
192 'AGP', *This Panel Business*, ch. III, p. 51.
193 *Ibid.*, ch. VI, p. 99, quote attributed to D.M. Simon and Nathan Sinai in a book called *The Way of Health Insurance* (provenance unknown).
194 Jan Blanpain, *National Health Insurance and Health Resources: The European Experience* (Harvard, 1978). p. 29.
195 *Ibid.*, p. 101.
196 *Medical World*, 27 November 1931, 'National Health Insurance,' p. 289.
197 Paul Starr, *The Social Transformation of American Medicine: The Rise of a Sovereign Profession and the Making of a Vast Industry* (New York, 1982). pp. 166–167 and 224.
198 'AGP', *This Panel Business*, p. 57.
199 Newsholme, *Medicine and the State*, pp. 81–86. See also comments of H.G. Dain in discussions with Ministry, *BMA Archive*, minutes of IAC meeting on 8 January 1931, Doc 18, Report of Deputation to Ministry of Health on 27 November 1930.
200 Webster, 'General Practice under the Panel', p. 20.
201 *Medical World*, 30 October 1931,'The cut and the Conference', p. 197.
202 Honigsbaum, *The Division in British Medicine*, p. 169.
203 Digby, *The Evolution of British General Practice*, p. 32.
204 Webster, 'General Practice under the Panel', p. 23.

9 Parallel developments

GPs and the 'mixed economy of care', 1914–1948

In 1920, Sir George Newman, the Chief Medical Officer of the Ministry of Health, informed the BMA's Annual Representative Meeting:

> In my view the State should never take out of the hands of the general practitioner – whether in contractual practice or otherwise – the patient whom he is willing and competent to treat, and on reasonable terms with which the patient can comply.[1]

GPs would no doubt have been pleased by such reassuring words from the most senior medical official in government service. Yet for many GPs, the period following the institution of NHI involved a war of attrition between would-be family doctors and forces they saw as determined to limit their role, deny them a living, and eventually subsume them within a government-mandated but locally administered State Medical Service. These forces were determined, it seemed, to compel GPs to relinquish their professional autonomy and become salaried employees of local authorities. The profession's representatives felt duty bound to prevent this and to resist therefore any attempt to establish or promote any non-insurance-based alternatives to GPs' private contract practice. The conflicts they consequently found themselves engaged in had a significant impact on the way GPs saw their changing situation in the interwar years. They served both to reinforce their previously described articles of faith and to determine their attitude to how health services might be reorganised in future.

In contrast to the paucity of recent historical research into the activities of GPs and their political activities in the interwar period, there has been a vast outpouring of research into what has been termed municipal medicine.[2] This encompasses the growing importance in the early twentieth century of the poor law infirmaries, and of health clinics and other specialist services under local authority control, which historians of this period regularly set alongside the changing character and fortunes of the larger voluntary hospitals.[3] This research has been supplemented by a host of local studies illustrating the 'mixed economy of healthcare' during this period in all its complexities, including municipal

DOI: 10.4324/9781003438274-9

general, provincial district, and cottage hospitals.[4] Other studies have focused on the importance of hospital contributory schemes and other forms of self-help, the increasing number of private pay beds in voluntary and public hospitals, and the extent to which charitable institutions were dependent on communal and individual philanthropy and/or local authority or central government funding.[5] Historians have sometimes sought to place these developments in the context of international debates about welfarism and the attitude of Liberal states towards public provision of personal healthcare generally.[6] Many of these works contain numerous, if often incidental, references to GPs and their national representations. This chapter attempts to tease out, reframe, and re-evaluate these references in light of the themes previously discussed in this book. An understanding of these issues is important for two reasons: firstly, in order to appreciate the political and administrative contexts in which both panel and private GPs operated and the extent of their involvement in, or detachment from, other forms of healthcare during this period; secondly, to understand the extent to which the changes occurring outside contract practice impacted GPs and influenced their thoughts, and insecurities, regarding the future of personal health services, and determined the way their representative bodies responded to these developments on their behalf. As will be demonstrated in later chapters, both these considerations had a direct bearing on the profession's response to proposals for a National Health Service in the 1940s.

GPs' involvement with the poor law hospitals

The justified distaste with which the public in the late nineteenth and early twentieth centuries viewed the workhouse and the general relief at its passing should not obscure the fact that, throughout their existence, the workhouse medical infirmaries provided much-needed medical and nursing care for the impoverished who were chronically sick, disabled, or elderly. The impetus for reform of the workhouse system came from a variety of sources. But the principal catalyst for change was the recognition in the early twentieth century that the system was completely unable to deal with the growing social problem of unemployment, which studies by social reformers like the young William Beveridge had shown to be a complex and concerning phenomenon.[7] The large number of unemployed could not be accommodated in the workhouses and were increasingly subject to 'outdoor relief' or doles, but in the early 1900s, the increasing cost of both outdoor and institutional relief had reached alarming proportions.[8] The Conservative Government's decision in 1905 to establish a 'Royal Commission into the Poor Law and Relief of Distress' coincided with government attempts to deal with the problem through the setting up of local distress committees under the Unemployed Workmen Act.[9] As the able-bodied were removed from the workhouse, the poor law medical officers (PLMOs) found it easier to elicit a more sympathetic response from Boards of Guardians towards the sick being care for there.

By 1914, few laymen could challenge the value of medical expertise in nutrition, sanitation, and therapeutics.[10] The resultant improvements in facilities and conditions were not universal but the range of equipment to be found in workhouse infirmaries was soon 'superior to some hospitals and some of the facilities (particularly sanitoria) available to the dependant poor were rather more advanced than those available to the labouring poor'.[11] Although the PLMOs' demands for the latest equipment were frequently declined by Guardians on grounds of cost, standards exceeded in some cases those of the private hospitals or nursing homes catering for the middle classes. Guardians sometimes complained therefore that they were providing a better medical service for paupers than they could afford for themselves.[12] Neither the Guardians nor the medical inspectors employed by the Local Government Board (LGB) found it easy, however, to accurately assess the competence of the PLMOs. The inspectors lamented the fact that in rural areas, the Guardians were still obliged to recruit from 'the lower ranks of the profession' and believed that the solution lay in improved salaries.[13] The battle for increased remuneration was intensified after 1911 when so many doctors took up contract practice under National Health Insurance.

The First World War proved a turning point in the history of the poor law hospitals. Many workhouse infirmaries were commandeered for use as casualty hospitals and centres for care and rehabilitation of injured servicemen. They and their seconded staff therefore became an essential part of wartime medical services.[14] The infirmaries' use as military hospitals exposed their deficiencies and led to profound changes, not just in the standard of facilities, but in the organisation of the hospitals and the conditions of staff working within them. They were supplied with new equipment, given access to visiting specialists, and the pay of nursing and medical staff was improved with lasting effect.[15] By the end of the war, more full-time infirmary doctors were being employed, especially in London, where the number of beds rose from more than 15,000 in 1905 to 21,000 in 1923.[16] Consultants from the voluntary hospitals were contracted to provide specialist services when required. By the 1920s, many of the larger institutions dropped the title 'union infirmary' and became, simply, 'hospital'.[17] The distinction between patients and paupers in these hospitals was ceasing to be important. The stigma attached to the workhouse infirmaries had by this time diminished to the extent that the Dawson Report in 1920 recommended that they, like the voluntary hospitals, be allowed to accept paying patients without deeming them paupers, and a number of poor law hospitals, such as the one in Bolton, did so.[18] By the 1920s, medical students were at last permitted to attend the infirmaries in London as a quid pro quo for access to Consultant advice.[19] Some infirmary doctors were now better paid than their equivalents in the voluntary hospitals and the experience they gained was often just as valuable.[20] In many cities, the outpatient departments of the infirmaries began to rival those of the voluntary hospitals. In rural areas by contrast, both standards and extent of provision in poor law infirmaries had not greatly improved and government restrictions on capital expenditure resulted in a significant shortage of beds in areas like North Yorkshire.[21]

The profession's experience of poor law medical services served to underline the problems and disadvantages of lay control, a fear of which lay behind their conflicts with the friendly societies over sickness insurance and hostility towards the concept of salaried employment. The Boards of Guardians' supercilious dismissal of the PLMOs' reasonable demands for things which would enhance the medical care of pauper patients or improve the PLMOs' pay and conditions represented an affront to GPs' sense of their own standing as medical experts.[22] It made the profession even more determined to resist anything which tended to increase lay influence over their activities. Lay people could not, in their eyes, be trusted to make sensible decisions about medical matters without the benefit of medical advice, a belief which lay behind the profession's subsequent insistence that, in matters relating to health, all public authorities be guided by professional advisory committees and that decision-making bodies always include medical representatives.[23] Although Boards of Guardians were answerable to the LGB rather than the county and county borough councils, GPs were just as strongly opposed to 'encroachments' made by the latter into the area of personal healthcare. The profession fully accepted local authorities' responsibility for maintaining public health in its broadest sense through the duties vested in them and their Medical Officers of Health (MOHs) by (mainly nineteenth-century) sanitarian legislation. They were increasingly concerned, however, at the blurring of the distinction between preventative and curative health services which occurred during and after the First World War. Before examining what these so-called encroachments entailed, it is important to explore the relationship between local authorities and the profession's understanding of the concept of a State Medical Service.

Local authorities and the chimera of a 'State Medical Service'

The Royal Commission into the Poor Law represented a watershed moment in thinking about the role of the state in provision of healthcare to its citizens. This was due to the widespread discussion within professional and governmental circles, of proposals within the minority report, drafted by the Webbs, which called for a unified public health service offering both preventative and curative medical services under local authority control.[24] The system they proposed would provide treatment for all that needed it, though free only to those below a predetermined income limit.[25] The National Insurance Act bore little resemblance to what the Webbs proposed.[26] However, many of the doctors actively supporting it, principally members of the State Medical Services Association, believed it to be a first step towards the goal which the Webbs and other socialist reformers envisaged.[27] While central government was expected to introduce the necessary legislation, it was the local authorities whom the reformers expected to exercise the responsibilities of the state in making healthcare in all its forms available to the population and who would employ the majority of doctors contracted to deliver it. They confidently expected the NHI Commission to be absorbed within the LGB and believed that standards of medical care would be improved by selective recruitment of doctors into local government service and by increased supervision and training of those doctors. The latter would be rewarded with security of tenure, state-funded pensions, and opportunities for promotion within a hierarchical system. When the prominent Fabian Sir John Collie, along with Dr Milson Russen Rhodes and others, outlined such ideas in medical journals and conferences of doctors in 1914, they met with outraged opposition from mainstream GPs who saw this as a restriction of their clinical freedom and re-pudiation of the patient's free choice of doctor.[28] Any notion of salaried service under the auspices of local government was thereafter condemned by a majority of the profession as intrinsically socialist in nature and inimical to British no-tions of individual freedom.

Even before the Royal Commission published its findings, legislation passed by, or with the support of, the Liberal Government had extended state responsi-bilities in matters of public health in ways which the profession saw as threaten-ing and likely to impinge on GPs' near monopoly of personal medical care. The compulsory inspection of schoolchildren under the Education (Administrative Provisions) Act of 1907 led to the creation in 1908 of the School Medical Ser-vice supervised by a medical department at the Board of Education under the control of Sir Robert Morant. In common with the provision of school meals for needy children, the Act was meant to address concerns about the poor physi-cal health of the population highlighted in studies by Rowntree and the Report of the Interdepartmental Committee into Physical Deterioration following the Boer War.[29] But it was also seen as a means of reducing the unacceptably high rates of infant mortality and morbidity which became a matter of increasing public concern before and during the First World War, when they were high-lighted by social reformers such as Benjamin Broadbent and the Association for the Prevention of Infant Mortality.[30] This concern led to the establishment of a number of charitably funded infant welfare centres, the first of which opened in St Marylebone in 1906 under the direction of Dr Eric Pritchard.[31] It was closely followed by similar centres in Finsbury, Leicester, and Sheffield.[32] By 1911, there were 100 such centres, including one in north Kensington established by the Women's Labour League in 1910 which was supervised by the Labour activ-ist GP and Panel Committee stalwart, Dr Ethel Bentham.[33] A pioneering scheme in Huddersfield aimed at educating and supporting new mothers in parenting and infant nutrition, which was sponsored by Broadbent and the local MOH, Samson George Moore, provided an example for other local authorities to fol-low.[34] The scheme explicitly eschewed medical treatment. However, Morant's department encouraged local authorities to provide free medical treatment to schoolchildren where appropriate. The first dedicated local authority clinic of this kind was established in Bradford in 1908 providing treatment for eye and ear problems, skin diseases, dental treatment, and control of vermin. In 1911, it provided treatment to 3,520 children out of 16,000 examined.[35] Following this example, metropolitan boroughs in London, Sheffield and Leicester established infant welfare clinics and by 1913, there were 260 in 139 local authority areas, 27 of which received grants from the Board of Education.[36] Between 1915 and 1918, the number of infant welfare centres grew from 650 to 12,787.[37] GPs viewed all of these developments with a growing sense of unease. In 1912, the Leicester education committee considered the idea of using the National Insurance Act to fund treatment of schoolchildren. Local GPs objected and a rival scheme was put forward by the local BMA division. The two sides finally agreed that a medical treatments subcommittee, which included representatives of local GPs and dentists, would manage a minor ailments clinic, while a school clinic committee was responsible for a clinic at the town hall to provide treatment for children with skin diseases. These became operational in 1912 when the profession took over the running of the local provident dispensary and established a new Public Medical Service. The local MOH insisted that these clinics were meant to supplement rather than supplant GP services and were strictly confined to the treatment of certain defects.[38] Here and elsewhere, the profession found it necessary to establish 'red lines' which local authorities were warned not to cross. In 1915, the vice chairman of the County Palatine of Chester Local Medical and Panel Committee (LMPC) spoke ominously of 'the undesirable and impolitic encroachment of public authorities on the field of medical practice'.[39]

Government efforts to address the issues of the infant welfare coincided with growing public concern about maternal health prompted by social reformers and groups within the Labour movement such as the Women's Cooperative Guild.[40] The GPs' response to their calls, however, was often indignant and protectionist. Fear of competition led GPs in the Greater Manchester area to oppose implementation of the Midwives Act of 1902 and for several years, on what now seem very questionable grounds, the Notification of Births Act 1907.[41] Following examples set in Liverpool, Cardiff, and St Helens, they eventually succeeded in persuading the local authority to pay them directly for emergency obstetric attendances on women too poor to pay for their services.[42] When NHI began, the medical profession immediately campaigned for benefits to be extended to dependents of the insured. Maternity benefits were available to insured workers' wives but were denied to women whose husbands were excluded from the scheme due to the irregular nature of their work or self-employment, and confinement itself was specifically excluded from the GP's responsibilities.[43] Pregnant women therefore had to decide if they could afford the services of a GP or one of the new qualified midwives as their birth attendant or rely on the cheaper expedient of an unqualified 'handywoman'. Though effectively outlawed by the Midwives Act 1902, these 'Nurse Gamps' were still commonly found in working-class communities. Mabel Ramsay describes those she encountered in the slums of Glasgow, the incongruously known 'dicky birds', as 'ghoulish'.[44] Proving that they were still to be found in the 1930s, Somerset GP Kenneth Lane provides an example in the less than helpful 'Granny Perkins'.[45] Usage of midwives increased significantly during the First World War due to the shortage of doctors and the Midwives Act of 1916 enhanced their status through efforts to ensure that they were adequately trained.[46] GPs in London at this time charged 1–2 Guineas for a confinement depending on the status of the woman and ability to pay. Midwives typically charged only 12s 6d for a first birth and 10s for subsequent births.[47] But neither GPs nor midwives were accustomed at this time to provide antenatal care. In 1915, at the instigation of its Chief Medical Officer, Sir Arthur Newsholme, the LGB encouraged local authorities to establish free antenatal clinics based in maternity centres which were sometimes combined with infant welfare services.[48] A significant number did so which many pregnant women were happy to make use of and attendance at clinics, in London especially, increased throughout the interwar period. However, a significant percentage of working-class mothers were resistant to using these and related services, viewing them, as they did the input of local authority-employed health visitors, as unwelcome state interference in their personal lives.[49]

The LGB accepted the BMA's insistence that the work of maternity and infant welfare clinics should be confined to diagnosis and advice and that if the need for treatment was identified, mothers and children should be referred to GPs or to an appropriate hospital facility.[50] But, as already noted, some local authorities were already providing a range of treatment services. For example, a special hospital for babies was opened in Manchester in 1914.[51] The BMA's Medico Political Committee took a negative view of such developments, stating that 'removing maternal and childcare from general practitioners would not only undermine income; it will also alter the relationship of the doctor to his patients by segmenting medical care into parts handled exclusively by specialists'.[52] The Association also insisted that medical posts in the new clinics remained part-time and therefore likely to be occupied by local GPs. Dr Christine Pillman Williams, a member of the BMA's Ministry of Health Committee, reported on efforts to ensure that the Maternity Centres remained 'advisory and preventative and not for treatment' and 'to work the clinics with part-time medical officers selected from the GPs of the district'.[53] It has been suggested that the School Medical Services and infant welfare and maternity centres provided a secure and relatively easy source of income for many GPs, particularly for women doctors.[54] Newsholme, however, made no secret of his desire to establish a full-time salaried service and encouraged local authorities' efforts to achieve this.[55] His actions were condemned by the BMA but the black listing of such appointments (or 'black boxing' when advertised in the *BMJ*) did not diminish their appeal.[56] In 1916, the responsibility for the care of patients with Tuberculosis (TB) under NHI was transferred from the NHI commission to the LGB and local authorities were encouraged to establish TB centres and sanitoria in which many of the medical staff were employed on a whole-time basis.[57] They were at the same time asked to establish municipal centres for the treatment of venereal disease sufferers. The BMA again objected to positions in these centres being whole-time salaried, but many GPs viewed these activities as specialist work for which they were happy to relinquish responsibility.[58] The Association therefore contented itself with persuading the LGB to appoint local GPs as members of the committees set up to oversee the establishment of these services.[59] One prominent LMPC disagreed with this policy. The County Palatine of Chester LMPC wrote to the LGB arguing that GPs should be allowed to prescribe Salvarsan and other new treatments for venereal disease which they believed to be well within the competence of the average GP. In responding, the LGB declared itself to be in favour of drawing up a list of GPs entitled to do so by dint of their experience. When the local MOH, Dr Meredith Young, explained the administrative difficulties this would entail, however, the LMPC was forced to concede that it was impracticable.[60] The LMPC continued to monitor the operation of venereal disease clinics and in 1918 organised a lecture by Colonel L.W. Harrison, a nationally recognised expert, on 'The treatment of Venereal Disease in General Practice'.[61] They were also dismissive of the work of TB clinics and use of tuberculin which they described as an 'already somewhat discredited' treatment for the disease'.[62]

Pressure for comprehensive medical cover for women and children during the First World War coalesced with the idea of a Ministry of Health to coordinate the disparate forms of healthcare provision which were spread at that time between the LGB, the Board of Education, and the NHI Commission.[63] This was a dream shared by Addison, Morant, and Newman. However, in 1915, when the president of the LGB, Lord Rhondda, submitted proposals for a Maternity and Infant Welfare Bill to extend provision of treatment services under LGB control, they were condemned by opponents within government and the profession, who rightly saw in them an attempt to forestall proposals for a Ministry and prevent the LGB's abolition.[64] In a meeting with BMA representatives, Rhondda himself acknowledged that 'the Board had very few friends', a situation he attributed to its association with 'our antiquated poor law system'.[65] After praising Rhondda's desire to save the lives of the 50,000 infants who died prematurely each year, the *BMJ* set out the profession's objections, stating that as GPs were responsible for the health of the adult population, it would be 'a departure from a desirable continuity of method if a different system were encouraged in earlier years'. There was no justification, it said, for a separate class of practitioners dealing with expectant mothers and children, still less for these posts to be whole-time salaried. Anxious to quell the growing controversy, the coalition Prime Minister, Lloyd George, replaced Rhondda but his successor, Hayes Fisher, pressed ahead with a modified version of the LGB's maternity service proposals. The Maternity and Child Welfare Act passed in 1918 sanctioned the expansion of maternity and child welfare clinics which were empowered to provide treatment where it was reasonably required. But, in deference to medical opinion, it excluded domiciliary care.[66] In Cheshire, the LMPC pointedly approved the County Council's local scheme 'subject to the definite provision that clinical treatment shall not be undertaken except by, or through, the patient's own doctor'.[67] The Act did not, of course, prevent the enactment of a separate Ministry of Health Bill which was pushed through parliament with the support of the profession, the trade unions, and the Approved Societies in June 1919.[68] With Addison at its head, all key posts in the new Ministry went to NHI figures and it has been described as 'practically the old NHI Commission under another name'.[69] To the GPs' relief, Newsholme, who had not distinguished himself by his handling of the recent influenza epidemic, was passed over for the post of Chief Medical Officer in favour of his protégé, Newman, who was equally committed to improving the availability of medical services but was more appreciative of professional concerns.[70]

Like Newman, most local authorities and their local MOHs were anxious to avoid conflict with the profession locally and, by and large, the BMA succeeded in ensuring that local authority clinics confined themselves to advice and diagnosis. 'At most centres, mothers and children were usually examined by a nurse and a doctor, and referred to their own GP, if they had one, or other medical agency, if any problem were detected'.[71] The BMA was not alone in wanting the maternal and infant welfare services to focus on advice. There were many within the charitable sector and voluntarist movement who opposed free treatment on ideological grounds. The Charity Organisation Society remained strongly of the view that voluntary hospital provision and other medical services provided by ratepayers should be available only to the truly necessitous and opposed anything which inhibited self-reliance and thrift.[72] Many conservative reformers believed that infant mortality was the result of maternal ignorance and neglect and felt that the prime objective of the new maternity and infant welfare centres should be to educate working-class mothers in 'mothercraft'. Thus, the philosophy delivered in these centres has been described as being 'as close to the ideals of earlier charitable endeavours as to those of a welfare state'.[73] In many parts of London, however, a more interventionist approach was taken, and the authorities were less scrupulous about intruding into the GP's domain. In April 1920, the infant welfare centre in Ladbroke Grove, Kensington run by the GP Ethel Bentham was transformed into a baby hospital at which a range of treatment, including minor operations, was provided.[74] While focused on childcare education, many of the new centres began to provide other social facilities and sold Cod liver oil and malt and, later, vitamins, and materials for making baby clothes. Many medical and social welfare experts criticised this development, arguing, as the BMA said in a report in 1921, 'the people who go to them mainly for what they can get very cheaply, or for nothing, are not as a rule people who value or will benefit from the educational work of the centre'.[75] In 1926, however, the MOH for the Borough of Kensington praised the work of these centres, stating that they were responsible for the health of mothers and children being better than 25 years previously and that many of these mothers were now 'better educated than many women of the middle classes'. The expansion of maternity and child welfare services in the interwar period was significant. Between 1918 and 1938, the number of health visitors rose by 72%, and the number of infant welfare centres by 131%. Between 1923 and 1938, the number of antenatal clinics increased by 200%, with the number of women attending rising from 200,000 (33.89% of notified births) to 366,000 (66.72% of notified births).[76] Lara Marks concludes, however, that despite this, local authority maternal and child welfare provision was never so complete as its advocates asserted and that 'even where there was an abundance of such services poor social and economic conditions could undermine the benefits they brought'.[77]

Views of the MOH and the BMA's report on 'encroachments'

GPs' concerns at the expansion of local authority medical services were, as has been shown, fuelled by a fear that it would eventually result in the replacement of independent contractors by salaried employees. They feared that this would render GPs subordinate to the much-maligned local authority MOH. In the early twentieth century, public health was not regarded as a clinical specialty its own right and great many, if not the majority, of those who became MOHs were themselves GPs at one time or another. Some were mindful of professional anxieties and were respectful of the boundaries between preventative and curative medicine. Others, fired with reforming zeal, were happy to exceed those boundaries, while some antagonised their medical colleagues in the officious way they exercised their public health duties. This was either by means of diligent pursuit of the community interest, or by negligence, or self-interest, depending on the local profession's perception of them. In 1922, the *Medical World* columnist 'Hereward' accused the MOH as 'having an attitude of complete disregard for the existence of the GP' and 'contemplating the economic abasement or destruction of the GP with equanimity'.[78] Charles Webster summed up many GPs' contemptuous view of the MOH when stating 'to other doctors the MOH was an officious and bullying bureaucrat, presiding over an empire of clinics and institutions run along inhumane lines and delivering services of proportionately small benefit, considering the costs involved'.[79] Contemporaries sometimes used less judicious language. In 1930, the TUC's medical adviser, H.B. Morgan, described the typical MOH as 'insensitive' and 'grasping' and 'in fact no good at all, even at his own job of directing dustmen and supervising plumbers' work'.[80]

But were these criticisms justified? John Welshman is among those who have sought to rehabilitate the reputation of the interwar MOH. As he points out, many MOHs were both conscientious in their duties and respectful of their peers, in many cases battling heroically the vested interests of their local authority employers and unsympathetic Ministry officials.[81] Drs Andrew Topping in

Rochdale and James Middleton Martin in Gloucestershire, for example, who were highly respected by medical colleagues, impressed on their local government colleagues the necessity of maintaining harmonious relationships with GPs and worked hard to mitigate professional concerns.[82] In Cheshire, by contrast, the LMPC scrutinised the activities of the long-suffering MOH, Dr Meredith Young, through regular meetings and correspondence and it was clear that he feared to do anything without their approval.[83] The introduction of local authority clinics and health centres, and the creation of district general hospitals, before or after the transfer of the poor law infirmaries under the Local Government Act of 1929 were policy decisions over which the MOH might sometimes have had little influence.[84] Yet, the interwar MOH was, by virtue of his office, complicit, in GPs' eyes, with these 'encroachments' which many of them believed to be inimical to their economic security. The perception of the interwar MOH by later generations has been heavily influenced by the negative image of them found in the popular fiction of A.J. Cronin. In *The Citadel,* the local MOH, Dr Griffiths, is portrayed as a lazy and incompetent placeholder who wilfully ignores the local GPs' calls to address issues of urgent public health concern, including a dangerous leaking sewer.[85] As a counterpoint to the criticisms levelled at MOHs by GPs, when Alfred Cox conducted a survey into encroachments for the BMA's private practice committee in 1928, the MOHs he encountered were happy to respond to his requests for information and to give him the opportunity to investigate, without hindrance, the services under their control. He was heartened, he reported, at finding in so many areas harmonious relations between public health and other branches of the profession and thanked the MOHs he had met for their honesty and courtesy.[86]

The BMA's 1928 report on 'encroachments', which drew on the evidence from Cox's survey, offers an illuminating insight into the mindset of the profession at this time. It acknowledged that the work of maternity and child welfare centres needed doing and that much of it was best done 'collectively at centres' where 'nursing service is available under the direction of a medical practitioner'.[87] It asserted that maternity work was, however, within the capabilities of the GP 'if he was willing to lay himself out for this kind of work'. It regretted that many GPs already felt this to be work that 'they cannot or ought not to do'. It was effectively up to GPs, the committee thought, to rise to the challenge especially as regards the 'comparatively new development' of antenatal work. The report welcomed the increase in institutional maternity facilities provided by local authorities but felt that GPs should be responsible for overseeing the care in maternity homes and that, where the mother was without means, the local authority should pay the GP's fee.[88] Cox's investigations revealed that in many cases, children had been referred to infant centres by the GPs themselves. In Swindon, even though half the population was covered by the trade union-sponsored Great Western Railway Medical Service, the municipal service handled everything connected with children up to the age of 16 with the apparent blessing of local GPs.[89] He found few GPs doing antenatal work because, being to some extent 'new work' as he put it, older GPs were not trained to do it and it was generally considered uneconomic in that poor patients either could not or would not pay for it. On the question of whether doctors in local public services should be employed on a part-time or whole-time basis, the report was clear that the advantages of part-time employment outweighed the disadvantages.[90] Many MOHs had informed Cox that whole-time service was preferable in their view, from both an administrative and an ethical perspective, whereas others felt that part-time GPs brought with them a greater breadth of medical knowledge. The report concluded that employment of private practitioners on a part-time basis increased those individuals' interest in preventative medicine, whereas whole-time posts represented a career cul de sac in which demotivated employees would quickly lose interest in their work and become deskilled. However, the report omitted Cox's conclusion that some of the profession's concerns about encroachments were 'wrong or are exaggerated' and his finding that much of the 'highly necessary' work which GPs saw as having been taken away from them was work which 'would never have come their way'. As a further indictment of the prevailing system, he explained that this was because the vast majority of patients 'simply cannot afford to go to the doctor except when they are ill'.[91]

GPs and the demand for a national maternity service

For all the profession's protests, the GPs' record in all aspects of maternity care during the interwar period left much to be desired. The training of GPs in obstetrics was poor, as was cooperation between midwives and doctors.[92] GPs who specialised in obstetrics, such as Dr William Francis Oxley, an obstetric surgeon in Stepney and a lecturer in midwifery who became the first GP member of the Royal College of Obstetricians and Gynaecologists, despaired at their colleagues' clinical inadequacies. Oxley's stress on minimal obstetric interference and a policy of 'wait and see' resulted in a remarkably low rate of maternal mortality. He was among those supporting the Ministry of Health's wish to confine GP obstetrics to those with proven skills and experience.[93] Tensions between midwives and GPs at this time were commonplace.[94] Midwives complained that many GPs declined their requests to attend births in which complications arose, due to fear of the consequences.[95] The BMA meanwhile objected to any expansion in the midwives' role, including the ability to deliver anaesthesia.[96] Throughout the interwar period, the BMA argued that all doctors were competent to undertake midwifery but objected to calls for a departmental investigation into maternal deaths, presumably through fear that it would reflect badly on the profession.[97] However, the inquiry into Maternal Mortality conducted by Dame Janet Campbell in 1924 confirmed their fears, suggesting that the high puerperal mortality rate 'might be primarily assigned to the inadequacy of…professional attention'.[98] This finding is confirmed by Irvine Loudon who found that, in a study covering more than a century, one in three maternal deaths in Britain was attributable to poor obstetric practice.[99]

In 1929, in response to the growing chorus of criticism, the BMA set out its own proposals for a national maternity medical service.[100] The BMA's scheme minimised the need for maternity beds and role of the midwife, which put them at odds with Consultants and with those like Oxley who believed that only specially skilled and trained GPs should be permitted to deliver babies.[101] The scheme proposed that GPs handle all antenatal care and, Lewis says, threatened to relegate the midwife to the status of maternity nurse.[102] However, the BMA's scheme was not totally regressive and was not as anti-midwife as Lewis suggests. It did not require the attendance of the GP the birth at unless the patient and midwife thought it appropriate. It was also supportive of better and 'less punitive' education for midwives and the establishment of a second tier of supervising midwives, anticipating the rapid phasing out of unqualified 'handywomen' as soon as there were sufficient qualified midwives to replace them.[103] The BMA ducked the issue of improved training for GPs, however, saying that it was for the GMC to determine what form that should take, and that it was already making the necessary changes.[104] The salient feature of the BMA's scheme is the emphasis on GPs assuming complete responsibility for antenatal care, thereby confining the local authority clinics' role to advice and education.[105] Publicly provided antenatal care was widely available in London in the 1920s and increasing numbers of pregnant women used it.[106] However, in 1924, the MOH for Sheffield reported in the *Lancet* that there was virtually no antenatal care given outside London. He and other MOHs blamed women for not taking advantage of the services offered.[107] Nevertheless, the number of clinics continued to expand, from 995 in 1931 to 1,307 in 1937, by which time the percentage of women attending them had reached 54%. In rural areas where it was impractical to run such clinics, some local authorities resorted to paying GPs for antenatal examinations.[108] One example was Cheshire where the LMPC secretary, Dr Lionel Picton, had introduced a GP antenatal care scheme in 1916 when he was the MOH for the Winsford district.[109] When the County Council became responsible for maternal health services, the LMPC lobbied hard for that scheme to be extended across the county and in 1934 saw fit to remind their constituents that, under the scheme they had negotiated, the local authority would pay GPs 10s 6d for every antenatal examination they undertook.[110] Elsewhere, practices, such as the Felstead practice in Essex, offered antenatal care to mothers on a purely private basis.[111]

The BMA's scheme was predicated on the assumption that funding for the service would be available as an extension of NHI.[112] It also presupposed a degree of cooperation between relevant parties which, if enacted, would have gone a long way to improving maternal and infant safety. According to Marks, 'effective antenatal supervision…relied on a high degree of cooperation between midwives, general practitioners and hospital consultants which was rare in the interwar period'. A survey in 1925 found that only 46% of clinics communicated directly with the expectant mother's GP and midwife.[113] Critics of the BMA's scheme objected that the standard of care aimed at was still not as good as the kind of service which, for example, women's groups, such as the Women's Cooperative Guild, were demanding. But, while the profession's attitude to improving maternity care was condemned as self-interested and protectionist, there were some good examples of collaboration between GPs and other agencies which showed how standards could be improved where there was sufficient goodwill. In Rochdale, for example, which at one time had the highest maternal mortality rate in England, the MOH, Dr Andrew Topping, worked with the BMA and local organisations to develop a collective multi-agency approach to antenatal care. This drastically cut the rate from 9 per 1,000 in 1921 to 1.76 in 1932. He stated that this was entirely due to 'good cooperation between the doctor, the midwife, the health department and the local authority'.[114]

Elsewhere, the lack of improvement in mortality rates was such that the Ministry of Health decided it had to take action, and in 1929, it established a departmental committee to look into its causes. In its report published in 1932, the committee estimated that 46% of the deaths investigated were preventable. Of these, around 19% were attributable to errors of judgement by midwives or doctors, 3% due to lack of facilities, and 15% due to the absence of antenatal care.[115] The main cause of these avoidable deaths, they concluded, was poor medical supervision before and during birth. The principal causes of death during or immediately after childbirth at that time were puerperal fever and haemorrhages.[116] The risk of puerperal sepsis was far greater outside the sterile conditions of the hospital and GPs and midwives were often the unwitting conduits of infection. Responding to the report, the GP MP and later Labour minister, Dr Edith Summerskill, accurately diagnosed the problems faced by the GP in these situations. The main problem was that GPs were unable to devote their sole attention to midwifery while being frequently interrupted by the need to attend other urgent patients during the delivery. This increased the risk of infection, already heightened by the fact that many poor homes had insufficient hot water facilities for doctors to wash themselves. Added to this was the rudimentary and fragmentary nature of their antenatal provision, which meant that GPs often missed the early detection of serious problems like toxaemia and albuminuria.[117] It should not be forgotten, of course, that GPs were usually called in by midwives only when there were complications and when mother and baby were already at risk, which goes someway to explaining both the higher mortality rate where they were involved and their occasional reluctance to attend. In hospitals, obstetricians were better able to adopt a cautious approach, allowing nature to take its course, whereas GPs were more likely to adopt the more immediate and brutal expedient of a forceps delivery. In 1933, the Chief Medical Officer, Sir George Newman, estimated that GPs used forceps in 60% of all their maternity cases.[118] Ironically, richer mothers in Hampstead who employed a GP as their accoucheur faced a greater risk of dying than the poor mothers of Stepney. This was because the

GP 'faced far less regulation and supervision than midwives or hospital-based doctors, was often less rigorous in practising antisepsis, and more likely to intervene unnecessarily'.[119] Statistics appear to bear out this assertion. The rate of maternal deaths in Stepney and other boroughs, like Woolwich, in which there was some equivalent public maternal facility declined accordingly during the interwar period, whereas there was no significant decline in the more affluent borough of Hampstead.[120]

The recommendations of the Ministerial inquiry failed to bring about any improvement in the standard of training for GPs. Despite the prompting of those doctors who in 1929 succeeded in founding the Royal College of Obstetricians and Gynaecologists, there was no major overhaul in obstetric training in the interwar period for GPs already in practice before the 1930s and undergraduate training remained rudimentary at best. Improvements were made in the education and supervision of midwives which paved the way for the establishment of a salaried midwife service under local authority control under the Midwives Act 1936. The London County Council (LCC) chose to develop its own maternity services scheme involving 50 salaried midwives and in the late 1930s had drawn up plans to employ salaried obstetricians and an obstetric 'flying squad' to deal with emergencies.[121] The situation in Scotland, however, was somewhat different. Following the recommendations of the Cathcart Committee, which had been set up to consider the possibility of extending NHI to dependents, the Scottish Health Board introduced its own maternity services scheme in 1937. But, while local authorities were permitted to employ salaried doctors, they were encouraged to use GP-independent contractors working alongside midwives. The Board saw it as an experiment to 'test the validity of founding public medicine upon a private contract basis'. The BMA recognised the significance of the experiment, but their endorsement did not ensure its success. A significant proportion of Scottish GPs declined to participate in the scheme because the fees were too low and midwives and other professionals involved complained about the GPs' shortcomings and declined to give the scheme their full support. The experiment was adjudged to be a failure therefore and in Glasgow the local authority later exercised its option to employ salaried obstetricians.[122]

Fortunately, the maternal mortality rate began to decline sharply both in Scotland and in the rest of Britain during the late 1930s. Experts generally ascribe this to the impact of the new wonder drug, Prontosil, and the highly effective sulphonamides which followed.[123] Another contributing factor was the increasing preference of women for hospital births. At the turn of the twentieth century, most women were delivered of babies in their own homes, but the situation was markedly different by the 1930s when increasing numbers of women were confined and delivered in hospitals and maternity homes and had little contact with GPs.[124] In 1925, the voluntary hospitals in London were admitting 10,000 pregnancies per year and in 1934 hospitals and maternity homes accounted for 51% of all births in the capital.[125] Across the country, the number of institutional deliveries rose from 15% in 1927 to 25% in 1937.[126] For working-class women, it was not just faith in the quality of institutional care which led to this rise. Over-crowding and poor housing made hospital seem a less stressful environment to have their babies. As early as 1913 Stepney's East End Maternity Home declared that 'the best place for a poor woman to be confined in is not her own home'.[127] Although specialist doctors, and even a good many GPs, agreed, the Ministerial inquiry concluded that, overall, the evidence suggested that home births were still safer and cheaper and that hospital admission should be reserved for high-risk cases and emergencies, and 'social admissions' in rare cases only.[128] In 1934, only 25% of 26,000 domiciliary confinements were attended by GPs and the trend towards hospital births continued up to and including the Second World War.[129] By that time, many GPs shared their Consultant colleagues' view that hospital was often the safest place for a woman to deliver her baby, but the GPs' leaders were determined that family doctors should be the main coordinators of the pregnant woman's care before and after childbirth and the individual respon-sible for ensuring that appropriate medical care was provided, directly or indi-rectly, whether the woman was delivered at home or in hospital.[130] In the revised version of their maternity scheme which they presented to the joint BMA/TUC joint committee on medical questions in 1937, the BMA continued to express a preference for home over hospital births except where there were complica-tions.[131] Looking at maternity care as a whole during the interwar period, how-ever, the number of variables makes it difficult to reach definitive conclusions, leading Jane Lewis to state: 'It is impossible to determine the relative safety of doctors versus midwives and home versus hospital during this period'.[132]

The Local Government Act 1929 and local authority hospital provision

As the BMA put together its Maternity Medical Services scheme, it did so know-ing that developments were taking place which greatly enhanced responsibilities of local authorities in the area of personal healthcare. Both the McLean Report of 1918 and the Betterton Committee of 1922 had called for the breakup of the poor law administration.[133] It was the inability of that administration to deal with the problems of unemployment in the 1920s, however, which finally persuaded government to replace it with a new system under the Local Government Act of 1929. The legislation finally disposed of the principle of less eligibility and transferred the poor law infrastructure to local authority control. Local author-ity care of the sick was now the responsibility of new public health committees, and the relief of poverty and unemployment was assigned to new public assis-tance committees. Clauses in the Act dealing with the appropriation of poor law medical infirmaries were, however, permissive rather than prescriptive in nature and the lack of centralised direction from the Ministry of Health meant that they were not universally acted upon.[134] It was the county Boroughs in England

and Wales which were most likely to seize the opportunity of changing hospital provision.[135] Elsewhere, the reluctance to appropriate the infirmaries could be put down to a host of variables including the (un)suitability of the accommodation, the availability of alternative provision under municipal voluntary schemes, the attitudes of the respective public health and public assistance committees, and the financial situation of the relevant authority.[136] With no effective power to enforce appropriation or improvement of facilities, the Ministry of Health could only guide and urge councils to act. Financial concerns were often a barrier to improvement, as expenditure on poor law infirmaries represented a heavy drain on borough coffers.[137] The system of central government block grants introduced in 1929 had little positive effect as the formula used to calculate them worked to the disadvantage of smaller authorities.[138]

In the 1930s, a Ministry survey found a wide variety of council-run institutions, some of which justified the description of them later given by Aneurin Bevan as 'monstrous buildings, a cross between the workhouse and a barracks – or a prison'.[139] In some areas, the public assistance committees were composed primarily of ex-Guardians who resisted appropriation by public health, preferring to maintain the link between the infirmaries and means-tested public assistance. In Stockport, for instance, the Ministry's inspectors regretted that 'the Guardians still reign supreme'.[140] Infirmaries with large numbers of chronically sick or elderly patients were often less likely to be appropriated as borough councils focused on improving provision for acute cases. There was therefore ample evidence of a two-tier municipal service for the sick poor. Sometimes, facilities for those who could be actively treated were improved at the cost of those who required palliative care only.[141] According to surveys conducted by the Ministry and the Nuffield hospitals trust in 1938, the unappropriated public assistance institutions housed around 15% of total hospital beds compared with 35% in the voluntary hospitals and 50% in the municipal hospitals. Alysa Levene comments that 'the poor law infirmaries could therefore be viewed pessimistically as a dumping ground for the least clinically interesting patients with the least chance of recovery, or optimistically as places specializing in the care of the chronically sick'.[142] Their facilities were undoubtedly poorer, with less equipment or staff. By 1937, only 37 county Boroughs, that is less than 50%, and nine county councils, less than 20%, had appropriated workhouse infirmaries.[143] Of the 22 infirmaries appropriated by county councils in England and Wales, half of those were in Middlesex and Surrey, while in Scotland, 'similar legislation produced little change outside Glasgow'.[144]

A historical research project on municipal medicine supported by the Wellcome Trust in the 2000s failed to identify conclusively the causes of variation in local authority provision, other than noting a strong correlation between expenditure and population size.[145] Local case studies highlighted the impact of, variously, the political outlook of key decision makers, the attitude of the Ministry of Health, the local existence of progressive institutions and energetic reformers, civic pride and competition, class, gender, and local attitudes towards charity, self-help, and community spirit.[146] Appropriation did not of itself signify a determination on the part of the local authority to invest in or development public hospital facilities. Some authorities were big investors, whereas others lacked the will or the means. Some evidenced intermittent progress, others stagnation of appropriated facilities which led to them being condemned by Ministerial surveyors along with those who had not appropriated at all.[147] In a study of local authority provision in Devon, Julia Neville found champions and opponents of intervention among councillors of every political affiliation. But while some saw their accountability as being to the community at large, others saw it as owing to the ratepayers; some were more inclined towards civic philanthropy, whereas others favoured self-help and a correctional approach.[148] Commenting on the standard of municipal hospital provision generally, Charles Webster stated:

> where permissive powers were applied to the utmost degree, when rate revenue was buoyant and where the local Medical Officer of Health was sympathetic to modern developments, the standard of service bore comparison with later counterparts in the National Health Service.[149]

The worst public services were, however, justly censured by the Labour MP Fred Messer as 'the last word in a despairing effort to dodge obligations'.[150] Cherry concludes therefore that 'the concept of the hospital as a supporting service for community care remained underdeveloped'.[151]

The greatest development of municipal medicine took place in London and especially after 1934 when the Labour party won a large majority of seats on the LCC and maintained its dominant position there until well after the Second World War. Encouraged by prominent doctors who in 1930 had formed the Socialist Medical Association (SMA), the LCC seized the opportunity to appropriate the best of the workhouse infirmaries and convert them into general hospitals while establishing de novo a number of new municipal general hospitals open to all and paid for largely out of ratepayer revenues. In its 1935 pamphlet 'London Under Socialist Rule', Labour's Council leader Herbert Morrison boasted that 30 London hospitals had now been enlarged, modernised, and improved and that they aimed to do the same for the remainder of the 74 existing.[152] This prompted Sir George Newman to comment that the LCC was now 'greatest Local Health Authority in the Empire' and 'the largest single provider of hospital beds in Britain if not the world'.[153] The ambitions of the LCC in this regard owed much to the efforts of the chair of its Hospitals and Medical Services committee, the SMA founder, Consultant physician, and Labour MP, Somerville Hastings.[154] Supported by his GP colleagues Charles Brook, Alfred Salter, and Edith Summerskill, and by the Consultant David Stark Murray, he sought to develop the LCC hospitals into a beacon of municipal excellence. Whether they achieved that goal is debatable. In the 1940s, the socialist GP, Labour MP and Peer,

Dr Stephen Taylor, the founder of Medical Planning Research, punctured Hastings' claims for the superiority of municipal medicine in London when describing his 'bitter experience' of an LCC hospital which he described as 'the worst-run in which he had ever worked'.[155] The mostly Conservative GPs and Consultants working in the London voluntary hospitals over which the LCC in the 1930s sought condominium were fearful of the latter's growing power. The formerly honorary Consultants had largely reconciled themselves to becoming part-time salaried but had done so without sacrificing one iota of their professional independence to their charitable trust employers.[156] They feared that this would not continue to be the case if the voluntary hospitals came under LCC control. Eckstein observes that 'class contempt' was an element in the profession's hostility towards local government, owing to the stereotyping of local councillors as power-hungry 'petit bourgeois'.[157] This was a view acknowledged in the 1940s by the Ministry of Health official Niven McNichol, who observed that the doctors' objection to control 'by the local butcher or baker' was 'partly snobbish and partly a genuine reaction against people who are not merely uniformed but have not allowed the expert to get on with his job'.[158] The vocal objections of GPs in London to the LCC's ambitions helped fuel the distrust of local government by GPs in other areas and, as will be seen in the next chapter, led to a general paranoia about the prospect of GPs working in local authority-built or managed health centres.

The distribution of acute hospital provision in Britain in the early twentieth century showed a noticeable bias towards London where the major teaching hospitals monopolised the services of leading specialists.[159] Following the First World War, they struggled to cope with increased demand for their free services in view of ever-rising costs and resorted to innovative means of fundraising in order to maintain their status as independent charitable institutions.[160] Similar institutions could be found in most major cities where the only alternatives were the poor law infirmaries and a small but increasing number of municipal general hospitals set up by local authorities. Of the poor law infirmaries appropriated by local authorities between 1929 and 1938, one-fifth (109) were redesignated general hospitals and 74 for special purposes.[161] With 2/3 of all hospital beds, the public sector had only 1/3 of hospital medical staffs and one teaching hospital, Hammersmith. London still had twice as many public hospital beds per 1,000 population as other cities and large towns in 1938 and four times more per 1,000 than in the county council areas.[162] Rising bed occupancy rates in the voluntary hospitals contributed to the fact that one in three hospital patients was treated in them in 1938 compared with one in four between 1891 and 1921.[163] The London hospitals experienced a tripling of costs over the period 1913–1938. Most of them therefore had chronic financial difficulties.[164] Faced with a decline in traditional subscription income, all the voluntary hospitals sought to abandon the subscriber recommendation system and introduced inpatient charges while embracing hospital contributory schemes which allowed individuals of modest means to afford and spread the costs of hospital treatment when needed.[165] Membership of these contributory schemes reached 6.3 million in 1933 and 10.3 million by 1938. In 1935, they provided 27% of provincial hospital income.[166] However in Cherry's analysis in more than half the hospitals studied, it was more than 50% in the late 1930s.[167] By the 1920s, private patients were admitted to the majority of voluntary, poor law, and municipal hospitals. Private wards, blocks, and insurance schemes for the middle classes rapidly followed, boosting hospital, and indirectly Consultant, incomes.[168] Pay beds allowed the voluntary hospitals to 'acquire a dual character'.[169] New and more regular sources of income were not enough, however, to rescue the large London teaching hospitals from debt. Faced with a continuing insufficiency, they sought support from the Ministry who directed them to initiate discussions with the LCC. These discussions were marred by a mutual distrust founded on widely differing ideologies and little progress was made.[170] As the Second World War approached, therefore, the threatened insolvency of the major London voluntary hospitals and the instability of their counterparts in the provinces due to the variation in funding sources represented a conundrum for central government to which hospital nationalisation seemed at that time the most unlikely and unappealing solution.

GPs in their element? Cottage hospitals and nursing homes

What did GPs collectively think of hospital services at this time and what contribution did they make, if any, to what they provided? At the turn of the twentieth century, GPs had largely come to accept the distinction between themselves and Consultants, the evident benefits of specialisation, and the utility of the referral system. The hostility some had shown towards Consultant colleagues following the rapid increase in outpatient numbers in the 1880s and 1890s, when they were accused of taking bread out of the GPs' mouths, rapidly abated after 1900 when efforts were made by the hospitals to restrict the 'misuse' of their charitable facilities. The increased use of hospital almoners enquiring into patients' personal circumstances helped reduce numbers of both inpatients and outpatients.[171] Moreover, when the National Insurance Act was introduced in 1913, it achieved, according to Keir Waddington, something hospital doctors and GPs had not been able to do 'by reducing admissions and making outpatient departments serve a more consultative role'.[172] Nevertheless, the continuing popularity of outpatients during the interwar period meant that in 1931, the BMA complained that this 'abuse' was still as pressing as ever and its Representative Body approved a report that year titled 'The Problem of the Out-Patient' in which it outlined further measures to curtail this development.[173] The BMA's support for Public Medical Services Schemes was boosted by concern at a report by the Outpatient Committee of the King Edward's Hospital Fund in 1933 which suggested that hospital doctors could manage the follow-up of patients in the community through delegated district nursing services.[174] GPs were largely powerless to prevent their gradual exclusion from hospital work but it was not as complete or as universal as Frank Honigsbaum and others have assumed. Honigsbaum admits that GPs specialising in specific areas of medicine continued to enjoy admitting rights to voluntary hospital beds, but were denied the title of Consultant, being sometimes described instead as 'Consultands' or 'Consultoids'.[175] While these had all but disappeared from the major teaching hospitals in London by the 1930s, these GP specialists continued to exercise a significant role in many provincial general hospitals up to and including the Second World War.[176] In the 1930s, however, the provident sickness insurance schemes on which the hospitals came to rely for income in respect of the increasing number of pay beds insisted on confining re-imbursement of the costs of treatment to that rendered by bona fide Consultants and not the GP sub-specialists.[177] When this was extended beyond the London hospitals, GPs began to relinquish the honorary hospital posts they had some-times occupied or were replaced in the provincial general hospitals by some of the expanding cadre of newly qualified Consultants. The number of Consultants and accredited specialists increased steadily throughout the twentieth century but before the Second World War, their number was still considered insufficient to meet the demand for their services and they were outnumbered by GPs by a ratio of 5:1.[178] This left plenty of scope for GPs to occupy the middle ground between family medicine and specialist practice.

The mixed economy of hospital care included many GPs keen to expand the boundaries of the practice, although sometimes venturing dangerously beyond the limitations of their personal skill and knowledge.[179] Their principal arena was the cottage hospital where GPs reigned supreme in an environment that was gen-erally less regulated than other medical institutions and where they were answer-able only to their peers and to (largely respectful) committees of middle-class charitable trustees and local benefactors. Between 1900 and 1936, the number of cottage hospitals in Britain doubled from around 300 to around 600 by which time they accounted for around 10,000 beds.[180] As an article in the *BMJ* in 1929 correctly asserted, these were very definitely GP hospitals.[181] About one in five GPs had access to beds in these institutions in the 1930s.[182] Initially funded by charitable donations from local benefactors and supported by community fund-raising initiatives, and later with the additional support of local or national con-tributory schemes, the cottage hospitals catered for patients needing emergency surgery or non-complex acute operations and short-term management of acute or chronic conditions within the competence of local GPs.[183] They were given a boost by the increasing volume of road accidents which occurred in the interwar period.[184] The Devon cottage hospitals described by Julia Neville were typical 'in developing a niche in emergency and elective surgery in addition to their origins as safe places for nursing of respiratory diseases or treatment of accidents'.[185] Appealing to their community spirit and civic pride, GPs persuaded governing committees to establish minor operating theatres where, with minimal scrutiny, they practised their surgical and diagnostic skills on an unsuspecting public.[186]

Many cottage hospitals enjoyed the kind of facilities advocated by the Dawson Report for putative primary health centres, like X-ray machines, electrotherapy, hydrotherapy, and massage, while a smaller number had laboratory facilities and ambulance services.[187]

As with the rest of the mixed economy, standards of care, equipment, and cleanliness were variable and perhaps lower than the standards of the larger voluntary hospitals. While GPs were hardly at the cutting edge of technological developments in medicine, the generation of doctors attending medical schools in the early decades of the twentieth century was sufficiently well versed in the use of anaesthesia and X-rays for those of them with appropriate skills and aptitude to undertake a great deal more surgery than many of their predecessors would have attempted. These included appendectomies, mastectomies, hysterectomies, and skin grafts.[188] In the novel *Dr Bradley Remembers*, the newly endowed cottage hospital is a place where the hero's younger rivals relish the opportunity to cultivate their reputation as surgeons. Bradley comments resignedly, 'In his day, surgery had been a special prerogative of the consultant; no ordinary practitioner like himself had ever dared to embark on a major operation'.[189] In his earlier novel, *My Brother Jonathan*, Young gives a good description of how cottage hospitals were administered in the interwar period, how access to beds and operating rights were apportioned, and were affected by petty jealousies and feuds between competing local doctors.[190] Kenneth Lane, himself one of the younger generation of GPs in the 1930s, comments in his memoir:

> The variety of our work was astounding. We were general and orthopaedic surgeons, physicians, obstetricians, gynaecologists and pathologists. We did our own blood transfusions with the antique method of tube and funnel, our own post mortems in primitive conditions and all our maternity in the homes of our patients.[191]

In 1938–1939, according to a later study by Bradford Hill, some 2.5 million surgical operations were performed by GPs in cottage hospitals, an average of three per doctor per week.[192] Thinking perhaps of Honigsbaum's contested hypothesis, Cherry states that, based on the number of operations performed in Cottage hospitals in the 1930s, 'descriptions of the GP as victim in the division of medical skills can be exaggerated'.[193]

Some observers, including the independent think tank PEP in their report on 'The British Health Services', were critical of the quality of care in these institutions.[194] Some claimed that it represented medical practice at its worst. On GP surgeons' reputation for poor quality work, Sir Arthur Newsholme commented, 'I suspect that a similar statement might truthfully be made about their work in the medical and specialist departments'.[195] In the *Lancet* in May 1930, E.W. Hay-Groves, professor of surgery at the University of Bristol, agreed that there was 'a great deal of bad surgical work in smaller hospitals', but added that 'this is really no reflection upon the professional attainments of the staff. They are being asked to carry out an impossible task, that of being general practitioners and also specialists at the same time'.[196] However, the continuing popularity of cottage hospitals suggests that outcomes cannot necessarily have been as bad as their critics alleged, and the historian of the cottage hospitals, Dr Emrys-Roberts, states, 'There was many a GP surgeon who, by carefully restricting his repertoire, achieved considerable competence within a certain range of operations'.[197] One such GP was Dr Hackney of Ongar who, with his assistant, in a four-year period from 1928 to 1932 admitted 1,086 patients and carried out 700 operations and 5,122 outpatient attendances.[198] Some cottage hospitals, for example, the Cromwell Hospital in Cromer, Norfolk, enjoyed an excellent reputation.[199] The cottage hospitals' GP staffs were accused of over-ambitious and bad surgical work but, like the workhouse infirmary MOs, they were usually prepared to call in specialists to assist, direct, or undertake more complex surgery when necessary, and referred their patients to the voluntary or municipal hospitals when the most complex operations were required.[200] However, they considered most emergency treatment well within their capabilities. When describing one such case, Kenneth Lane admits in his memoir:

> It may seem strange that we didn't telephone the nearest major hospital twelve miles away and ask them to admit the perforation. The answer is that such an idea would never occur to us. We had an operating theatre, a hospital bed, we did our own surgery and that was that.[201]

Cherry states that 'small children, along with women in childbirth, were probably most affected by adverse results of overzealous medical intervention'.[202] Today, removal of tonsils and adenoids is considered largely unnecessary but was considered by the bulk of the profession at that time as entirely appropriate and advisable.[203] Consultants were just as likely, however, to undertake unnecessary surgery and their criticisms of the quality of work performed by GPs in cottage hospitals may have been influenced by a perceived loss of income.[204]

From the outset, cottage hospitals had admitted a small number of private patients.[205] As Cherry has shown in his study of cottage hospitals in East Anglia, in the 1930s, many found it beneficial to establish contributory schemes which ensured that their services were accessible to a wider section of the local community.[206] This encouraged links with large hospitals such as the Norfolk and Norwich as it enabled subscribers to the schemes to benefit from something more like complete secondary care provision.[207] The same was true of the trade union-run schemes in South Wales where, as Steven Thompson has shown, doctors in Medical Aid Society-run cottage hospitals referred patients for specialist treatment at the municipal hospitals of Cardiff, Newport, Swansea, and even Bristol and London.[208] Admission to cottage hospitals was determined by a host of variables and was not infrequently denied to both the rich, who were excluded from contributory schemes and might instead choose to occupy a private room in a voluntary hospital or nursing home, and the destitute, who were obliged to make use of the workhouse infirmary. With their lack of accommodation for the chronically sick and the most acute cases, the cottage hospitals were, however, of limited significance as regards welfare provision in its most general sense. Their role was consequently marginal to the consideration of provision under the National health Service (NHS) and did not feature in discussions between the BMA and the government over the nationalisation of hospitals.[209]

Cottage hospitals were not the only form of institutional care with which GPs were involved. While hospitals tended to address the need for acute medical care, individuals needing longer term medical or nursing care, convalescence or rehabilitation and who could afford to pay for it were accommodated in nursing homes. Medical oversight of patients in nursing homes was not exclusively the preserve of GPs – Consultants also accommodated their recuperating private patients in them. According to Harry Eckstein, they were 'frequently nothing more than adjuncts to the offices of eminent specialists'.[210] However, nursing home attendances boosted GPs' income from private practice and a significant number of GPs saw the benefit of opening their own nursing homes, among the most successful of these being BMA Council member E. Rowland Fothergill.[211] Despite being poorly staffed, under-equipped, and housed in often inappropriate accommodation, nursing homes catered almost exclusively for the wealthy middle and upper classes who, due to class considerations, 'zealously avoided hospitalization'.[212] The number of nursing home beds grew steadily during the early twentieth century and almost certainly exceeded the number of pay beds in hospitals. In 1928, there were 3,000–4,000 in the London area compared with only 1,000 pay beds in the voluntary hospitals and in 1921 there were estimated to be around 26,000 nursing homes beds in England and Wales.[213] Legislation introducing inspection and monitoring of nursing homes in 1927 led to many homes changing their designation from nursing to convalescent homes. This contributed to the increase in the number of beds in the latter from 13,000 to 26,000 between 1921 and 1938 and the smaller decrease in the number of nursing home beds from 26,000 to 22,500 during the same period.[214] Some GPs, including Fothergill, saw this development as another means by which the economic stability of general practice was being slowly undermined and this spurred his frequent yet ultimately unsuccessful attempts to challenge the Consultants' efforts to deny GPs hospital admitting rights and specialist recognition.

Conclusion

GPs in the interwar period continued to feel insecure about their position within the mixed economy of healthcare. Having seen off and largely neutralised the Approved Societies' attempts to control them within the field of NHI, they were unnerved by the efforts of local authorities and their supporters within government and within the profession itself, to provide publicly funded alternatives to their services for the poor and those excluded from NHI. Doctors feared that if this trend continued, as it showed every sign of doing in London and other large metropolitan areas in particular, the days of the independent contractor GP were numbered and that their professional autonomy would be eradicated. This was at a time, moreover, when, due to advances in medical practice and public expectations of healthcare, GPs were being gradually shut out of hospital medicine. Their discomfiture was alleviated by the control they continued to exercise over the not inconsiderable part of the healthcare economy occupied by the cottage hospitals and nursing homes. This was perhaps more important than many historians, with their eyes fixed on the expansion of secondary care under the subsequent NHS, may have appreciated.

Cherry states that when viewing this period, it could be argued that in the best cases, the cottage hospitals allowed GPs to group and develop some specialist skills and overcome their professional isolation.[215] As PEP, echoing the BMA, had noted, here was a potential place for group practice or community healthcare without the implied threat of local government control.[216] In his obituary in 1948, the Cheshire LMPC secretary Lionel Picton was hailed as a champion of the cottage hospital who 'held that for many areas properly equipped cottage hospitals would constitute the organised method of group practice called for in the National Health Service proposals'.[217] Some historians focusing on interwar hospital provision have suggested that the criticisms of it by centralising reformers have been overstated, and that the municipal hospitals in particular had the potential to evolve into an equally comprehensive, efficient, yet locally controlled, alternative to the NHS.[218] While stretching the point a little, the same argument could perhaps be applied to cottage hospitals and Public Medical Services run by GPs. This assumes, of course, that whatever alternatives to a State Medical Service the profession itself could put forward encompassed appropriate links between GPs, hospitals, and public health services. This, as will be seen in the next chapter, was something which most of the profession had difficulty coming to terms with during the interwar period, though, as will be shown, their collective vision was by no means as narrow or as self-interested as their critics alleged.

Notes

1 *BMJ*, 10 July 1920, Report of BMA Annual Meeting, Proceedings of Medical Sociology section, Sir George Newman, 'The Future of Medical Practice', p. 35.
2 Of special significance is the Wellcome project on Municipal medicine in the early 2000s involving, *inter alia*, Alysa Levene, Becky Taylor, Martin Powell, and John Stewart (see references below and bibliography).
3 See, *inter alia*, Paul Bridgen, Stephen Cherry, Margaret Crowther, Martin Gorsky, George Gosling, Steven King, Jane Lewis, Lara Marks, Keir Waddington, and John Welshman (see references below and bibliography).
4 These comprise works by Cherry, Gorsky et al., Gosling, Powell, and Waddington; and by Barry Doyle, Nick Hayes, Donnacha Lucey, Esyllt Jones, Hilary Marland, Lara Marks, Angela Negrine, Julia Neville, John Pickstone, Jonathan Reinarz, Sally Sheard, Steven Thompson, and Tim Willis (see references below and bibliography).

5 See, *inter alia*, Paul Bridgen, Geoffrey Finlayson, Gorsky et al., Gosling, Levene, John Mohan, and Keir Waddington (see references below and bibliography).
6 See, for example, essays by Roger Cooter and John Pickstone, Paul Weindling and Charles Webster in R. Cooter and J. Pickstone (eds) *Companion to Medicine in the Twentieth Century, Production, Community and Consumption: The Political Economy of Twentieth Century Medicine* (London, 2000).
7 Jose Harris, *William Beveridge: A Biography* (2nd edn., Oxford, 2003). pp. 143, 148.
8 Pat Thane, *Foundations of the Welfare State* (2nd edn., Harlow, 1996). p. 68.
9 *Ibid.*, p. 67.
10 Margaret Anne Crowther, *The Workhouse System, 1934–1929: The History of an English Social Institution* (London, 1981). p. 173.
11 Steven King, 'Poverty, Medicine and the Workhouse,' in Jonathan Reinarz and Leonard Schwarz (eds) *Medicine and the Workhouse* (Rochester, NJ, 2013). p. 238.
12 Crowther, *The Workhouse System,* p. 173.
13 *Ibid.*, p. 171.
14 *Ibid.*, p. 182.
15 Steven Cherry, *Medical Services and the Hospitals in Britain, 1860–1939* (Cambridge, 1996), p. 55; Crowther, *The Workhouse System,* p. 182.
16 Crowther, *The Workhouse System,* p. 183.
17 *Ibid.*, p. 184.
18 *Ibid.*
19 *Ibid.*, p. 185 and King, 'Poverty, Medicine and the Workhouse', p. 238.
20 Crowther, *The Workhouse System,* pp. 185–186.
21 *Ibid.*, p. 186.
22 Rosemary Stevens, *Medical Practice in Modern England: The Impact of Specialization and State Medicine* (New Haven, CT, 1966). p. 286.
23 See *BMJ*, 13 July 1918, Sir Bertrand Dawson, 'The Future of the Medical Profession' (The Cavendish Lecture). p. 25.
24 See Beatrice & Sidney Webb, *The State and the Doctor* (London, 1910). pp. 211–227.
25 *Ibid.*, p. 257.
26 See Chris Renwick, *Bread for All: The Origins of The Welfare State* (2nd edn., London, 2018). p. 58.
27 See *Medical World*, 21 August 1913, Editorial 'The Future of the Panel Doctor', p. 103.
28 *Ibid.*, 15 January 1914 'The Medical Man and National Health Insurance', Lecture by Sir John Collie, and 'Defects in the Act and their Remedy', pp. 94–99. *BMJ*, 24 January 1914, Supplement, pp. 38–40, letter from Dr Milson Russen Rhodes and the response by Dr J. Charles, *BMJ*, 14 February 1914, Supplement, p. 82.
29 Seebohm Rowntree, *Poverty: A Study of Town Life* (London, 1901). *passim*; Bentley B. Gilbert 'Health and Politics: The British Physical Deterioration Report of 1904.' *Bulletin of the History of Medicine*, 39 (2) (1965). pp. 143–153.
30 Frank Honigsbaum, *The Division in British Medicine: A History of the Separation of General Practice from Hospital Care* (London, 1979). p. 34.
31 Lara Marks, *Metropolitan Maternity: Maternal and Infant Welfare Services in Early Twentieth Century London* (Amsterdam, 1996). p. 177.
32 Cherry, *Medical Services and the Hospitals,* p. 50.
33 Marks, *Metropolitan Maternity,* p. 72.
34 Hilary Marland 'A Pioneer in Infant Welfare: the Huddersfield Scheme, 1903–1920.' *Social History of Medicine*, 6 (1) (1993). pp. 25–50.
35 Thane, *Foundations of the Welfare State,* p. 72.
36 Jane Lewis, *The Politics of Motherhood: Child and Maternal Welfare in England 1900–1939* (London, 1980). pp. 409–410.

37 Marks, *Metropolitan Maternity*, p. 178.
38 John Welshman, *Municipal Medicine: Public Health in Twentieth Century Britain* (Oxford, 2000). pp. 175–176.
39 *Cheshire County PRO*, NHL 7135/1/, Minutes of a meeting of the County Palatine of Chester LMPC on 6 August 1915.
40 Frank Honigsbaum, *The Struggle for the Ministry of Health, 1914–1919* (London, 1970). p. 31.
41 John Mottram, 'State Control in Local Context: Public Health and Midwife Regulation in Manchester, 1900–1914,' in Hilary Marland and Anne Marie Rafferty (eds) *Midwives, Society and Childbirth: Debates and Controversies in the Modern Period* (London, 1997). pp. 136–139.
42 *Ibid.*, pp. 140–141.
43 Honigsbaum, *The Struggle for the Ministry of Health*, p. 33.
44 Mabel Ramsay, *The Doctor's Zig-Zag Road*, Unpublished autobiography, Royal College of Physicians, London, p. 49.
45 Kenneth Lane, *Diary of a Medical Nobody* (London, 1982). pp. 119–123.
46 Thane, *Foundations of the Welfare State*, pp. 126–127; Frank Honigsbaum, *The Struggle for the Ministry of Health, 1914–1919* (London, 1970), p. 33.
47 Lewis, *The Politics of Motherhood*, p. 141.
48 Honigsbaum, *The Division in British Medicine*, p. 33.
49 Lewis, *The Politics of Motherhood*, pp. 106–107.
50 Marks, *Metropolitan Maternity*, p. 181.
51 Cherry, *Medical Services and the Hospitals*, p. 50.
52 *BMA Archive*, B/231/1/2, minutes of the Medico Political Committee meeting on 8 January 1915.
53 Joyce Cockram 'The Federation and the British Medical Association.' *Journal of the Medical Women's Federation*, 49 (1967). pp. 77–78.
54 John Welshman, *Municipal Medicine Public Health in Twentieth Century Britain* (Oxford, 2000), p. 274.
55 Honigsbaum, *The Division in British Medicine*, p. 35.
56 Jay Winter, *The Great War and the British People* (2nd edn., Basingstoke, 2003). p. 174.
57 Honigsbaum, *The Division in British Medicine*, p. 35.
58 *Ibid.*
59 Winter, *The Great War and the British People*, p. 177.
60 *Cheshire County PRO*, NHL 7135/2, minutes of a meeting of the County Palatine of Chester LMPC on 7 October 1917, pp. 1–2.
61 *Ibid.*, NHL 7135/3, minutes of special meeting on 14 September 1918.
62 *Ibid.*, NHL 7135/1, minutes of County Palatine of Chester LMPC meeting on 6 August 1916, letter to LGB, p. 5.
63 Honigsbaum, *The Division in British Medicine*, pp. 23–25.
64 Honigsbaum, *The Struggle for the Ministry of Health*, pp. 37–44.
65 *BMJ*, 31 March 1917, 'Maternity, Child Welfare and a Ministry of Health, pp. 430–431.
66 Honigsbaum, *The Struggle for the Ministry of Health*, p. 37. Bernard Harris, *The Origins of the British Welfare State: Social Welfare in England and Wales, 1800–1945* (Basingstoke, 2004). pp. 324–235.
67 *Cheshire County PRO*, NHL 7135/2, Minutes of a meeting of the County Palatine of Chester LMPC on 16 September 1917, resolution 4.
68 Honigsbaum, *The Struggle for the Ministry of Health*, p. 39.
69 *Ibid.*, p. 56.
70 *Ibid.*, p. 51.
71 Marks, *Metropolitan Maternity*, p. 181.

72 Keir Waddington, 'Unsuitable Patients: The Debate Over Outpatient Admissions, the Medical Profession and the Late Victorian Hospitals.' *Medical History*, 42 (1998). p. 28.

73 Lewis, *The Politics of Motherhood*, p. 220.

74 Marks, *Metropolitan Maternity*, p. 72.

75 *Ibid.*, p. 180. Lewis, *The Politics of Motherhood*, p. 105.

76 Harris, *The Origins of the British Welfare State*, p. 235.

77 Marks, *Metropolitan Maternity*, p. 191.

78 *Medical World*, 6 January 1922, 'Hereward', p. 439.

79 John Welshman 'The Medical Officer of Health in England and Wales, 1900–1974: Watchdog or Lapdog?' *Journal of Public Health Medicine*, 19 (4) (1997). p. 443, note 4.

80 Quoted by Honigsbaum, *The Division in British Medicine*, p. 219.

81 Welshman, 'The Medical Officer of Health', p. 446.

82 Lewis, *The Politics of Motherhood*, pp. 152–153. Martin Gorsky, 'The Gloucestershire Extension of Medical Services Scheme: An Experiment in the Integration of Health Services in Britain before the NHS.' *Medical History*, 1 (2006). p. 502. However, Topping was later unequivocal in condemning GPs for their obstetric shortcomings, see Honigsbaum, *The Division in British Medicine*, p. 139.

83 *Cheshire County PRO*, 7135 1/8; see, for example, minutes of meetings of the County Palatine of Chester LMPC on 3 September 1915, 15 July 1917, and 16 September 1917.

84 Alysa Levene, Martin Powell and John Stewart, 'The Development of Municipal General Hospitals in English County Boroughs in the 1930s.' *Medical History*, 50 (2006). p. 13.

85 A.J. Cronin, *The Citadel* (London, 1937) Vista edn, 1996, pp. 30–33.

86 *BMJ*, 3 November 1928, 'Private Practice Committee, Interim Report on Encroachments on the Sphere of Private Practice by the Activities of Local Authorities' Appendix, 'Report by Medical Secretary on Investigation into the Operation of Maternity and Child Welfare Centres and School Clinics in Certain Areas.' Supplement, p. 195, para 57.

87 *Ibid.*, 'Private Practice Committee, Interim Report…', p. 186, para 6.

88 *Ibid.*, p. 187, paras 9–11.

89 *Ibid.*, Appendix, p. 191, para 15.

90 *Ibid.*, Interim Report, pp. 187–188, paras 14–19.

91 *Ibid.*, Appendix, p. 194. paras 50 and 54.

92 Marks, *Metropolitan Maternity*, p. 226.

93 *Ibid.*, pp. 76–77.

94 Lewis, *The Politics of Motherhood*, pp. 144–145.

95 *Ibid.*, p. 149.

96 *Ibid.*, p. 146.

97 *Ibid.*

98 Ernest Muirhead Little, *History of the British Medical Association, 1832–1932* (London, 1932). p. 132.

99 Irvine Loudon 'Death in Childbed from the Eighteenth Century to 1935.' *Medical History*, 30 (1986). p. 26.

100 *BMJ*, 29 June 1929, Supplement, Appendix 1, 'Memorandum Outlining a National Maternity Service Scheme for England and Wales.' pp. 259–262.

101 Honigsbaum, *The Division in British Medicine*, p. 188.

102 Lewis, *The Politics of Motherhood*, p. 145.

103 *BMJ*, 29 June 1929, Supplement, Appendix 1, p. 260, paras 25–26.
104 *Ibid.*, p. 259, para 10. The introduction of undergraduate teaching in obstetrics became compulsory for medical students from 1930. Lewis, *The Politics of Motherhood*, p. 147.
105 *BMJ*, 29 June 1929, Supplement, Appendix 1 pp. 258, paras 4–7, and 260, para 28.
106 Marks, *Metropolitan Maternity*, p. 183.
107 Lewis, *The Politics of Motherhood*, p. 155.
108 *Ibid.*, p. 152.
109 *BMJ*, 27 November 1948, Picton Obituary, p. 960.
110 *Cheshire County PRO*, NHL 7135/8, Minutes of a meeting of the County Palatine of Chester LMPC on 13 September 1934, Appendix.
111 Anne Digby, *The Evolution of British General Practice, 1848–1948* (Oxford, 1999). p. 203.
112 *Ibid.*, para 49.
113 Marks, *Metropolitan Maternity*, pp. 215–216.
114 Lewis, *The Politics of Motherhood*, p. 118.
115 *Ibid.*, p. 118.
116 *Ibid.*, pp. 122–124.
117 Marks, *Metropolitan Maternity*, p. 227.
118 Lewis, *The Politics of Motherhood*, p. 149.
119 Marks, *Metropolitan Maternity*, p. 294.
120 *Ibid.*, p. 232. See also Irvine Loudon, 'Midwives and the Control of Maternal Care,' in Hilary Marland and Anne Marie Rafferty (eds) *Midwives, Society and Childbirth: Debates and Controversies in the Modern Period* (London, 1997). p. 183.
121 John Stewart, *The Battle for Health: A Political History of the Socialist Medical Association, 1930–1951* (Abingdon, 1999). pp. 93–94.
122 Honigsbaum, *Health, Happiness and Security*, p. 11.
123 *Ibid.*
124 Marks, *Metropolitan Maternity*, p. 200.
125 *Ibid.*, pp. 201–202.
126 Lewis, *The Politics of Motherhood*, p. 120.
127 Marks, *Metropolitan Maternity*, p. 211.
128 *Ibid.*, p. 213.
129 Marks, *Metropolitan Maternity*, p. 203.
130 *BMJ*, 29 June 1929, Supplement, Appendix 1, p. 259, paras 12–13, and p. 261, paras 36–37.
131 Ray Earwicker 'A Study of the BMA-TUC Joint Committee on Medical Questions.' *Journal of Social Policy* 8 (3) (1979). p. 344.
132 Lewis, *The Politics of Motherhood*, p. 121.
133 Thane, *Foundations of the Welfare State*, pp. 131–132 and 173.
134 Alysa Levene 'Between Less Eligibility and the NHS: The Changing Place of Poor Law Hospitals in England and Wales, 1929–39.' *Twentieth-Century British History*, 20 (3) (2009). p. 323.
135 *Ibid.*, p. 328.
136 *Ibid.*, p. 329.
137 *Ibid.*
138 Harris, *The Origins of the British Welfare State*, p. 235. See also Harry Eckstein, *The English Health Services: its Origins, Structures and Achievements* (Cambridge, MA, 1958). p. 3.
139 Quoted by Levene, 'Between Less Eligibility and the NHS', p. 332.

140 Alysa Levene, Martin Powell, and John Stewart 'The Development of Municipal General Hospitals in English County Boroughs in the 1930s.' *Medical History* 50 (2006). pp. 3–38. p. 14.
141 Levene, 'Between Less Eligibility and the NHS', p. 338.
142 *Ibid.*, pp. 340–341.
143 Julia Neville, 'Explaining Local Authority Choices on Public Hospital Provision in the 1930s: A Public Policy Hypothesis.' *Medical History*, 1 (vi) (2012). p. 48.
144 Cherry, *Medical Services and the Hospitals*, p. 63.
145 See Levene, Powell and Stewart, 'The Development of Municipal General Hospitals', pp. 18–19 and 24.
146 Neville, 'Explaining Local Authority Choices', p. 49. Her summary is borne out by local studies of municipal medicine, including those by Steven Cherry, Angela Legrine, and herself on Leicester; Barry Doyle on Middlesbrough, Leeds and Sheffield; Martin Gorsky, on Aberdeen and Northeast Scotland; Gorsky, George Gosling, and others on Bristol and the west country; Nick Hayes on Nottingham; Hilary Marland on Wakefield and Huddersfield; John Pickstone on Manchester; Jonathan Reinarz on Birmingham; Steven Thompson on South Wales; and Tim Willis on Bradford – see bibliography.
147 Neville, 'Explaining Local Authority Choices', pp. 21–23.
148 *Ibid.*, pp. 55–61.
149 Charles Webster, *The Health Services Since the War, Volume 1: Problems of Healthcare: The National Health Service Before 1957* (London, 1988). pp. 8–9.
150 Harris, *The Origins of the British Welfare State*, p. 233.
151 Cherry, *Medical Services and the Hospitals*, p. 64.
152 Stewart, *The Battle for Health*, p. 91.
153 *Ibid.*, p. 96.
154 John Stewart 'Socialist Proposals for Health Reform: The Case of Somerville Hastings.' *Medical History*, 39 (3) (1995). pp. 347–348.
155 Stewart, *The Battle for Health*, p 140.
156 John Pater, *The Making of the National Health Service* (London, 1981). p. 22. Frank Honigsbaum, *Health, Happiness and Security, The Creation of the National Health Service* (London, 1989). p. 16.
157 Eckstein, *The English Health Services*, p. 150.
158 Honigsbaum, *Health, Happiness and Security*, p. 54.
159 Eckstein, *The English Health Services*, p. 40.
160 George Campbell Gosling, *Payment and Philanthropy in British Healthcare, 1918–1948* (Manchester, 2017). pp. 20–22.
161 Cherry, *Medical Services and the Hospitals*, p. 63.
162 *Ibid.*, p. 64.
163 *Ibid.*, p. 61.
164 *Ibid.*, p. 72.
165 Gosling, *Payment and Philanthropy*, pp. 20–22. See also Steven Cherry 'Financing the Voluntary Hospitals 1900–1939.' *The Economic History Review*, 50 (2) (1997). pp. 317–321.
166 Gosling, *Payment and Philanthropy*, p. 73.
167 Cherry, 'Financing the Voluntary Hospitals', p. 320.
168 *Ibid.*, p. 74.
169 Eckstein, *The English Health Services*, p. 36.
170 Honigsbaum, *Health, Happiness and Security*, pp. 16–17.
171 Waddington 'Unsuitable Patients: The Debate Over Outpatient Admissions, the Medical Profession and the Late Victorian Hospitals.' *Medical History*, 42 (1998). pp. 44–45.

172 *Ibid.,* p. 46.
173 *BMJ,* 21 February 1931, Supplement, pp. 53–55.
174 *BMA Archive,* Minutes of the Medico Political Committee's PMS subcommittee on 27 January 1933.
175 Honigsbaum, *The Division in British Medicine,* pp. 141–142.
176 Honigsbaum, *Health, Happiness and Security,* p. 113.
177 Honigsbaum, *The Division in British Medicine,* pp. 142–143.
178 Honigsbaum, *Health, Happiness and Security,* p. 51.
179 Digby, *The Evolution of British General Practice,* pp. 194–195.
180 *BMJ,* 19 September 1936, C.E.S. Flemming, 'Cottage Hospitals', Supplement, pp. 177–178.
181 *Ibid.,* p. 177.
182 Lewis, *The Politics of Motherhood,* p. 140.
183 *Ibid.*
184 Honigsbaum, *The Division in British Medicine,* p. 141.
185 Julia Neville, 'Cottage Hospitals and Communities in Rural East Devon, 1919–1939', in Donnacha Sean Lucey, and Virginia Crossman (eds) *Healthcare in Ireland and Britain from 1850: Voluntary, Regional and Comparative Perspectives* (London, 2014). p. 137. (check)
186 *Ibid.,* pp. 137–138.
187 Meyrick Emrys-Roberts, *The Cottage Hospitals 1859–1990: Arrival, Survival and Revival* (Motcombe, Dorset, 1991). pp. 161–167. Accordingly, a great number of these institutions were absorbed into the NHS when it was established in 1948. *Ibid.,* pp. 185–189.
188 Steven Cherry 'Change and Continuity in the Cottage Hospitals circa 1859–1948: the Experience in East Anglia.' *Medical History,* 36 (1992). p. 280.
189 Francis Brett Young, *Dr Bradley Remembers* (London, 1938). p. 538.
190 Francis Brett Young, *My Brother Jonathan* (London, 1928). pp. 374–404.
191 Kenneth Lane, *Diary of a Medical Nobody* (London, 1982). p. 46.
192 A Bradford Hill 'The Doctor's Day and Pay.' *Bulletin of the Royal Statistical Society,* Series A (General) 114 (1) (1951). p. 17.
193 Cherry, *Medical Services and the Hospitals,* p. 32.
194 Political and Economic Planning, *Report on the British Health Services* (London, 1937). pp. 243 and 262.
195 Quoted in Emrys-Roberts, *The Cottage Hospitals,* p. 160.
196 Quoted in Sir Arthur Newsholme, *Medicine and the State* (London, 1932). p. 93. (Unfortunately his citation on p. 88 is erroneous!)
197 Emrys-Roberts, *The Cottage Hospitals,* p. 161.
198 *Ibid.,* p. 168.
199 Cherry, 'Change and Continuity in the Cottage Hospitals', p. 277.
200 Cherry, *Medical Services and the Hospitals,* p. 61.
201 Lane, *Diary of a Medical Nobody,* p. 93.
202 Cherry, *Medical Services and the Hospitals,* p. 26.
203 Cherry, 'Change and Continuity in the Cottage Hospitals', pp. 279–280.
204 *Ibid.,* pp. 280–282.
205 *Ibid.,* p. 284.
206 Cherry, 'Change and Continuity in the Cottage Hospitals', pp. 282–283.
207 *Ibid.,* pp. 283–284.
208 Steven Thompson, 'The Mixed Economy of Care in the South Wales Coalfields, c.1850–1950', in Donnacha Sean Lucey and Virginia Crossman (eds) *Healthcare in Ireland and Britain from 1850: Voluntary, Regional and Comparative Perspectives* (London, 2014). p. 152.

209 Cherry, 'Change and Continuity in the Cottage Hospitals', p. 285.
210 Eckstein, *The English Health Services*, p. 41.
211 Honigsbaum, *The Division in British Medicine*, p. 145.
212 Eckstein, *The English Health Services*, p. 41.
213 Honigsbaum, *The Division in British Medicine*, pp. 144–145.
214 *Ibid.*, p. 144.
215 Cherry, 'Change and Continuity in the Cottage Hospitals', p. 287.
216 PEP, *Report on the British Health Services*, p. 164.
217 *BMJ*, 27 November 1948, Picton Obituary, p. 960.
218 See, for example, Alysa Levene, Martin Powell and John Stewart 'Patterns of Municipal Health Expenditure in Interwar England and Wales.' *Bulletin of the History of Medicine,* 78 (3) (2004). pp. 635–669.

10 Utopian visions

GPs and interwar debates about the future of health services in Britain, 1920–1939

Despite their complaints about insufficient remuneration and diminishing status, GPs in the interwar period have been portrayed by their critics as comfortable, complacent, and largely disinterested in changing the status quo. But it would be incorrect to deduce from their generally conservative outlook an unwillingness to embrace change or to improve or broaden the range of medical services available to the public. As will be made clear, most panel GPs wished to see National Health Insurance (NHI) extended, and by the 1930s, many GPs, including the profession's political leaders, were convinced of the desirability of developing it into something like a comprehensive National Health Service (NHS). The extent of their interest in and support for such ideas can be gauged from an analysis of the various plans to improve and eventually replace NHI which were put before the profession and the public during the 1920s and 1930s. These were, principally, the Dawson Report, the Royal Commission on NHI, the BMA's policy document, *A General Medical Service for the Nation*, Political and Economic Planning's *Report on the British Health Services*, and a variety of proposals put forward by the Labour party and the Socialist Medical Association (SMA). These are considered sequentially in this chapter in the context of contemporary debates about health, medical services and their organisation, and the role and aspirations of the country's medical practitioners. Such debates involved all elements of society, from politicians, civil servants, and the Approved Societies, to trade unions, the press, and even writers of popular fiction. What this analysis seeks to demonstrate is GPs' continued willingness to embrace the development of NHI medical services, while acknowledging that their enthusiasm for reform was tempered by fears of state control and the need to maintain their social status and financial security. It also considers the extent to which the profession's leaders were prepared, to lead debates about the shape of publicly subsidised health services, and subordinate professional interests to the public good.

GPs' determination to bring about improvements in the NHI scheme, it will be shown, led them to acknowledge the need to incorporate the scheme within a more comprehensive and integrated healthcare system catering for all sections

DOI: 10.4324/9781003438274-10

of society. It also led them to accept the increasing separation of general practice from specialist care and to embrace a vision of a family doctor service whose chief virtue was continuity of care for the patient. This analysis therefore challenges the assumptions of historians who have been critical of the profession's motives and sceptical of GPs' commitment to improving state-funded services.[1] In endeavouring to explain the moral dilemmas which the GPs faced, note is taken of the symbiotic relationship between public and private medicine and the dangers of determinism when looking at how health services were configured or evolved during this period. As has been shown, by the end of the 1930s, many panel patients were as likely as private patients to view their panel GP as their family doctor. This convinced the GPs' leaders and other influential groups that the family doctor should lie at the heart of any future NHS' however, it was organised and funded.

The Dawson Report: the organisation of health services and a collectivist vision of general practice

Discussions about improvements in health services and their organisation had begun as soon as NHI was established, with Addison informing a dinner organised by his supporters in 1914 of his hopes of adding to it a domiciliary nursing service. He also stated that, 'It might be of great value...for medical men to work in groups where for certain purposes they could combine at a common centre for mutual help and have access to better means for confirming diagnosis'. This would, be said, 'help to keep men up to date'.[2] In May the same year, the newly established London Panel Committee noted proposals made in Lloyd George's budget for 'the establishment of centres for the cooperation of practitioners on the panel'. Fearing that local authorities would be put in charge, the committee resolved that panel committees should decide the scope of what these centres would provide, concluding that they should be accessible to all panel doctors, and provide consulting rooms for up to five GPs and accommodation for a trained nurse, X-ray operator, clerk, and dispensing chemist, under the joint control of the local Insurance and Panel Committees.[3] In thinking about health centres, it seems that Addison may have taken his cue from ideas put forward in 1912 by Charles Parker and other prominent members of the State Medical Services Association.[4] The outbreak of the First World War nullified any prospect of implementing such proposals. But during the war, arguments about future provision of state-funded medical services continued, influenced by the progress of efforts by the Local Government Board to establish municipal health clinics offering maternity and child welfare services, and separately, community-based clinics for venereal disease sufferers.[5] As has been seen, the profession's representatives fought hard to ensure that as many as possible of the salaried medical officer posts in the new municipal clinics were part-time and therefore open to panel GPs in order to prevent the growth of a whole-time salaried service.[6]

As a Minister of Health in 1919, Addison looked forward to realising his dream of creating a comprehensive, integrated medical service from the myriad of separate and often overlapping services for which he was now responsible, about which he hoped to build consensus through his Consultative Council. Addison rejected the idea of the Council being directly elected by their colleagues and showed a determination to harness the best ideas from those he considered the brightest and most respected members of the profession. He may have hoped that the advice they provided would be objective but he could not expect it to be untainted by professional interest, and in choosing Sir Bertrand (later Lord) Dawson as the chairman, he must have been aware that he was relying of an individual who had made no secret of his belief in the supremacy of medical over lay advice and the desirability of medical leadership of organised health services. Dawson strongly supported doctors' autonomy and freedom from bureaucratic influence, as he demonstrated in his Cavendish lecture in 1918 in which he stated that 'the practice of putting the skilled under the control of the unskilled must cease'.[7] Places where doctors worked should be controlled by doctors, Dawson had maintained, and, when established, the Ministry of Health should be peopled by a mix of medical and lay officials while strictly medical matters should be subject to the advice of a central medical board.[8]

For Frank Honigsbaum, the origins of the *Interim Report of the Consultative Council on the Future of Medical and Allied Services*, to give Dawson's report its full title, and its reception by the profession, were intricately bound up with concerns about a salaried medical service. This assertion is central to his explanation of the separation of general practice from hospital care which took place while NHI was in force. But his argument is somewhat overstated. Neither the Minister nor Morant was especially wedded to the idea of salaried service at this time, and their key medical advisers, Whitaker and Newman, had each put forward arguments as to why it was not desirable.[9] Honigsbaum admits that Addison had ruled out the idea by January 1919 but repeatedly claims that the prime minister, Lloyd George, favoured a salaried service, even though he was dissuaded from that view in 1911. His argument rests entirely on the existence of contingency plans to introduce salaried service in areas, like Bradford, in which the profession had threatened to boycott NHI.[10] Dawson was, in any case, motivated by much more lofty ideals. His experience as a Major General in the Royal Army Medical Corps had convinced him of the benefits of doctors and ancillary professions working together in teams under an organised structure and, as a leading specialist, he was aware of the difference which new diagnostic and therapeutic equipment and technology could make, if only doctors generally had access to them. The proposals set out in the interim report were principally concerned therefore with organisation. They involved what later health planners would have referred to as a 'hub and spoke' model involving primary, secondary, and tertiary medical centres whose number and location would be determined by geography and the extent to which existing estate could be modified and utilised for the purpose.[11] The report cites as an example of this model the scheme established by Gloucestershire County Council under the leadership of its Medical Officer of Health, Dr J. Middleton Martin.[12] Dawson's scheme was to be available for all classes of society but not 'free to all'. Although the Consultative Council stated that their remit did not extend to the question of how the new system should be funded, they made it clear that they expected preventive, public health, and 'communal' services to be provided free to users at public expense, but those 'curative' services would be means-tested as under NHI.[13] This meant that, as with NHI, the majority of the population would access services under some kind or provident or insurance arrangement and individuals earning more than a specified amount would be expected to pay for their treatment and the usual privileges which that guaranteed.[14]

At the heart of Dawson's proposals was the health centre, 'an institution wherein are brought together various medical services, preventive and curative, so as to form one organisation'.[15] The primary health centre (PHC) would vary in size and scope but would form the basis of 'domiciliary services' provided by GPs, nurses, and others. While the GP would continue to attend patients at their homes or at the surgery and carry out such treatment as fell within the GP's competence, the PHC would provide a base from which GPs could obtain for patients when needed a range of facilities such as a minor operating suite, radiography, and laboratory facilities. The PHCs would also house a dispensary, hydrotherapy baths, therapeutic massage, and physiotherapy, together with clinical records storage and a common room in which doctors could meet and share in postgraduate instruction.[16] The centre would include maternity beds for more complex labour cases and other services already available in local authority clinics such as antenatal, child welfare, school medical inspections, and medical examination of infectious diseases and occupational disease.[17] GPs would be paid to provide these services under separate contracts, the report suggested, and PHCs might also provide a place for dental clinics and ambulance services. The socialist doctor, David Stark Murray, later claimed that what Dawson was proposing was not a 'true' health centre because 'it showed no inkling of group practice'.[18] This is not quite correct. The Council hoped that the establishment of PHCs might encourage GPs to work in large groups just as Addison had hoped but they did not want to be coercive. They stated that

> the custom whereby every GP has his own consulting rooms in his own house should continue but where it is impossible for a doctor to provide adequate accommodation at his own expense…it should be possible for the health authority (which is described later in the report) to provide such accommodation at the Primary Health Centre or elsewhere on such terms as are reasonable.

They continued that where medical opinion favoured the plan, 'collective surgeries might with advantage be tried, either attached to the Primary Health

Centre or set up elsewhere'.[19] 'Collective surgeries' can be viewed as shorthand for group practice or at the very least a necessary stage in their development.

Under the plan, the more numerous PHCs would feed into a smaller number of Secondary Health Centres at which Consultants and specialists would deal with more complex cases. These 'would of necessity be based in towns' and would be linked to a small number of teaching hospitals in cities with attached medical schools. They would provide the 'highest skill available' for patients and facilitate postgraduate instruction.[20] Consultants would also attend patients' homes in cases of emergency or 'special summons' by the GP.[21] The PHC would be the 'home' of the health organisation and of 'the intellectual life of the unit'. It would overcome the professional isolation experienced by most GPs who would thereby commune with specialists and Consultants and develop 'an intellectual traffic and camaraderie to the great advantage of the service'.[22] These proposals would provide the advantage of better organisation while ensuring 'the preservation of liberty of thought and action'.[23] While the question of salaried service was incidental to their proposals, the Council was clear that they saw no benefit in GPs working in PHCs being whole-time salaried employees because choice of doctor was necessary, the report says, 'to win the confidence so vital to the treatment of illness'. The report adds that the 'voluntary character of the association between patient and doctor' stimulates the latter 'to excel in skill and helpfulness', whereas whole-time service would tend 'to discourage initiative, to diminish the sense of responsibility and to encourage mediocrity'.[24] Securing the efficient working of the new system would require a new type of health authority, the report said, but the Council were divided as to its form or location.[25] They were clear, however, that one of the conditions of efficient service was that the medical profession 'should come into organic relation with the health administration' as success was dependent on their 'cooperation and enthusiasm'.[26]

Dawson was careful to anticipate and acknowledge the profession's fears and possible objections to the Council's proposals.[27] The report's conclusions were carefully qualified, but its critics were reluctant to accept its provisos at face value. The cautiously favourable response in the *BMJ*'s editorial and the endorsement of the much-venerated Sir James Mackenzie, who acknowledged similarities between the PHC and the successful clinic he had established in St Andrews, were quickly superseded by a succession of admonitory diatribes in the medical press.[28] Ignoring the report's carefully rehearsed arguments, Dr Blackhall-Morrison thought that the report provided ammunition for the supporters of salaried service, while Dr W. Gordon feared that GPs would become 'mere first aiders' under Dawson's scheme.[29] Others had more principled objections. Dr Michael Dewar questioned the need for its recommendations, stating that 80–95% of illness 'was amply and carefully attended to by GPs already', while Dr J.L. Halstead considered the whole thing 'extravagant' and unnecessary.[30] Others rose to defend the report. Dr J.W. Marshall offered another example of a successful PHC already in existence in Scotland, showing how cottage hospitals could be transformed in the way the report envisaged.[31] A report to Kent LMPC welcomed Dawson's proposals as 'a sane and practical statement of the lines along which the reconstruction of public health administration may best proceed'.[32] When in July 1920 the BMA invited Dawson to speak to its Representative Meeting, he was evidently frustrated by the debate in which many speakers voiced concerns based on a misreading or misunderstanding of the report's intentions. Typical of these was Dr John Stevens of Edinburgh who thought it meant healthcare was to be 'free to all'.[33] Reflecting the unrestrained comments of the anti-government lobby, Sir James Barr stated that the proposals were completely unaffordable and, repeating his objections to NHI voiced in 1913, said, provocatively, that it was not the duty of the state to look after sick people.[34] Although there was little likelihood of such reactionary views being supported, Dawson urged the meeting not to follow Barr's 'evil path' and was no doubt grateful when Brackenbury pointed out that the proposed PHCs corresponded in many respects to 'a cottage hospital with improvements'.[35] He was supported by another of the report's authors, his fellow IAC member, H. Guy Dain, who said that it would be the GPs' own fault if, by not embracing the health centre concept, the growth of local authority clinics staffed by whole-time salaried doctors was thereby allowed to continue unchecked.[36] Ignoring the critics, the Representative Body confirmed support for the principles behind the report and instructed its Ministry of Health Committee to consider it further. The committee was to present its conclusions to a special Representative Meeting convened for the purpose, but this did not take place.

The fact that Dawson's proposals were not taken forward, and no final report was ever published, was down to a combination of institutional inertia and the hostility of anti-government forces led by the press, for whom the report was very epitome of the Coalition Government's overweening ambition and extravagance. Typical of press criticisms is *The Times* article which denounced Dawson's scheme as 'fantastically costly'.[37] The ambitious scope of the programme raised fears of significantly increased public expenditure at a time when the economy was struggling to cope with the effects of post-war debt and dislocation and was heading inexorably into depression. The Anti-Waste campaign championed by the Northcliffe and Rothermere press combined with ideological opponents of state intervention to denounce the Council's proposals.[38] The death of Morant, moreover, signalled a change on the part of the officials dealing with the report. Robinson was of a more prosaic mind than his predecessor and had none of his passion to effect social change, and when Addison was replaced by Sir Alfred Mond, a Minister more interested in reducing rather than enhancing the state's role in health, the plan itself was quickly buried and GPs' attention turned once more to their familiar grievances. Sir George Godber, the NHS Chief Medical Officer, noted with regard to the plan that, 'The British did not really believe in the capacity of government at any level to run such human health services in 1920'.[39] However, the ideals Dawson articulated and his vision of a truly integrated and comprehensive health service remained a cherished, if elusive, objective for many within the profession and outside it and continued to exercise considerable influence in debates about the extension or expansion of NHI and about what might replace it.

Honigsbaum cites evidence that Dawson was primarily interested in extending the range of services to the public, rather than extending existing NHI coverage to dependants of the insured and argues that this put him at odds with Brackenbury.[40] But there is nothing in the report to suggest the exclusion of women and children from its proposals. It offers no view on the issue of coverage and how services should be funded, only that they should be available, though not free, to the entire population.[41] Honigsbaum suggests that the expansion in the scope of services which Brackenbury vainly attempted to persuade the LMPCs Conference to accept in 1919 was somehow 'in opposition to the Dawson report' but this conclusion lacks substance.[42] So too does his suggestion that the BMA's leaders, Cox and Brackenbury, were at odds at this time because Cox favoured the inclusion of specialist work by GPs over the care of dependants, whereas Brackenbury strongly favoured the latter.[43] Certainly, Brackenbury wanted GPs to provide a complete family medical service to the insured and their dependants and felt that they could not do this effectively while becoming part-time specialists. But he was not averse to GPs continuing to undertake minor surgery in cottage hospitals, maintaining interest in maternity care, or administering any form of treatment that was within their competence to perform outside hospitals. The only real point of departure between Dawson and the BMA's leadership was over the importance of GPs working in groups, an idea for which, despite its obvious merits, the individualistic nature of general practice at that time guaranteed a lukewarm response.[44] With Dawson's utopian vision side-lined, the profession subsequently pinned its hopes for beneficial changes to health services on the Royal Commission on NHI which had been conceded by a reluctant government as a condition of the settlement of the GPs' grievances in 1924.

The Royal Commission on NHI: conflicting expectations of future development

When it came to improvements to medical benefits under NHI, the regular discussions between the Approved Societies and the IAC which had begun in September 1920 at the Ministry's instigation showed that there was actually much common ground between them. Both sides wanted a better service for the insured and for dependants to be covered by it. But although they differed about how much the doctors should be paid to deliver a more adequate service, both recognised that this would require a great deal more money which, in the worsening economic climate, the Government was unlikely to provide. The antagonism between the profession and the Approved Societies was based on the issue of who should control the evolving system. The Societies' desire for more control was frustrated by the doctors' newfound confidence and influence with government officials. The inevitable showdown between the two sides took place within the context of the Royal Commission into NHI in 1926. When the Commission met, it was against a background of orchestrated and politically inspired criticism of the panel system in the popular press. Typical of these was the *Daily Express* article entitled 'A fraud on the patients'.[45] Angered by the *Express* campaign against NHI, the IAC was incensed by comments in it attributed to a member of the BMA's Non-Panel Doctors Committee, Dr Blackhall-Morrison.[46] Having taken copious evidence from all parties, however, the Commission concluded that it had received 'very little evidence directed against the scheme as a whole, nor have we any reason to think there now exists any considerable body of opinion adverse to the principle of National Health Insurance'.[47]

Regarding the critics of NHI, the Commission agreed with the Ministry which stated in its evidence that 'with few exceptions, those persons who speak to the detriment of the Insurance Medical Service have never been under treatment of the panel practitioner'.[48] Indeed, the fiercest critics of the scheme were the National Medical Union (NMU). Although the aforementioned *Daily Express* article spoke of the NMU as representing the 16,000 doctors not on the panel (of which, of course, a significant proportion were specialists), the NMU were forced to admit to the Commission that their membership numbered only 247![49] Alban Gordon was among a small number of witnesses who accused GPs of providing a better service to their private patients than to their panel patients, echoing views previously given credence by the MP Sir Kingsley Wood.[50] However, the Commission stated:

we are glad to say that, except from some rather contradictory evidence given by witnesses from the national conference of friendly societies…we have found no support for this allegation. On the contrary there has been a great body of evidence not only from interested parties – the doctors and chemists – but from the societies and representative bodies, showing that no such distinction is made.

The Commission noted, moreover,

a growing tendency among practitioners to be more scrupulous to avoid giving offence in the case of insured patients than in the case of private patients, since the former are, in a sense, protected by the machinery under the Act for the investigation of complaints.[51]

The Commission saw its main task as being to decide how the present system could be improved. Their first priority was to expand the scope of services to include access to (essentially outpatient) specialist advice but not, it must be emphasised, to allow inclusion of hospital treatment. Then, in descending order of priority, they recommended extension of the insurance system to dependants, improved maternity services provision, and improved dental service provision.[52] They decided that the inclusion of hospital inpatient treatment was unafford-able and were concerned that it would leave non-insured persons 'of moderate means' at a great disadvantage.[53] They were clearly thinking of the Dawson Re-port when they sought to justify their outpatient proposal, saying that the panel GP 'suffered great disadvantages in the maintenance of his professional effi-ciency' due to their professional isolation. Regretting that GPs had few opportu-nities of coming into contact with those at the leading edge of developments in medicine and surgery, the Commission argued that 'a more systematised refer-ral process would aid GP diagnosis and learning' and that specialist feedback would 'act as a valuable form of postgraduate instruction that would probably be welcomed by the isolated general practitioners'.[54] The Commission was care-ful to avoid expressing any opinion on what GPs should be paid. It was with the administration of NHI that it was principally concerned. They were therefore highly critical of the Approved Societies whose involvement had been 'justified by the necessity of retaining, under a system imposed by the state, a system of insurance that had 'been evolved by the people themselves'. The Insurance Act was thus 'an experiment in democracy, no less than in the domain of social bet-terment' but in some of the larger societies associated with industrial insurance companies 'there was no effective means whereby the members could exercise control over the societies' affairs'.[55]

Despite these shortcomings, the majority report did not propose that the Ap-proved Societies be stripped of their role. It proposed instead that Insurance Committees be abolished and that their work 'pending any radical remodelling and unification of Health Services' should be handed over to committees of 'the appropriate local authorities'.[56] It was not that the Insurance Committees had been inefficient, they argued, but that their role was currently so narrow that it did not justify their existence as independent administrative authorities.[57] Al-ban Gordon had argued that 'the continued existence of Insurance Committees within their present limitations is, except for one single function, pure farce'. The exception he referred to was the Medical Services Subcommittee which, he acknowledged, 'performs useful work'.[58] The Commission spent some time looking at the NHI complaints machinery and it was to this that the Medical Practitioners Union (MPU) directed most of its evidence. It completely failed to impress the Commission, however, who commented that 'the privileged position which the MPU argues should be granted to practitioners under the complaints procedure is one that we do not think could be conceded or any grounds public policy'.[59] The BMA fared little better when they argued that complaints about behaviour rather than the quality of treatment should not be disciplinary mat-ters. To the argument that the patients' remedy was already to hand in the ability to change doctor, the Commission responded that it was not a remedy in areas where the shortage of panel doctors left patients with no choice of alternative

GP and dismissed the idea that the LMPCs be left to adjudicate on such matters as 'highly undesirable'.[60]

It was clear that in the Commission's summation, the Approved Societies' reputation was more tarnished than the doctors'. The minority report even went so far as to call for local authorities to take over insurance funds from the Societies on the grounds that their lack of accountability 'negated parliament's original intentions in involving them in the administration of NHI' and that they were 'a hindrance to further development'.[61] The doctors were particularly pleased to see the Commission accept their opinion, supported by Ministry officials, of Medical Aid Institutes. This was confirmed by the statement that 'the treatment given to members of these institutions is generally of inferior quality to that provided under the normal panel arrangements'. The Commission concluded that medical institutes were an anomalous feature of the scheme and that no more be established.[62] The fall of the Labour government and the changing political and economic situation of the country, however, meant that the Commission's recommendations, like those of the Consultative Council, remained unimplemented. While they continued to consider improvements to and expansion of the service, the Ministry focused its attention instead on trying to reduce the cost of medical benefits by tightening up the rules on certification. The IAC eventually decided therefore to take the initiative and offer its own views on what the ideal national medical service should comprise.

The BMA's vision: 'A General Medical Service for the Nation'

Dissatisfied with the slow progress of discussions about reform of NHI, the IAC decided in early 1929 to set out their own proposals for the future of health services and established a committee for that purpose, the General Medical Services Scheme Committee, under the chairmanship of Guy Dain. It listed among its reference documents the Dawson Report, the Royal Commission report, and extracts from recent *Lancet* articles on modern hospitals in Sweden and Denmark.[63] The Committee's remit, explained in a memorandum from Alfred Cox, was to address the following questions: (1) What kind of medical service should be at the disposal of every member of the community? (2) Under what conditions should the service be placed? (3) What were the financial and administrative details of such a scheme? Cox noted that there would be no need for the committee to consult with the profession before drafting a scheme addressing these questions 'since there will be nothing very new to the medical profession in the plan, it being an attempt to synthesise those separate policies which have already received the approval of the Representative Body'.[64] What was unique about the report, published in 1930 under the title *A General Medical Service for the Nation*, was the emphasis it gave to the importance of the family doctor.

As has been noted, prior to the mid-1920s, the terms 'insurance practitioner' and 'family doctor' were not synonymous. By 1926 however, the Royal

Commission noted, NHI had become an established and appreciated part of the social fabric of the nation and those of the panel patients' families who could afford to were generally happy to make use of panel doctors' services and regarded them as their family doctors. The BMA therefore felt able to state much more strongly than Dawson had done that 'the family doctor is the foundation of any complete and efficient medical service' and insisted on provision for every individual, regardless of status or ability to pay, of 'a personal practitioner or family doctor'.[65] The report extolled the virtues of the GP not just as a medical attendant but as 'guardian of the health interests of the family' and 'home doctor' who was uniquely conversant with the patient's personal environment.[66] It contrasted this with the situation in the USA where the supply of specialists far exceeded that of generalists and family medicine was now fast disappearing.[67] It equated the GP's role in helping patients access the services of specialists when needed to that the solicitors helping clients choose a barrister. Consequently, the specialist was always to be a Consultant brought in by and acting in concert with the GP as family doctor and consultant service and all ancillary forms of diagnosis and treatment should be available to the patient only through the medium of the GP.[68] The relationship between the patient and doctor was sacrosanct, the report argued, and consequently while the service envisaged might be a state-coordinated or state-subsidised service, the interposition of any third party between doctor and patient 'should be as limited as possible'.[69] 'The patient needs to think of the doctor as *his* doctor', the report stated, not a representative of the state which might be the case in other European countries where there was interference 'for political reasons' and which is 'alien to the British experience'. This is one of a number of references by GPs leaders at this time to citizens' choice of doctor being more restricted in other countries, though they fail to cite any definite evidence.[70]

The report put forward a modified version of Dawson's health centre idea in the form of the 'home hospital'. Where domiciliary care and treatment was needed and the patient's home was not best suited to such care, and the patient could not afford 'good nursing home care', patients could be safely and efficiently catered for in beds in a home hospital, or home hospital ward, located at or adjacent to existing hospitals, either voluntary or municipal. The description 'Home Hospital' had first been employed by Sir Henry Burdett in 1877 when referring to a hospital run by GPs.[71] Patients would be cared for there by nurses, or midwives in maternity cases, under the overall supervision of their GP, with Consultants brought in only where needed. Utilising existing buildings meant that the costs of these new establishments could be minimised.[72] The report noted that as the poor law infirmaries had recently come under the control of local authorities as a result of the Local Government Act of 1929, it was a propitious time to make such suggestions. While not explicit about the role local authorities might play in future health service provision, it may be inferred from the report that the BMA saw the municipal hospitals being subsumed at some point within a more unified hospital service supported by compulsory hospital contributory schemes like the one described in the report's appendix.[73] Such proposals, the report stated, would help GPs maintain an interest in institutional care and ensure that the convalescing patient benefited from continuity of care from the doctor who knew them best. Dawson's PHC was not completely abandoned, however. 'Local Medical Centres' with consulting rooms, nursing services, diagnostic equipment, and laboratory facilities 'would be very useful', the report noted, stating that many forms of treatment could be carried out at such centres by the family doctor more satisfactorily then at the patient's home or the doctor's surgery.[74] In some cases, home hospitals and local medical centres could be combined, and here too, it adds, the doctor would be given the opportunity of cooperation with professional colleagues and the help of nursing and all ancillary facilities.[75]

Echoing Dawson's views about team working and education, the report opines that these facilities would widen the GPs' experience and knowledge and bring them into closer contact with their colleagues. They would learn from each other and 'be stimulated by the sense of fellowship and common purpose'.[76] The report reiterates the conclusions of the BMA's maternity services scheme issued in 1929 which suggested that GPs assume control of antenatal and postnatal care while working in collaboration with midwives and suggested that while local authority child health clinics should continue 'their admirable work of instruction in mothercraft', they should, under these proposals, be free to refer children needing treatment to GPs, safe in the knowledge that parents would not be discouraged by inability to pay.[77] This was because dependants of the insured, under the BMA's proposals, would be included under NHI, which would be enhanced by the addition of nursing, midwifery, diagnostic, laboratory, and possibly dental, services in community settings.[78] This would, of course, benefit GPs indirectly. While the inclusion of dependants might initially increase demand, GPs would be more likely to offer treatment before illness became acute and thereby prevent the need for longer term care. They would also be spared the necessity of chasing patients for payment of bills they could not afford. Those who could afford to pay for the services directly, however, would continue to do so, and local authorities would pay into NHI to ensure provision for what would formerly have been poor law patients now subject to public assistance.[79] Recognising the prohibitive costs involved, hospitals or specialist services would be available to all via a separate contributory scheme for which, in an appendix, the report helpfully provided a model.[80] The report strongly favoured the contributory system which 'helps preserve self-reliance and independence and promote thrift'. It also helped preserve 'the most valuable features of private practice', including free choice of doctor and 'reasonable competition'.[81]

It is easy to see in the BMA scheme, as some historians have done, a self-interested attempt to justify the continuance of a mixed practice system. Thus, Anne Digby claims that the BMA 'missed an opportunity to work towards a social health service' and that they 'privileged doctors' remuneration over other concerns'.[82] There is likewise more than a hint of disparagement in Brian Abel-Smith's comment that 'the scheme gave full payment to doctors for all services but preserved their position as independent entrepreneurs who were responsible only to their professional code of honour'.[83] These comments reflect a failure to appreciate the moral complexity of medical opinion at that time and in particular the doctors' attachment to the 'professional social ideal'. They fail to acknowledge that GPs, both the rank and file and the IAC leadership, sincerely believed that what they were proposing would be of equal benefit to themselves, their patients, and the wider society at a time when the idea of an entirely tax-funded system was dismissed by all but a minority of socialist idealists. They also ignore the indirect benefits which private practice brought to panel patients. The fees earned from middle-class patients could be seen as subsidising the care of the poorer sections of the community by helping GPs maintain their income at a reasonable level. Dain was reported to have described this as 'climbing over the backs of the poor into the pockets of the rich'.[84]

But private practice was at the same time a place in which GPs were free to experiment with innovative techniques, procedures, and drugs not available or permitted under NHI. As Digby herself notes, mixed practices began to invest in equipment like X-ray machines, ophthalmoscopes, and blood-pressure monitors and experimented with new drugs like sulphonamides, and vaccines which private patients were willing to pay for relating to influenza, typhoid, catarrh, rheumatism, scarlatina, cholera, and whooping cough.[85] They were thus able to acquaint themselves with new drugs, therapeutics, and diagnostic devices which only private patients could afford, and in time share the benefits of this experience with their panel patients. It was in this less accountable arena also that enterprising GPs had the freedom to pursue interests in fringe medicine or specialist areas like psychotherapy. Rhodri Hayward details the development of a special interest in psychological medicine and psychotherapy among many GPs in the interwar period. He notes, 'Psychology and General Practice enjoyed a symbiotic relationship. Each derived a new significance from its association with the other' and that 'Health Insurance encouraged psychological approaches' particularly as regards functional illness.[86] He concludes, 'As even Consultant Psychiatrists recognised, by the late 1930s the family doctor played a key role in the achievement of mental health'.[87]

In 1930, under Dain's leadership, the IAC was clear that the inclusion of dependants within NHI was of far greater importance than any other development of it, and the LMPCs conference agreed, resolving that 'the time is now ripe for the medical profession to ask for the inclusion for the purposes of medical benefit…of the dependants of insured persons'.[88] Their pragmatic caveat – 'provided that such an extended scheme includes adequate safeguards respecting remuneration and conditions of service' – does not detract from their idealism. When a delegation led by Dain met with the Ministry in November 1930, he acknowledged that 'from a financial point of view a more inconvenient moment possibly could not have been chosen for bringing the matter forward'.[89] The delegation persevered, however, stating that the alternative was the continued expansion of local authority maintained clinics catering for women and children which would fatally undermine general practice.[90] This fear was heightened as the Local Government Act of 1929 gave local authorities direct responsibility for the poor law infirmaries, a number of which were thereafter developed as generously equipped municipal hospitals with an increasing complement of salaried staff.[91] As has already been shown, GPs' leaders feared that the expanding scope of municipal medicine would reduce demand for their services, forcing impecunious GPs to accept the security of local authority employment as subordinates of the hated Medical Officers of Health.[92] 'If the public did not wake up', Dain complained, 'the time was coming when the general practitioner…would cease to exist', as was the case, he was given to understand, in some parts of the USA. For the Ministry, Robinson appeared to agree with the thrust of Dain's argument and said that while 'the time had not yet come' for the inclusion of dependants, he would bring the Conference's resolution to the Minister's attention.[93] In 1932, the IAC established a Dependants Subcommittee. After some deliberation, this concluded that the financial situation of the country meant any extension of medical benefit to dependants of insured persons under NHI 'had been placed at the time being outside the bounds of practical politics'. The subcommittee therefore proposed that 'other means be made available for all classes under consideration to obtain domiciliary medical attendance from private practitioners through arrangements incorporating the choice system'.[94] It thereby made explicit its preference for dependants being treated through Public Medical Services (PMS) and recommended that the BMA's model scheme be updated accordingly.[95]

The alternative expedient of Public Medical Services (PMS)

In 1932, the BMA's Medico Political Committee set up a PMS subcommittee.[96] Its principal functions were to bring the BMA's model scheme up to date and approve PMS schemes as deserving of loans from the Defence Trust, as recommended by the Conference of LMPCs.[97] This proved to be something of a poisoned chalice, as the majority of schemes, being designed to suit local circumstances, contained features at variance with the model scheme or charged rates which the BMA deemed 'uneconomic'. The extent to which PMS schemes were beginning to take off can be gauged from the survey which the IAC's Remuneration Subcommittee conducted as a data-gathering exercise in 1933. In addition to cities like Birmingham, Dundee, Reading, Nottingham, Coventry, Swansea, Norwich, and Newcastle, there were schemes covering rural areas such as Lincolnshire and Hampshire. Demonstrating the autonomous nature of such schemes, the survey of 26 schemes revealed wide variations in policies and criteria for membership. Some involved a flat rate per family, while others charged separately for uninsured males, females, and juveniles and many charged for children on a sliding scale.[98] A memorandum by the BMA's Deputy Secretary George Anderson in 1932 revealed a similar variation in the size and popularity of the schemes. They were particularly popular in the Northeast of England where there were schemes in Gateshead, Jarrow and Hebburn, Middlesborough, Stockton on Tees, Tynemouth and Northumberland. Elsewhere, Essex and Warwickshire were among the largest with over 22,000 subscribers, whereas Nottingham had only 1,350.[99] Figures for the largest schemes, namely Birmingham and Leicester, were not included.

One of the first applications considered by the subcommittee was from Midlothian whose request for a loan of £150 was denied because, under its scheme, the patient contracted with the scheme instead of an individual GP as the BMA recommended.[100] Despite a spirited and reasoned defence of the constitution and operation of the scheme by its Secretary, Dr Hamilton, the subcommittee declined to change its decision. Hamilton pointed out that the scheme was so perfectly suited to conditions in Scotland that it was to be replicated in East and West Lothian and, with a hint of nationalist pique, criticised the subcommittee for viewing matters from an English perspective.[101] At the same meeting, the subcommittee approved the constitution of the London PMS and recommended that the National Insurance Defence Trust award this scheme £1,000 to facilitate its expansion.[102] Another scheme considered by the subcommittee in 1933 was a South London PMS called The Medical Contributory Service which the subcommittee felt unable to approve because it was managed by a limited company rather than, as the BMA recommended, a trust. In correspondence in 1934, the proposers of the scheme subsequently explained that it was designed to meet 'a public need' in providing services for middle-class subscribers.[103] This need was appreciated by others in the capital. In 1935, the subcommittee considered a request for approval by The London Provident Medical Service. This was allied to the existing PMS scheme and established for the benefit of people earning above the NHI income limit but under £550 per annum yet which in all other respects corresponded with the model scheme.[104] Seeing that the BMA's Representative Meeting had resolved in 1920 to prohibit the treatment under contract of any person earning over £250 per annum, the subcommittee approved the scheme 'in principle' while asking the Medico Political Committee to recommend that the ARM resolution be rescinded.[105] In 1936, the Representative Meeting accepted the recommendation and the Association's model scheme rules were modified accordingly.[106] An alternative view of the origins of this scheme is offered by the anonymous author of *This Panel Business*, published in 1933. He said that it was necessary because many subscribers to the existing PMS lied about their income and acerbically declared his opinion that 'the London Public Medical Service has been a failure'.[107]

In discussing NHI capitation fees, the IAC negotiating committee had been embarrassed and wrongfooted when Ministry officials drew attention to the subscription rates for families charged by PMS schemes, which were in many cases considerably below what the IAC alleged to be 'economic'.[108] PMS schemes which prided themselves on adhering to rates recommended by the BMA, principally London, drew attention to this problem in the *BMJ*. They were said to be particularly concerned at the cheapness of rates charged in Birmingham but were unable to persuade the PMS subcommittee to penalise the offenders.[109] A number of PMS scheme operators, including those in Reading, called for a conference as a means to establish a national coordinating body for PMS.[110] The subcommittee agreed to the request and arranged a conference which met for the first time in December 1935 and thereafter became an annual event. Representatives or 43 different areas attended to hear papers on advertising of services and business aspects of PMS, and on the use of PMS to combat encroachments on private practice presented by Alfred Cox.[111] Cox became the Secretary of the London PMS on his retirement as BMA Secretary in 1933.[112] As a sign of their expectation of the continued expansion of PMS, the conference resolved that the BMA should establish a PMS Committee as a standing committee 'analogous to the IAC'.[113] However, the subcommittee considered this action premature and decided instead to co-opt on to the subcommittee the conference chairman-elect, Alfred Cox.[114] When the next PMS conference was being organised, London representatives vainly urged that any PMS scheme not approved by the subcommittee be denied the privilege of BMA support and the right to attend the conference.[115] The proposal, however, was self-defeating. A document prepared by PMS subcommittee chairman H.W. Pooler in 1936 contained an analysis of existing schemes and their comparative charges. It revealed that of 38 areas for which data was available, only ten had been fully approved plus two provisionally, and there were an additional 12 for which there was insufficient data.[116] It was clear therefore that the majority of schemes could not qualify for BMA endorsement. The analysis showed the highest rates in the country to be in Thornaby and Middlesborough which charged around 12s per person per annum, and the cheapest to be Reading which charged only 5s 6d, exclusive of medicines.[117] With or without BMA approval, many GPs believed that PMS would grow in popularity and would become an essential part of national healthcare provision. In a paper on advertising of PMS services, which the BMA Council had concluded in 1933 was not in any way unethical, subcommittee member Solomon Wand had stated the objective of making PMS a 'byword' and of making the public 'PMS-minded'.[118]

The extent to which this was achieved can be gauged from the study of NHI conducted in 1938 by the American physician Douglass Orr and his wife Jean. They found that GPs considered PMS 'a most valuable adjunct to NHI' and 'the most satisfactory form of contract practice'.[119] The London scheme had made a slow start they noted, having enrolled only 50,000 families.[120] The more successful Birmingham scheme was highly regarded even by the local MOH, Dr H.P. Newsholme.[121] Starting in 1923, they noted that it initially had 250 doctors and 250,000 subscribers. Commenting on its success, the *Birmingham*

Medical Review opined in 1936 that the popularity of PMS around the country was demonstrated by the numbers represented at the recent Conference of PMS schemes and its call for a national representative body equivalent to the IAC.[122] A Dr A, whose practice was in the West End of London, described the benefits of PMS to GPs prosaically, stating that without it, 'the wife is likely to run off to a hospital or a clinic where she and the children might get less intelligent care than can be given by a family doctor'.[123] In answer to those who viewed PMS as being purely a matter of economic survival, Orr notes that doctors in PMS schemes 'cooperated to maintain standards' and 'were arranging refresher courses in paediatrics, infant feeding and the like in order to be able to compete with the public clinics'.[124]

On speaking to Alfred Cox, Orr learned that in London the BMA had brokered an arrangement whereby Consultants would see PMS patients for one-third of their normal fee.[125] Cox states in his memoirs that he was anxious to develop the 'professional side of PMS work', emphasising that 'it was not a mere collecting agency'.[126] Assisted by Dr Frank Gray, a GP from Wandsworth, he laid great stress on the PMS family doctor being an adviser in health as well as sickness. Cox and the London PMS Chairman Edward Gregg strongly urged their members to take on the responsibilities of managing infant welfare and to follow the recommendations of the IAC's maternity scheme.[127] In 1936, they submitted a paper to the PMS subcommittee which mentioned that Drs Eric Pritchard and W.F. Oxley were advising them on leaflets circulated to members of the PMS regarding the treatment of expectant mothers and that 200 PMS GPs in London were providing child welfare and maternity services.[128] The Orrs observed another possible motive behind the GPs' enthusiasm for PMS. After declaring that PMS was 'definitely a good thing', a Dr Wilson of Oxford said that the BMA was assuming that the government would eventually extend NHI to include the dependants of wage earners and so 'for this reason they are promoting PMS both as a temporary stopgap and as a means of getting in on the ground floor when the government extends medical benefits to include the worker's family group'.[129] As was the case with the Leicester scheme from its inception, the friendly societies were often happy to contract with PMS schemes, thereby surrendering the control they once had over the doctors as far as the families of insured workers were concerned.[130] The number of subscribers to PMS continued to grow therefore throughout the 1930s. In a survey conducted by the BMA in 1943, returns from 70 out of 80 known PMS schemes allowed them to postulate a minimum estimate of 650,000 subscribers from which Green deduces that they could have been catering for as many as 1.2 million individuals.[131]

Despite their support for PMS, the IAC maintained its commitment to seeking extension of NHI to dependants and in its report to the LMPCs Conference in June 1933 stated that it had responded to a request from the Conference of Friendly Societies to cooperate with them in preparing the way for such an extension.[132] In 1934, the IAC reappointed its General Medical Services Scheme

Subcommittee asking it to determine if there was any reason to revise its previous proposals in the light of changes to legislation relating to Public Assistance and NHI.[133] No substantial changes were recommended though the subcommittee took careful note of a memorandum from the chair of the BMA's hospitals committee, Peter Macdonald, who made a plea for GP to be given access to beds in which to treat their own cases in hospitals. In light of recent changes such as the increased use of nursing homes by the middle classes and the need for more expensive equipment, it would be 'disastrous' for all concerned, he said, were increased use made of hospitals 'to further separate the patient from the family doctor'.[134] It is clear from the preceding comments that GPs favoured the extension of insurance-based services to workers' dependants, expecting that at some point they would be so included under a state-sponsored scheme. They wanted and expected the wealthy to continue paying directly for private consultations. They also wanted ready access to hospital services for all sections of the community and, recognising that charity was insufficient to sustain the demands of modern medicine and that the costs of intensive treatment were beyond what even middle-class families could afford, that hospital contributory schemes should be universally available. Only a minority of socialist doctors considered a non-contributory, tax-funded system to be a realistic option. Alfred Welply was one of these. 'Why devise an elaborate and expensive administrative machinery to exclude the twenty per cent who could afford to pay?' he asked. As was the case with schools, he told the Orrs, 'the rich would always make their own arrangements'.[135] Welply's MPU colleague Alfred Salter shared this view, opining that the BMA proposals for a complete medical service were 'quite incomplete' and that such a service would have to await a Labour majority in parliament.[136] To explain this comment, it is necessary to understand the contributions to the debates about health services made during the interwar period by the various elements of the Labour movement.

The Left's contribution: the Socialist Medical Association and the BMA/TUC accord

The State Medical Services Association went into abeyance in the 1920s. According to David Stark Murray, this was because, following the Dawson Report, many of its members felt that 'the job was finished' but mostly it was because left-wing doctors preferred to devote their energies to the activities of the Labour party or the MPU.[137] The foundation of the SMA in 1930 has been attributed to a variety of factors but is largely due to the initiative of one man, the Consultant physician and Labour MP, Somerville Hastings.[138] Webster suggests that an additional catalyst was the publication that year of *A General Medical Service for the Nation*, whose precepts were so markedly at variance with the views of Hastings and his confederates.[139] The new organisation aroused a disproportionate amount of, mostly hostile, interest from the press. Following its first AGM in May 1931, the SMA decided to affiliate to the Labour party and its chairman, Hastings, gave a keynote speech at the party's conference in 1932 entitled 'The Medical Service of the Future'.[140] From the outset, Hastings supported salaried service by local authorities and dismissed free choice of doctor, believing that the public were 'extremely bad judges of a doctor's worth'.[141] He was passionate about removing economic barriers to healthcare and expatiated his views in *The People's Health* published by the Labour Party in 1932 and in the SMA leaflet, *A Socialist Medical Service*.[142] Both these documents argued for the absorption of the voluntary hospitals into a unified and coordinated health service. They also advocated primary healthcare centres housing teams of GPs whose duties would include preventative as well as curative medicine. Both were clear that the health service of the future would be administered by local authorities under the auspices of the Ministry of Health.[143] John Stewart says that the SMA realised the importance of not alienating GPs, but Hastings was contemptuous of independent contractor status which he felt had 'failed lamentably' and was not in keeping with the spirit of the age, which demanded 'collective action'.[144] He contrasted the Soviet Union, where there were no economic barriers to a career in medicine, with Britain where the profession was predominantly drawn from the middle and upper classes and where 'the outlook of doctors was shaped by the nursery and the public school'.[145]

In 1934, the SMA presented its views to the Labour Party conference, condemning the commercial insurance industry and the BMA as having a vested interest in sickness rather than health.[146] It was not until 1937, however, that the SMA achieved any real influence over Labour policy when the Party reestablished its Public Health Advisory Committee of which the SMA ultimately constituted half the membership.[147] By then, however, the SMA found itself operating in 'a contested area' as a result of a new political alliance, based on a blossoming relationship between the BMA and the Trades Union Congress (TUC). This relationship arose from a determination by the TUC leadership, spearheaded by its General Secretary, the urbane and politically astute Walter Citrine, and its blunt but sagacious chairman, Ernest Bevin, to move the policy of the organisation from one of 'advocacy' to one of 'administration'.[148] The crisis affecting the Labour movement after the establishment of the National Government in 1931 had left the TUC anxious to establish a new role for itself and its leaders hoped to achieve this by forging constructive relationships with important interest groups like the BMA. They recognised and admired the BMA's corporate power and influence. Bevin hoped that he could enlist their support for the TUC's campaign to reform the Government's workmen's compensation scheme.[149] The opportunity to establish a productive relationship with the BMA came from the need for an arbitrated settlement of the bitter dispute which erupted in the mid-1930s between GPs and the miners' Medical Aid Society in Llanelli in South Wales.[150] The dispute centred on the unilateral decision by the workmen's committee in 1934 to employ a whole-time salaried specialist paid for by a deduction from the remuneration paid to the GPs for the treatment of the workmen's dependants. The strenuous opposition to this by the local GPs prompted the workmen's committee to terminate the existing doctors' contracts and establish their own salaried GP service and other specialist services.[151] After attempts at mediation failed, the town found itself split between rival camps in an affair described as 'sordid' by the local newspaper, *The Llanelly Mercury*.[152] Doctors on both sides of the dispute were referred to the GMC for canvassing.[153]

The profession's attempts to neutralise the workmen's efforts led to the establishment of a PMS for the area which was hastily approved by the PMS subcommittee committee in 1934.[154] The stalemate was broken when the BMA's Deputy Secretary Charles Hill approached the TUC medical adviser H.B. Morgan to propose a jointly arbitrated settlement.[155] Their joint efforts resulted in a lasting resolution for which both sides congratulated themselves.[156] According to Ray Earwicker, each side 'was surprised at the practical approach of the other and at the cordial relations that developed in the arbitration of this dispute'. This led to a decision to establish in 1936 a 'Joint Committee on Medical Questions' at which 'the whole question of the relationship between doctors and the general public could be gone into'.[157] The MPU immediately objected to this proposal. The Union had affiliated to the TUC in 1934 but angered both the TUC and the BMA when, after declining to become involved in the Llanelli dispute, it tried to claim credit for its resolution.[158] Rejecting the MPU's claim that it alone should be allowed to speak on behalf of medical practitioners, the TUC's social insurance committee decided that the proposed joint committee on medical questions could not be properly representative or authoritative unless the BMA was involved. It also noted that the BMA was not 'antagonistic towards trade unions'.[159] Both Earwicker and Stewart disagree with this statement, but they have perhaps not appreciated the subtlety of the BMA's position.[160] The largely Conservative and middle-class doctors were certainly fearful of the power of organised labour, but the profession had for decades been engaged in and supported what amounted to trade union activity though they could not quite bring themselves to call it that. Their leaders therefore found it easy to engage with 'responsible' trade unionists like Bevin and Citrine with whom they shared a distaste for the ideological extremism exhibited both by militant miners and by fellow medical practitioners in the MPU and the SMA. A BMA member of the joint committee, Harry Pooler, summed up their feeling when stating: 'We had found out that official Labour was more liberal minded and amenable than we had imagined; and Labour had discovered that doctors were not so very far from its ideals as they thought'.[161]

Bereft of TUC support, the SMA concentrated its efforts on influencing Labour party policy on health, buoyed by its apparent successes in reforming health services in London following Labour's victory in the LCC elections of 1934. But, as Stewart points out, the municipal socialism of the LCC proved divisive for those on the left with strong ties to the GP world.[162] Hastings' colleague

Charles Brook was among several doctors concerned at the varying efficiency of local government health services.[163] His doubts were shared by the Fabian Society which in a paper published in 1943 went so far as to condemn local authorities like the LCC as 'at best described as bourgeois and at worst...almost fascist in their methods, and with petty corruption by no means always distant'.[164] The initial focus of the joint BMA/TUC committee was on a scheme for a national maternity service for which both sides agreed there was an urgent need. The proposals the BMA presented were based on three basic tenets: firstly, that the GP would be the prime mover and coordinator of the medical care of the pregnant woman; secondly, that apart from difficult cases, births should take place at home rather than in hospital; and thirdly, that such a service should be funded by an extension to NHI. The scheme approved and presented to the TUC by the joint committee, is described by Earwicker, echoing the views expressed by many in the Labour movement at the time, as 'a complete capitulation by the TUC to the BMA point of view'.[165] The consensus was welcomed by many sections of the press but the scheme was condemned by Hastings who questioned the ability and willingness of GPs to fulfil the promise of continuous maternity care.[166]

Although the joint scheme eventually secured the backing of the MPU, many in the Labour movement believed that local authority maternity clinics offered a better alternative. The growing chorus of criticism, led by unions representing women workers, eventually resulted in the Labour Party and many individual trade unions distancing themselves from the TUC's scheme.[167] The TUC leaders were therefore already questioning the wisdom of proceeding with it when the outbreak of war in 1939 provided the excuse to consign the proposals to 'the back burner' from whence they were never to return.[168] When the joint committee met again in 1944, it was to discuss published proposals for a state medical service of which maternity services were but one component. The meeting showed how much each side's views had evolved in the interim and no longer seemed to be in alignment.[169] However, Earwicker's judgement that the BMA 'was not really interested in cooperation with the TUC' and was intent on pursuing its own interests is wide of the mark.[170] When the joint committee was established, there was genuine mutual respect and a shared enthusiasm for consensus on the future of health services between the BMA and TUC.[171] But, like any trade union, the BMA was reluctant to sacrifice its members' economic security for the public good, and its proposals suffered from an unrealistic assessment of GPs' capacity to deliver what society expected of them.

The PEP Report and contemporary experiments in primary healthcare provision

In the late 1930s, all shades of political opinion were greatly influenced by a report from another source, namely the non-partisan lobby group, Political and Economic Planning (PEP).[172] This independent think-tank published their hugely influential *Report on The British Health Services* in 1937.[173] Its influence with the public increased when a summary of it, *Britain's Health*, was published in paperback by Penguin in 1939 with a foreword by Lord Horder.[174] Generally considered to be the most thorough and authoritative assessment of medical services in Britain at that time, PEP's dispassionate analysis of the existing system is based on a clear understanding of its problems to which it acknowledges the contributions of the individual and wider society. Like the Webbs in 1910 and the Royal Commission in 1926, the report describes the inefficiency of uncoordinated and overlapping services.[175] It confirms many of the conclusions of the Royal Commission but is also at one in many respects with the BMA's proposals in *A General Medical Service for the Nation*, particularly in its appreciation of the role of the GP who, 'with his essential knowledge of the patient's background should be recognised as the specialist in diagnosis'. They also acknowledged the GP's gatekeeper role, stating that their function included seeing that 'best use is made of specialist services by the patient under his care'.[176] The authors deprecate excessive use of specialist services which 'is bad for those services and for the public, lowering standards, increasing congestion and often wasting time and money', and state that

> We consider that the making universal of general practitioner services is one of the most urgent conditions of an adequate National Health policy and that the most practical way of securing this object is by a reform or extension of National Health Insurance.[177]

The report argues for extension of NHI to dependants, juvenile workers and low-earning self-employed, and the addition to it of both a comprehensive maternity service and hospital services. It suggests that these can all be provided via increased insurance contributions into a centrally administered compulsory National Insurance scheme in which the Approved Societies and the voluntary organisations managing hospitals would no longer play any part.[178] However, PEP do not go so far as to say that the system should be open to all regardless of income and they reject the idea of it being fully tax-funded.

The report's conclusions are therefore remarkably similar to the BMA's which, as previously noted, some historians have been perhaps unfairly critical. Indeed, the PEP report, while acknowledging the deficiencies of the GP service, is remarkably sympathetic to the panel doctor's problems. 'The present status of the general practitioner is unsatisfactory', it states, 'because he is too overburdened with routine work to exercise judgment and to act as an effective health adviser'. PEP's proposed 'reorientation' of the service would involve increased efforts to reduce the GPs' workload to manageable proportions. Echoing the Royal Commission's views that NHI had provided much needed treatment to many in society who would otherwise not have received it, it says that 'the original service is much improved in quality'.[179] Rejecting those authorities who felt that GP services were stagnating, they quoted the Ministry's Chief Medical Officer who stated that:

> The vast majority of insurance practitioners interpret the terms of their contract in no niggardly spirit, and undoubtedly the standard of service they give is not only high but is yearly rising as fresh advances in medical science add to the general practitioner's armamentarium in diagnosis and treatment.[180]

However, the service, they admit, is not as good as it could be, especially in working-class areas of large towns where the GP has neither the facilities or the equipment necessary to provide an adequate service and as a result passes on more patients to hospital and 'tends to become little more than an agent for signing certificates'. These tendencies are strengthened where 'owing to the low remuneration he receives and the circumstances of the area in which he lives, the practitioner is forced to undertake more work than he can conscientiously perform'.[181] The solution, the report concludes, is to do what Dawson and the Royal Commission recommended, that is, facilitate opportunities for local groups of doctors to operate from well-equipped centres or 'central dispensaries', offering the latest diagnostic and therapeutic equipment, a small operating theatre, a pathology laboratory, etc., and housing ancillary health professionals under the same roof.[182] Ironically perhaps, given the profession's views of Medical Aid Institutes, PEP believed that those run by the GWR Medical Fund Society in Swindon and the Llanelly and District Medical Service offered the most obvious model for such centres.[183]

The BMA was clearly conscious of the influence of the PEP report when compiling the revised version of *A General Medical Service for the Nation* in 1938. According to Honigsbaum, the only major change between this and its original was that while home hospitals still featured prominently, all mention of health centres had been dropped.[184] There is no doubt that the majority of panel GPs were at best ambivalent and at worst openly hostile towards Dawson's 'big idea'. The hostility was due to fears that local authorities would inevitably seize control of these centres and that this would lead inexorably to the demise of GP independent contractor status. Dawson hoped that the sharing by GPs of facilities in such centres would crystallise into some form of group practice. Unfortunately, the spirit of individualism was too great for GPs at this time to really trust each other enough to want to work side by side, other than when compelled to do so, as in wartime. That is not to say that they were blind to the benefits of having access to improved facilities or the support of other professionals in their day-to-day tasks. In the 1920s, the East End GP Harry Roberts had become something of a celebrity and visiting dignitaries were invited to inspect the 'state of the art' premises he had established in Stepney.[185] He had paid for these premises himself, making no secret of the fact that this was made possible by his having the largest panel list in the capital, if not the country, a situation which had earned him some notoriety. Roberts employed a dentist, and a medical masseur qualified in electrotherapy and soon had four partners, one of whom was female. He expanded his premises by acquiring the property adjacent to his original house in Harford Street and then the three adjoining ones.[186] He had thereby created a local health centre of sorts, but it was not open to use by GPs from other practices.

Roberts' experience was similar in many ways to that of the Bermondsey GP Alfred Salter, who formed a partnership with other GPs sharing his socialist convictions.[187] Being intricately bound up with local politics, he found his proposals for a health centre in Bermondsey blocked by the Conservative Party-controlled LCC in 1929 but the proposal was given the go ahead following a Ministerial inquiry and the centre eventually opened its doors in 1936.[188] It was one of a number to be opened in Labour-controlled boroughs in the capital. No discussion of health centres can fail to mention the Pioneer Health Centre in Peckham which opened in 1926 and in purpose-built premises in 1935. But while this centre, the brainchild of the pathologist, Scott Williamson, and his GP wife, Innes Pearse, offered many of the benefits which Dawson had envisaged, it was effectively a healthy living centre and consequently did not house or facilitate GP treatment.[189] However worthy its intentions therefore, and however great its influence on future health centre design, it cannot be said to represent a realisation of Dawson's vision. Nor could that be said of the of the other ground-breaking health centre of the period, the Finsbury Health Centre designed by the Russian architect Berthold Lubetkin which was opened by the local authority in 1937. For many, this iconic building offered an inspiring example of modernity – it featured in posters in the 1940s offering war-weary Britons a vision of the kind of health services and public buildings they could expect to see once victory had been achieved. Its futuristic façade was a world away from the wholesomely suburban and backward-looking designs for PHCs featured in the Dawson Report. But the vision it offered proved to be just as illusory. It housed all the facilities Dawson envisaged other than what he considered the most essential, the GPs, who remained steadfastly opposed to any thought of becoming local authority tenants. By 1946 the centre was already needing to be expanded and the MOH, Dr Stewart, expressed the hope that GPs could at last be persuaded to set aside their hostility to local authority involvement and play a part in it in order that 'the general practitioner can lose his present partial isolation and regain some of the atmosphere of his hospital days'.[190]

Despite their support for more comprehensive health services, the spirit of individualism continued to dominate GPs' thinking and outlook. This was perfectly illustrated in the novel which many commentators considered to be as influential as the PEP report in changing the tide of public opinion in favour of an NHS, that is, *The Citadel*, by the GP turned novelist A.J. Cronin, published in 1937.[191] In his illuminating study of Cronin's portrayal of the 'medical hero', Ross McKibbin notes that *The Citadel* proved an enormous hit with the public, being the best-selling hardback of the decade and, according to a survey by Gallup, 'impressing more people than the Bible'.[192] However, the medical profession's reaction to *The Citadel* was invariably hostile. This is hardly surprising, given its unflattering portrait of medical practice, in all its forms, and its governing institutions. *The Citadel* is not, however, as McKibbin points out, a direct plea for an NHS. Cronin appears ambivalent about any service which, like the miners medical institute at which he had worked in Tredegar, South Wales, allows patients carte blanche to call for medical attention day or night.[193] Though *The Citadel* is often viewed as the touchstone of growing public support for the idea of an NHS in the late 1930s, Cronin himself seems sceptical of the benefits of a central government-managed health service.[194] At one point, his hero Manson, contemplates the idea only to reject it for the same reasons cited by most of his peers at that time, namely that it would be mired in suffocating bureaucracy which would stifle individual initiative.[195] The socialist GP Julian Tudor Hart criticises Cronin's failure to specify solutions to the problems he described in *The Citadel* and questions Cronin's motivation for writing the book, stating that 'he only wanted to get rich and comfortable'.[196] But whatever its author may have intended, what the novel did do most effectively was expose the ramshackle nature of medical organisation at that time and the adverse consequences of it for patients and doctors. The profession's leaders may have deprecated the effect which Cronin's novel may have had on their public reputation, but they could not and did not disagree that the need for root and branch reform of the healthcare system as a whole was now long overdue.

Conclusion

By 1939, some 21 million workers in Britain were covered by NHI and about 19,000 GPs participated in the scheme.[197] In his book, *Patient and Doctor*, Brackenbury described the period in which he practised as one of 'transition', that is from the experiment of NHI covering part of the population to one in which doctors looked forward to a more comprehensive, state-sponsored NHS covering all sections of society.[198] There was little disagreement during the interwar period about the need for NHI to be improved, both in scope and in quality, but the worsening economic situation in Britain following the First World War forced the government, professional leaders, and other interested parties to list possible improvements in order of priority, according to cost and ease of implementation. To later sensibilities, Dawson's bold vision may have seen both logical and deliverable, given sufficient political will. It was meant to begin the debate about the future of health and allied services but changing economic and political circumstances, and the reactionary nature of the response to it in certain quarters of the profession, the Government, and the press, closed down discussion of it prematurely. The report was, however, to exert a powerful influence on future health service planning up to and including the early days of the NHS.

For a variety of reasons, the ideal of group practices and primary healthcare teams set out by Dawson failed to appeal to the generality of GPs, who saw the growth of local authority clinics during the 1920s and 1930s as a threat to their autonomy and economic status. This was despite the fact that they struggled to meet the demand for their services, from both patients insured under NHI and the considerable number, including dependants, who remained outside it. The benefits of group practice could not for most GPs outweigh the loss of personal freedom of action which that appeared to entail.

Honigsbaum is correct to identify two distinct and occasionally competing objectives for development of NHI: extension, to include dependants, or expansion in the range of services, to include specialist care.[199] For the reasons documented in his book, GPs found themselves gradually excluded from specialist hospital work in this period even though, as has been shown, their involvement in cottage hospitals and nursing homes was significant and requires greater acknowledgement. While some GP leaders hoped to prevent or mitigate what Honigsbaum calls 'the division in British medicine' others, including Brackenbury, viewed it more philosophically, believing that the future of general practice lay in the realisation of the old nineteenth-century ideal of the family doctor.[200] Extending the benefits of NHI to dependants was thus of paramount importance and it was only when the economic crisis of 1931 rendered that 'beyond the bounds of practical politics' that the profession's leaders actively promulgated PMS schemes as the most acceptable alternative.

It is easy from a late twentieth- and early twenty-first-century viewpoint to criticise the GPs' determination to hold on to private practice. But, prior to 1945, only a small number among the minority of socialist doctors thought a non-contributory, fully tax-funded scheme feasible or desirable and, however selfish it might seem, the panel GPs' attachment to the mixed practice model was one which they found easy to justify. In general practice at this time there was a symbiotic relationship between private and state-funded healthcare. The fees GPs charged to middle-class patients who could afford them helped maintain the level of income GPs needed to continue to undertake panel practice and compensated for the government's refusal to increase their remuneration from it. It should not be forgotten that many so-called private patients were actually dependants of insured workers for whom charges for medical cover had to be set at affordable levels. When it came to hospitals, the profession recognised that the costs of treatment were becoming unaffordable even for the middle classes and that increasing numbers of patients were opting for some kind of insurance to protect them from ruinous bills. What they were not able to agree on was what organisational structure would be needed to bring hospitals within a national scheme, ensuring that they were able to provide the best and most up to date clinical services accessible to all, without compelling doctors to forfeit any of the professional freedoms and privileges they held dear. Few imagined that the necessities and perils of a war of unprecedented dimensions and dangers to the British public would help provide the answer.

Notes

1 Such as Anne Digby and Brian Abel-Smith. See notes 82 and 83 below.
2 *Medical World,* 12 February 1914, 'Complimentary dinner to Dr C. Addison', p. 254.
3 *BMA Archive*, LMC1/1, minutes of the London Panel Committee meeting on 26 May 1914, Report of the Panel Service Subcommittee (meetings on 5 and 12 May 1914) min. 3.
4 John Stewart, *The Battle for Health: A Political History of the Socialist Medical Association, 1930–1951* (Aldershot, 1999). p. 20.
5 Frank Honigsbaum, *The Division in British Medicine: A History of the Separation of General Practice from Hospital Care 1911–1968* (London, 1979). pp. 34–35, 46, 120. Jane Lewis, *The Politics of Motherhood: Child and Maternal Welfare in England 1900–1939* (London, 1980). p. 97; Helen Jones, *Health and Society in Twentieth Century Britain* (London, 1994). pp. 37 and 76.
6 Attested by the reports of Dr Christine Pillman Williams, a member of the BMA's Ministry of Health Committee. Joyce Cockram, 'The Federation and the British Medical Association.' *Journal of the Medical Women's Federation,* 49 (1967). pp. 77–78.
7 *BMJ,* 13 July 1918, Sir Bertrand Dawson, 'The Future of the Medical Profession' (The Cavendish Lecture). p. 25.
8 *Ibid.*
9 *National Archive/Public Record Office Kew,* MH 62/116, Undated memorandum assumed to be by Whitaker 'Developments necessary for provision of a complete medical service for insured persons'; and *BMJ,* 23 October 1920, Sir George Newman, 'Preventive Medicine and the Ministry of Health', p. 635.
10 Honigsbaum, *The Division in British Medicine,* pp. 88, 79. *Hansard,* HC, 1 August 1911. col. 318.
11 *Interim Report of the Consultative Council on the Future Provision of Medical Services,* Cmd. 693, London 1920, paras 10, 17 and 46.
12 *Ibid.,* para 16.
13 *Ibid.,* paras 7, 71–72.
14 *Ibid.,* paras 69–72.
15 *Ibid.,* para 9.
16 *Ibid.,* paras 19 and 37.
17 *Ibid.,* paras 19 and 39.
18 Stewart, *The Battle for Health,* p. 20.
19 *Interim Report of the Consultative Council on the Future Provision of Medical Services,* para 21.
20 *Ibid.,* paras 12 and 13.
21 *Ibid.,* para 47.
22 *Ibid.,* para 50.
23 *Ibid.,* para 51.
24 *Ibid.,* para 52.
25 *Ibid.,* paras 93–94.
26 *Ibid.,* para 96.
27 *Ibid.,* para 17.
28 *BMJ,* 29 May 1920, Editorial, 'The Future Provision of Medical Services', pp. 756–757; 5 June 1920, Sir James McKenzie, p. 783.
29 *Ibid.,* 12 June 1920, p. 812.
30 *Ibid.,* 19 June 1920, p. 850; 26 June 1920, p. 882.
31 *Ibid.,* 17 July 1920, pp. 93–94.
32 *Kent LMC Archive,* minutes of meeting of Kent County LMPC on 13 January 1921.
33 *BMJ,* 3 July 1920, 'Report of Annual Representative Meeting', Supplement, p. 19.

34 *Ibid.,* p. 19.
35 *Ibid.,* p. 19, and p. 21.
36 *Ibid.,* p. 21.
37 *The Times,* 15 December 1920, 'The Health Bill Rejected', p. 13.
38 See James E. Cronin, *The Politics of State Expansion: War, State and Society in Twentieth Century Britain* (London, 1991). pp. 87–90, Kenneth O. Morgan, *Consensus and Disunity: The Lloyd George Coalition Government 1918–1922* (Oxford, 1979). p. 290. and Peter Clarke, *Hope and Glory: Britain 1900–2000* (2nd ed., London 2004). pp. 108–109.
39 Sir George Godber 'The Domesday Book of British Hospitals.' *Bulletin of the Society for the Social History of Medicine,* 32 (1983). p. 4.
40 Honigsbaum, *The Division in British Medicine,* p. 74 and pp. 122–125.
41 *Interim Report of the Consultative Council on the Future Provision of Medical Services,* paragraphs 7, 71–72.
42 Honigsbaum, *The Division in British Medicine,* pp. 131, 122.
43 *Ibid.,* pp. 126–128.
44 *Ibid.,* pp. 101–109.
45 *Daily Express,* 4 September 1924.
46 *BMA Archive,* B/252/1/5, minutes of meeting of Non-Panel Doctors' Committee on 25 September 1924, min 10.
47 *Report of Royal Commission on National Health Insurance,* Cmd. 2596 (1926). p. 12, para 20.
48 *Ibid.,* p. 34, para 68.
49 *BMJ,* 20 June 1925, Supplement, p. 269.
50 *The Times,* 21 March 1923, p. 11.
51 *Report of Royal Commission,* pp. 36–37, para 72.
52 *Ibid.,* Recommendations, ch. XIV, p. 280, para 42.
53 *Ibid.,* p. 124, para 263 and p. 126, para 126.
54 *Ibid.,* pp. 130–131, para 280.
55 *Ibid.,* p. 93, para 199, p. 92, para 197, and p. 107, para 231.
56 *Ibid.,* p. 173, para 396.
57 *Ibid.,* p. 60, para 125 and pp. 166–167, paras 375 and 379.
58 *Ibid.,* pp. 171–172, para 395.
59 *Ibid.,* p. 187, para 437.
60 *Ibid.,* p. 188, paras 430 and 440 and p. 189, paras 442–443.
61 *Ibid.,* Minority report, p. 304, para. 26 and p. 310, para 54.
62 *Ibid.,* p. 261, para 642.
63 *BMA Archive,* B/177/1/1, General Medical Services Scheme Committee, 1929–1930, minutes of meeting on 29 October 1929.
64 *Ibid.*
65 *BMA Archive,* B/177/2/1, BMA, A *General Medical Service for the Nation* (1930), para 8.
66 *Ibid.,* para 9.
67 *Ibid.,* para 10. See Paul Starr, *The Social Transformation of American Medicine: The Rise of a Sovereign Profession and a Vast Industry* (New York, 1982). pp. 165–167, 210–213, and 224.
68 BMA, *A General Medical Service for the Nation,* paras 8 and 13.
69 *Ibid.,* para 25.
70 *Ibid.,* para 26–27.
71 See Brian Abel-Smith, *The Hospitals 1800–1948: A Study in Social Administration in England and Wales* (London, 1964). p. 350.

72 BMA, *A General Medical Service for the Nation*, para 50–55.
73 *Ibid.*, para 53.
74 *Ibid.*, para 44.
75 *Ibid.*, para 51.
76 *Ibid.*, para 54.
77 *Ibid.*, paras 65–66.
78 *Ibid.*, Appendix A, A. (1) (i)–(iv) and B, (1) (i)–(iii).
79 *Ibid.*, Appendix A, B, (1) (iii).
80 *Ibid.*, Appendix B.
81 *Ibid.*, para 31 (a) and (c).
82 Anne Digby, *The Evolution of British General Practice, 1850–1948* (Oxford, 1999). p. 326.
83 Abel-Smith, *The Hospitals*, p. 350.
84 Charles Webster, 'General Practice under the Panel: The Last Phase.' *Bulletin of the Social History of Medicine,* 32 (1983). p. 26 (no citation).
85 Digby, *The Evolution of British General Practice*, pp. 213–214.
86 Rhodri Hayward, *The Transformation of the Psyche in British Primary Care, 1870–1970* (London, 2014). p. 35.
87 *Ibid.*, p. 57.
88 *BMA Archive*, B/203/1/22, minutes of IAC meeting on 20 November 1930, Doc M23; Minutes of the Annual Conference of Representatives of LMPCs, min 40.
89 *Ibid.*, B/203/1/22, minutes of IAC meeting on 8 January 1931, Doc 18, Report of Deputation to Ministry of Health on 27 November 1930.
90 *Ibid.*
91 See Becky Taylor, Martin Powell and John Stewart 'Central and Local Government and the Provision of Municipal Medicine 1919–1939.' *English Historical Review,* 122 (2007). pp. 397–426, and Martin Gorsky, 'Local Government Health Services in Interwar England: Problems of Quantification and Interpretation.' *Bulletin of History of Medicine*, 85 (3) (2011). pp. 384–412.
92 John Welshman 'The Medical Officer of Health in England and Wales 1900–1974: Watchdog or Lapdog?' *Journal of Public Health Medicine*, 19 (4) (1997). p. 443, note 4.
93 *BMA Archive*, B/203/1/22, minutes of IAC meeting on 8 January 1931, Doc 18, Report of Deputation to Ministry of Health on 27 November 1930.
94 *Ibid.*, B/203/1/24, minutes of the IAC Dependants Subcommittee meeting on 5 May 1932, p. 9, item (10).
95 *Ibid.*, item (11).
96 *Ibid.*, B/231/1/20, minutes of Medico Political Committee meeting on 19 October 1932.
97 *Ibid.*, minutes of PMS subcommittee on 9 December 1932; B/203/31/21, minutes of Annual Conference of Representatives of LMPCs, 20 October 1932, minute 51.
98 *Ibid.*, B/203/1/25, minutes of the IAC Remuneration Subcommittee meeting on 1 June 1933, Doc 92.
99 *Ibid.*, B/231/1/20, minutes of meeting of Medico Political Committee on 19 October 1932, Memorandum by Deputy Secretary, p. 7.
100 *Ibid.*, minutes of meeting of PMS Subcommittee on 9 December 1932, min. 13.
101 *Ibid.*, B/231/1/22, agenda of meeting on 15 November 1933, and min. 20.
102 *Ibid.*
103 *Ibid.*, B/231/1/21 minutes of meeting of 27 January 1933, min. 29 and B/231/1/22, agenda for meeting of 21 February 1934, letter from H.E. Rowley and H. Wentworth Grist.

104 *Ibid.,* B/231/1/23, agenda of meeting on 4 January 1935, Doc. MP38 and min. 21.
105 *Ibid.,* min. 21.
106 *Ibid.,* B/231/1/26, minutes of meeting of PMS Subcommittee on 16 April 1937, min. 32, which notes the resolution recorded as minute 84 of the BMA's ARM of 1936.
107 'AGP', *This Panel Business* (London, 1933). pp. 49 and 275.
108 *BMA Archive,* B/231/1/22, agenda for meeting of PMS Subcommittee on 21 February 1934, item 7, 'Fundamentals of Public Medical Services', p. 3.
109 *Ibid.*
110 *Ibid.,* B/231/1/21, minutes of PMS subcommittee meeting on 27 January 1933, min. 32.
111 *Ibid.,* B/231/1/24, minutes of Conference of Representatives of Public Medical Services on 19 December 1935.
112 Alfred Cox, *Among the Doctors* (London, c.1949). p. 199.
113 *BMA Archive,* B/231/1/24, minutes of Conference of Representatives of Public Medical Services on 19 December 1935, min. 22.
114 *Ibid.,* minutes of PMS Subcommittee on 26 February 1936, min. 7 (2).
115 *Ibid.,* B/231/1/25, minutes of 15 May 1936, min. 23.
116 *Ibid.,* Doc. MP 84.
117 *Ibid.*
118 *Ibid.,* B/231/1/23, minutes of PMS Subcommittee meeting on 4 January 1935, Appendix, 'Advertising of Public Medical Services', p. 4.
119 Orr and Orr, *Health Insurance with Medical Care,* p. 48.
120 *Ibid.*
121 *Ibid.,* p. 136.
122 *Ibid.,* p. 159.
123 *Ibid.,* p. 160.
124 *Ibid.*
125 *Ibid.,* p. 158.
126 Cox, *Among the Doctors,* p. 200.
127 *BMA Archive,* B/231/1/25, minutes of the PMS Subcommittee meeting on 15 May 1936, Doc. MP77.
128 *Ibid.*
129 Douglass W. Orr and Jean Walker Orr, *Health Insurance with Medical Care in Great Britain* (New York, 1938). p. 159.
130 David B. Green 'Medical Care in Britain Before the Welfare State.' *Critical Review,* 7 (4) (1993). p. 490.
131 *University of Leicester, David Wilson Library Medical Archive,* E1/2/13 BMA Report, 'Analysis of Reports from Public Medical Services 1943.' Green, 'Medical Care in Britain Before the Welfare State', p. 490.
132 *BMA Archive,* B/203/1/25, minutes of the IAC meeting on 2 May 1933, Draft report to LMPCs Conference, p. 17.
133 *Ibid.,* B/178/1/1, agenda for the General Medical Services Scheme Committee meeting on 23 May 1934.
134 *Ibid.,* Memorandum (undated) from Dr Peter Macdonald, p. 2.
135 Orr and Orr, *Health Insurance with Medical Care,* p. 181.
136 *Ibid.,* p. 180.
137 John Stewart, *The Battle for Health: A Political History of the Socialist Medical Association, 1930–1951* (Aldershot, 1999). p. 21.
138 *Ibid.,* p. 37.
139 *Ibid.,* p. 38.

140 *Ibid.*, pp. 38–39.
141 *Ibid.,* p. 41.
142 *Ibid.*, p. 48.
143 *Ibid.*, pp. 53–54.
144 *Ibid.*, p. 56.
145 *Ibid.,* p. 58.
146 *Ibid.*, p. 64.
147 *Ibid.*, p. 66.
148 Ray Earwicker 'A Study of the Joint BMA-TUC Joint Committee on Medical Questions, 1935–1939.' *Journal of Social Policy*, 8 (3) (1979). p. 335, 341.
149 Honigsbaum, *The Division in British Medicine*, pp. 233–238, 239–242.
150 Earwicker, 'A Study of the BMA-TUC Joint Committee', pp. 335–356.
151 *BMA Archive*, B/231/1/23, minutes of the PMS subcommittee meeting on 30 November 1934, Medico Political Committee Draft Report on Llanelly Dispute, MP 33, 1934–1935, pp. 2–3.
152 Steve Thompson, 'A Proletarian Public Sphere: Working-Class Provision of Medical Services in South Wales, 1900–1948', in Anne Borsay (ed) *Medicine in Wales, 1800-200: Public Services or Private Commodity?* (Cardiff, 2003). pp. 97–98.
153 Harry W. Pooler, *My Life in General Practice* (London, 1948). p. 169.
154 *BMA Archive*, B/231/1/32, minutes of the PMS Subcommittee meeting on 30 November 1943, min. 9.
155 Pooler, *My Life in General Practice*, p. 169.
156 *BMJ*, 30 November 1935, Supplement, 'Report on the Llanelly Dispute', pp. 236–237.
157 Earwicker, 'A Study of the BMA-TUC Joint Committee', p. 336.
158 *Ibid.*, p. 338.
159 *Ibid.,* p. 339.
160 *Ibid.*, 340. Stewart, *The Battle for Health*, p. 73.
161 Pooler, *My Life in General Practice*, p. 170.
162 *Ibid.,* pp. 71–72.
163 *Ibid.*, pp. 139–140.
164 *Ibid.*, p. 172.
165 *Ibid.,* p. 347.
166 *Ibid.*, p. 348.
167 *Ibid.*, pp. 348–352.
168 *Ibid.*, p. 352.
169 *Ibid.,* p. 353.
170 *Ibid.*
171 See Pooler, *My Life in General Practice*, pp. 169–170.
172 Virginia Berridge, Mark Harrison and Paul Weindling, 'The Impact of War and Depression, 1918–1948,' in Charles Webster (ed) *Caring for Health: History and Diversity* (3rd ed., Buckingham, 2001). p. 141.
173 Political and Economic Planning (PEP), *Report on The British Health Services* (London, 1937).
174 S. Mervyn Herbert, *Britain's Health* (Harmondsworth, 1939).
175 *Ibid.*, p. 25.
176 *Ibid.*, p. 10.
177 *Ibid.,* pp. 10, 15.
178 *Ibid.*, p. 16.
179 *Ibid.,* p. 162.
180 *Ibid.,* p. 146.

181 *Ibid.*, p. 162.
182 *Ibid.*, p. 164.
183 *Ibid.*, pp. 151–152.
184 Honigsbaum, *The Division in British Medicine*, p. 148.
185 Winifred Stamp, *Doctor Himself: An Unorthodox Biography of Harry Roberts MD* (London, 1949). p. 76.
186 *Ibid.*, p. 87.
187 A. Fenner Brockway, *Bermondsey Story: The Life of Alfred J. Salter* (London, 1949). pp. 25 and 149.
188 *Ibid.*, pp. 168–169. See also Esyllt Jones 'Local Labour and London's Interwar Health Centre Movement.' *Social History of Medicine*, 25 (1) (2011). pp. 87–90.
189 Jane Lewis and Barbara Brookes 'A Reassessment of the Work of the Peckham Health Centre, 1926–1951.' *Health and Society*, 61 (2) (1983). pp 307–350.
190 A. B. (Alexander Bernard) Stewart 'Health Centres of Today.' *Lancet,* 16 March 1946, pp. 392–393.
191 A.J.(Archibald Joseph) Cronin, *The Citadel* (London, 1937).
192 Ross McKibbin 'Politics and the Medical Hero: A.J. Cronin's 'The Citadel'.' *English Historical Review*, 123 (502) (2008). pp. 651–678.
193 *Ibid.*, p. 676. See also Cronin's autobiographical novel, *Adventures in Two Worlds* (London, 1952), Bello edn, London, 2013, ch.18, p. 160.
194 *Ibid.*, p. 675.
195 Cronin, *The Citadel*, Vista edn, p. 224.
196 Julian Tudor Hart, 'Storming the Citadel', in Pamela Michael and Charles Webster (eds) *Health and Society in Twentieth Century Wales* (Cardiff, 2006). p. 212.
197 Bernard Harris, *The Origins of the British Welfare State: Social Welfare in England and Wales, 1800–1945* (Basingstoke, 2004). p. 234; PEP, *Report on the British Health Services,* p. 142.
198 Sir Henry B. Brackenbury, *Patient and Doctor* (London, 1935), p. 162.
199 Honigsbaum, *The Division in British Medicine*, pp. 122–129.
200 Compare Irvine Loudon 'The Concept of the Family Doctor.' *Bulletin of the Society for History of Medicine*, 58 (3) (1984). pp. 347–352.

11 For victory and health

*The Second World War, the
Beveridge report, and the
coming of the NHS, 1939–1945*

Some recent studies have suggested that the UK was not as ill prepared militarily for the advent of the Second World War as many contemporaries assumed.[1] Some, seeking to rehabilitate the reputation of Prime Minister Neville Chamberlain and his colleagues, the so-called 'guilty men', have even argued that the ill-fated policy of appeasement bought the country valuable time in which to effect measures necessary to put the country back on a war footing, though this is not a widely held view.[2] What is clear is that during the mid to late 1930s, many within the Government and outside it feared that some kind of war was inevitable, and the medical profession was among those involved in actively preparing for it by considering how health, and particularly hospital, services would need to be organised to deal with the prospect of mass civilian casualties. The bombing of civilians perpetrated by the Japanese in Manchuria in 1931 and by Franco's fascist allies in the Spanish Civil War in 1936 offered a perfect illustration of how the anticipated wider conflict was expected to be conducted.[3] Members of the Socialist Medical Association (SMA), who had witnessed first-hand the effects of this new type of warfare when supporting the Republican cause in Spain, were among the most vocal of those advocating a plan by which the various types of hospitals could be brought within a unified and effective system in the event of war.[4] The BMA was similarly concerned and discussion of air raid precautions (ARP) featured in the *BMJ* from the early 1930s.[5] The Association welcomed the news that the Home Office had established a department for ARP in 1935 which was given legislative authority in the ARP Act of 1937.[6] In 1936, the BMA reactivated its Central Medical War Committee (CMWC) which had existed in name only since the mid-1920s, as the Central Emergency Committee (CEC) and the Association was heavily involved in organising ARP classes and anti-gas instruction for doctors and officials – to such an extent that there were complaints that it had over-burdened medical professional volunteers. By January 1938, some 10,000 doctors had received appropriate instruction.[7]

DOI: 10.4324/9781003438274-11

The mobilisation of medical personnel and the impact on civilian health

The function of the CEC was to facilitate medical mobilisation, eradicating the 'confusion and inconvenience' evidenced during the First World War. It soon involved representatives of the Royal Colleges and other medical groups and was attended by officials from the Ministry of Health and the Home Office.[8] The BMA Secretary, Dr George Anderson, was invited to join a subcommittee of the Cabinet Committee on Imperial Defence set up to examine medical arrangements in the event of war. In 1937, the subcommittee recommended a survey to ascertain the number of medical personnel who could be placed at the Government's disposal which the CEC agreed to undertake with the aim of compiling a war emergency medical register. Respondents were asked to indicate their willingness to serve abroad or at home and in what capacity.[9] By 1938, the details of 80% of the medical profession had been entered into a card index maintained by the BMA, and by the time war broke out, the details of 98% of the profession had been obtained.[10]

The CEC's other function was to oversee the terms and conditions of service for those accepting emergency commissions in the armed forces which began as soon as war had been declared in 1939.[11] Learning lessons from the First World War, the BMA devised a scheme, which was formally adopted in 1940, to protect those accepting service in the forces from the consequences of financial loss (the 'Protection of Practices' scheme).[12] Once again, the colleagues of those given commissions in the Royal Army Medical Corps (RAMC) and its service equivalents were enjoined to provide care for those doctors' patients without accepting any of those patients on to their practice lists. There was also a moratorium, which the Insurance Committees were expected to police, on GPs accepting any patients of a doctor away on military service for a period of 12 months until after that doctor had returned to civilian practice. When membership of the CEC was widened to ensure that it was more truly representative of the profession as a whole, the Government conceded in the autumn of 1939 that it should have full authority, in consultation with the appropriate government organisations, to advise on all questions of medical personnel during the emergency. Shortly after, it assumed responsibility for the supply of medical personnel both for fighting forces and for the civilian population.[13] Impressed by the BMA's industry and resolve, the wartime Coalition Government decided that henceforward the CEC, which from 1939 onwards was once again called the CMWC, would decide on allocations of personnel in consultation with local emergency committees established, as they had been in the First World War, in BMA divisions. Personnel were 'earmarked' for certain duties to which they would be allocated when required. In practice, all doctors below the age of 35 were earmarked for service within the armed forces. The local emergency committees dealt with local demands for medical support to first aid posts, hospitals, and home guard units. Geoffrey Barber gives a vivid description of how involved local GPs not enlisted in the forces were in all of these and, given the demands on them for medical care of absentee doctors' patients, how little time it left those doctors for rest and relaxation.[14] The committees were soon recommending the retention of a disproportionate number of practitioners for local service.[15] Bartrip concludes however that the arrangements for managing medical personnel demonstrated a good deal of 'muddling through' and a total absence of communication between the CMWC and some of the official committees charged with overseeing the safety, health, and welfare of the civilian population. In particular, the CMWC was almost totally lacking information about evacuation plans and the BMA rightly complained that no single body was responsible for medical arrangements for the civilian population.

Arrangements for deployment coincided with planning for the Emergency Medical Service (EMS). Fearful of the effects of bombing raids, the Ministry of Health embarked on an active programme of improving and extending hospital facilities, recruiting staff, organising supplies, and planning evacuation procedures and set about establishing a pool of beds sufficient to meet expected need. What began as an improvised casualty scheme for air raid victims had, by the summer of 1940, been transformed into a national hospital service for increasing numbers of the population. As Webster pithily puts it, 'The Luftwaffe achieved in months what had defeated politicians and planners for at least two decades'.[16] The CMWC was not involved in the organisation of the EMS other than negotiating the terms and conditions of the medical personnel working within it. The voluntary system of medical recruitment worked well in the early stages of the war, and some 2,500 volunteers had enlisted by February 1940. Thereafter additional personnel were deemed necessary and women, retired, newly qualified, and 'alien' or refugee doctors, whose temporary registration was overseen by the CMWC, were drafted in to replace those in the services.[17] Even so the number of patients per GP doubled or trebled. Geoffrey Barber covered his absent partner and the rest of his district with one another remaining GP who was, like himself, 'overworked'. He notes that the local medical war committee occasionally sent him a locum, including a retired orthopaedic surgeon 'who had no clue', two 'fairly advanced drug addicts' and another GP who was 'marvellous…when sober'. His most consistent support came from a formidable and efficient female GP who, he notes with obvious disapproval, was 'a red-hot socialist'.[18]

The medical personnel priorities committee was established by government in 1941 to devise quotas which the CMWC was to implement. Unable to meet the quotas supplied, the CMWC eventually recommended medical conscription. From April 1940, all male practitioners in England, Wales, and Scotland below the age of 41 were liable to call up.[19] Following the evacuation from Dunkirk in June 1940, the CMWC was also concerned to protect the livelihoods of GPs threatened by the mass evacuation of civilians from the southeast of England and agreed to them being made whole-time employees of the EMS. The resumption of military recruitment resulted in another 1,900 doctors being allocated to the forces in 1941 and in March 1942, it was agreed that any male doctor under 46 and any single female doctor under 31 would be subject to immediate compulsory recruitment. By September 1940, 100 doctors a week were being recruited and the number was still deemed insufficient. It was not until January 1945 that the CMWC concluded that no more GPs could be spared and, as was the case in the First World War, the forces were obliged to rely on the newly qualified as the only significant source of medical personnel, some being called up after only three months into their first house jobs. Doctors continued to be recruited into the forces even after Victory in Europe (VE) day. By 1945, a total of 15,701 doctors had been recruited during the course of the war and the numbers available to provide medical support to the forces exceeded those available on the home front by a ratio of 4:1. This massive deployment had been achieved according to Bartrip 'without inflicting any serious damage on the health of a civilian population subjected much more than in 1914–18 to the strains, privations and dangers of war'.[20]

The Ministry of Health was thus right to applaud the efforts of the CMWC and its local committees. As in the First World War, it was the BMA which provided the bulk of membership of these bodies and the staff supporting them. During the war, the Insurance Acts Committee (IAC) considered reports suggesting that the Association's protection of practices schemes, which were expected to be policed by the profession with support where appropriate from Insurance Committees, were not always working as expected. There were significant variations in how these were implemented and the payments made to the covering doctors but the IAC claimed that it would be impractical to enforce a uniform payment structure across the country.[21] In Torquay, a decision was taken to create an 'emergency panel centre' in which local GPs, including wholly private GPs, volunteered to treat the patients of absentee doctors on a rota basis in clinic premises operated by the local authorities. These were well organised and were generally appreciated by patients, but the acting doctors were left with a 'meagre dividend' to cover out of pocket expenses.[22] The effectiveness of the Association's efforts to protect the livelihood of doctors absent in the forces, however, may be gauged by statements made in BMA Council reports. During a discussion in November 1945, they acknowledged evidence of failure to abide by undertakings given which in one instance had resulted in a case being taken to the high court and judgement being given against the acting practitioner.[23] The following year, Council concluded:

> That a large number of acting practitioners faithfully discharged their obligations is not open to doubt, but it must regrettably be admitted that there were others who did not loyally carry out their agreement to protect the practices of those of their colleagues on whole time war service.[24]

But what of the civilian population for which the GPs were responsible? It is generally agreed that the mass evacuation of civilians was badly organised, and it led to a great deal of ill feeling among those evacuated and those with whom the evacuees were billeted. Geoffrey Barber describes with kindly amusement the clash of cultures evident when his well-off family agreed to accommodate two evacuees from a poor area of London. These children were, to his relief, returned to their parents when the worst of the initial bombing of the capital had abated.[25] Medical provision for the evacuees was decidedly haphazard. The constant upheaval and movement of population and the recruitment of doctors into the armed forces which led to the number of GPs available for the civilian population being reduced by one-third, led to inevitable delays in treatment and civilian health undoubtedly deteriorated. As an indication of the level of disruption GPs had to contend with, it should be noted that over the course of the war, there were 60 million changes of addresses in a civilian population of 38 million.[26] Health was initially at least detrimentally affected by working conditions which in the munitions industry in particular were often hazardous and there was a significant amount of mental illness resulting from wartime privation and the trauma of bombing and evacuation.[27] Evacuee children from inner city areas were presented to GPs with the familiar illnesses of poverty like rickets and ringworm but, Barber notes, 'tuberculous joints once again made their appearance in quite appreciable numbers and every sore throat was a suspected case of diphtheria unless I was reasonably convinced otherwise'.[28] While priority was given to the EMS, health-related welfare schemes for pregnant women, children, and the elderly were severely curtailed. Many elderly patients were discharged from hospitals to free up beds for the expected flood of air raid casualties.

Although the number injured by bombing raids was thankfully less than expected, those discharged suffered neglect, many being sent to public assistance institutions, the old workhouses, where conditions were roundly criticised in a report for the Nuffield Foundation in 1943. Nevertheless, the number of chronic sick requiring institutional care reached alarming proportions. At one point, they occupied 6,200 of the 9,915 hospital beds operated by the London County Council (LCC).[29] Under the EMS, hospitals based in local authority buildings were established in a ring 30–40 miles outside London, some of which were maternity hospitals from which women returned to their home districts after giving birth.[30] Gaps in health and social services were filled to some extent by organisations like the women's voluntary service. From 1942 however, evidence suggests that the health of the nation began to improve. This was most likely due to rising living standards as a consequence of full employment, intelligent rationing, the institution of workplace canteens, and reliance on home grown food, all of which resulted in improved nutrition.[31] It is generally accepted that people were better fed by the end of the war than they had been when it started. The need to maintain productivity for the war effort also led to a renewed interest in rehabilitation although the coalition government was slow to respond to the recommendations relating to this by its Minister of Labour, Ernest Bevin.[32]

The Medical Planning Commission: 'deceptive radicalism'?

It may seem astonishing that, in the midst of an existential struggle to protect the nation and indeed Western democracy from the onslaught of the Nazi war machine, members of the British medical profession should have taken the time to plan the shape of a future National Health Service (NHS). It was the BMA, of its own volition, however, which, with what Paul Vaughan called 'incongruous sang-froid' did precisely that in 1942 when it established a body called the Medical Planning Commission (MPC).[33] Webster says that the BMA did this 'to update its image and seize the initiative'.[34] Now retired, but still actively seeking to influence BMA opinion, Alfred Cox was among those urging the BMA to take action to help determine the shape of future health services. *A General Medical Service for the Nation* was no longer sufficient, he suggested, to meet the needs of the profession and the public and a more expansive vision was required.[35] The successful organisation of the EMS had already demonstrated the benefits of medical planning and coordination. In 1941, Political and Economic Planning (PEP) had published a broadsheet urging transformation of it into a national hospital service, something which many specialists now desired.[36] The time was therefore propitious for the profession itself to set out a new vision for a unified health service of the future. As Bartrip correctly points out, the MPC was 'less of a departure, more of a continuum of planning and discussion in which the BMA had been involved for a decade or more.[37] It was buoyed by a feeling that, should the Allies emerge victorious, public expectations of social transformation would demand changes which the profession should aim to be in a position to influence. Reflective perhaps of the solidarist mood of the nation during those perilous times, the BMA had sought to make the membership of the Commission as wide and inclusive as possible. One admirer described it as 'the most representative body ever established by the medical profession'.[38] It included representatives of the Royal Colleges and a number of interest groups, including the SMA but not, it should be noted, the Association's old antagonists the Medical Practitioners Union (MPU), who had recently renewed their attacks on the BMA with their familiar lack of restraint. They were foremost among those who questioned the MPC's representativeness, alleging that it contained 'too many old men, too many consultants and not enough GPs to do any good'.[39]

In June 1941, a group of left leaning 'under forty-year-old' doctors led by Dr Stephen Taylor formed an alternative caucus called 'Medical Planning Research' to explore a more radical approach to health services reform.[40] The contents of the Commission's interim report, however, surprised a great many of its readers in both the profession and government by its boldness and lack of deference to the prevailing orthodoxy.[41] Webster comments that 'its Liberal tone suggested greater receptivity to change within the medical profession than was previously evident'.[42] The 'questions for decision' the report contained represented 'striking, even revolutionary ideas' according to their supposed author, BMA Deputy Secretary Charles Hill. These included the unification of hospitals under regional bodies, the grouping of GPs in health centres and paying them partly by salary, and the gradual disappearance of the custom of buying and selling practices.[43] The MPC opined that the comprehensive new service should be available to around 90% of the population.[44] Michael Foot, in his biography of Aneurin Bevan, described the interim report of the MPC as 'an imaginative breakthrough' and 'the boldest document ever produced by the BMA'.[45] Harry Eckstein avers that the Commission's 'principles, if not its program, were practically at one with those of the more radical reformers'.[46] This led Conservative critics of the Commission to surmise that it had been unduly influenced by its socialist members. However, the historian of the SMA, John Stewart, points out that of 66 members of the Commission, only four were paid up members of the SMA though they were supported a number of influential fellow travellers.[47]

The Commission did list many SMA documents among those it considered in addition to the SMA's official submission, 'The Socialist Programme for Health'. Their main influence was felt to lie in the Commission's adoption of the idea of health centres as the locus of grouped GP provision. The Commission's debates exposed differences of opinion, however, between Hastings and other prominent SMA members over the issue of how hospitals should be managed and by whom.[48] In his autobiography, the Commission's secretary Charles Hill, later a Tory cabinet minister, dismissed the idea of left-wing influence as 'a form of imperfect hindsight'.[49] His failure to properly explain, however, what Honigsbaum later christened 'the profession's deceptive radicalism' at this time may be due to the fact that, as the report's principal author, he may have supported if not initiated some of its most radical ideas, ideas he was later to criticise so effectively when they were repudiated by the bulk of the profession.[50] The contents of contemporaneous correspondence with Ministry officials certainly suggest that Hill and his superior, George Anderson, were more open to some of these ideas than Hill's later public utterances would imply. Honigsbaum cites an unsigned paper from the MPC's 'GP committee' which not only advocated statutory health centres but called for abolition of the sale of practices and medically controlled appointments to vacancies in place of free entry to the service for all GPs.[51] He suggests that the BMA's ulterior motive may have been to wrest control of all the existing health centres from local authorities, something the Ministry was unlikely to accede to given that municipal control of health services had been, according to Honigsbaum and other historians, the established policy aim of successive administrations in the interwar period.[52]

Considering the profession's later reaction to government proposals for the NHS, some historians have puzzled over the BMA's willingness to consider such a broad range of options as the MPC did at this time. It is not, however, completely surprising. The BMA was happy to put any number of ideas on the table for discussion, never once anticipating that professional consensus would be reached so easily, or that the Government would thereafter seek to develop proposals for the NHS so speedily and with such determination. In 25 years, the

Government had never once been persuaded to take the necessary steps to extend the benefits of NHI to dependents of the insured. Even the impetus of victory over the Nazis was not thought likely to result in major changes to the structure of health services without a great deal of professional and public consultation and discussion, and a good deal of time-consuming parliamentary manoeuvring. Doctors had little to fear, it was thought, from initiating a debate which, on past experience, was likely to take place over several years if not decades. Gradualism, that is 'evolution rather than revolution', had proven to be 'the British way' and this would allow the profession the necessary time and opportunity to see that its interests were protected.[53] It is possible that willingness to consider radical ideas owed much to the eminent Consultants on the Commission who were less defensive than their GP colleagues because they had little to lose and potentially much to gain from their proposals. It is also possible that the Commission believed reports from a variety of sources, including the Ministry, that support for the idea of salaried service was growing, not just among Consultants, most of whom by now were comfortable with the idea of receiving part of their remuneration as salary, but also among the younger generation of GPs.[54] This was especially felt to be the case with those who had recently experienced employment, and the benefits of teamwork, in the disciplined hierarchy of the armed services.[55] Pater speculates that a memorandum to that effect shared by the Ministry with BMA secretary George Anderson may have influenced the Commission in its final deliberations.[56] Historians are agreed that the MPC and the BMA's leaders at this time were guilty of misinterpreting the mood of the profession. However, the initial reaction to the Commission's report was largely positive. The *BMJ* spoke glowingly of it and when it was presented to the BMA's Annual Representative Meeting (ARM) in September 1942 the meeting went much further than anticipated in its endorsement, actually voting, by the narrowest of margins, in favour of the new health service being available to 100%, instead of the MPC's cautious 90%, of the population.[57] Their decision may just have been influenced by the fact that, following the inclusion of juvenile workers in 1937 and the increase in 1942 in the income limit for eligibility, the percentage of the working population left outside NHI had already been significantly reduced.[58]

In any event, the Ministry seems to have taken this decision as a sign that the profession had effectively abandoned its old protectionist attitudes and to have assumed, incorrectly, that belief in the articles of faith that had lain behind the GPs' political activities for the previous 30 years had crumbled. Had they paid more attention to the discussion of the proposals taking place at the LMPCs Conference in November they would have been less confident. Pater notes laconically that the Conference 'was less warm in its welcome'.[59] However, when the IAC surveyed LMPCs about the report earlier in the year, most agreed with the object of a complete medical service for the public and whereas they were evenly split on the '100% principle', that is, whether the service should be universal or exclude the affluent, LMPCs approved of group practice and a small number, namely Derbyshire, Doncaster, Dundee, Preston, and Kent (with significant caveats), were not even opposed to a whole-time salaried service![60] The atmosphere of the Conference may have changed the minds of some of those who had initially looked favourably on the report. While the ARM had endorsed the idea of GPs working in health centres, the LMPCs conference which, in Eckstein's words, 'included most of the men who would actually have to staff (them)' turned the proposals down.[61] They also rejected the 100% principle. It did not take long for the profession's leaders and the Ministry to realise their mistake and, as the wider profession digested and ruminated on the MPC's proposals, a rising tide of criticism overwhelmed the BMA and swept away the principal reformers, including the Commission chairman, the thoughtful and altruistic Henry Souttar, in its wake.[62] He was eventually forced to relinquish the chairmanship of the BMA's Council just as Ewen Maclean had been forced to do in 1912. By this time, however the much-anticipated publication of the Beveridge report had transformed the nature of the debate and with it the relations between the profession's representatives and the Government. Before considering that momentous chain of events it is appropriate to consider how the GPs' concerns were manifested during the war years and where they and their leaders stood in relation to the reformist agenda.

Remuneration woes: the GPs' continuing grievance

At the outbreak of war the panel GPs were in the process of pursuing a pay claim for which they considered they had an unquestionable justification and which nothing less than the national emergency and threat of invasion forced the IAC to suspend.[63] The suspension was only temporary, however, as in late 1940 the IAC once again took their case to the Ministry.[64] The increased workload and the rising tide of suffering among the civilian population they were obliged to attend to during the war years merely served to reinforce their sense of grievance over the way their claims for increased remuneration had been treated by government. It emboldened them to take a surprisingly militant approach in which the threat of mass resignation was once again to raise its head. Panel GPs were incensed to discover that lack of parliamentary time had not prevented the Coalition Government from increasing the qualifying income limit for NHI to £420 per annum without even consulting the profession's representatives.[65] Amid calls for a special LMPCs Conference and a vote on mass resignations, the Minister, Malcolm MacDonald, reluctantly agreed to institute a increase in the capitation fee to 9s 9d.[66] Given the continued danger in which the country found itself in, the Conference in July 1941 accepted this offer 'without prejudice', emphasising its belief that such an award was inadequate and reiterating its support for the IAC in its attempts to secure a further increase when the outlook was more propitious.[67] Interestingly, in a complete departure from the normal course of relations between the IAC, the LMPCs Conference, and the BMA, the Association's

Representative Body subsequently took a different view and condemned the IAC's decision, accusing the Conference of being unrepresentative.[68] Such comments point to the emergence of militant elements within some of the BMA divisions sympathetic to the criticisms levelled at the IAC by the MPU. No doubt infuriated by their exclusion from the MPC, the MPU had resumed its attacks on the IAC, prompting the latter to write to panel committees defending its efforts to obtain a war bonus and asserting that the MPU was 'a body of small size, little responsibility and less authority'.[69] The new leadership of the MPU evidently regarded Edward Gregg, the chairman of the IAC, as a turncoat and accused him of the same timidity and ineptitude with which they had tarred his predecessors. He responded, as they had done, with the same withering contempt. But, however strongly the bulk of the profession felt about the inadequacy of their remuneration, Gregg and his colleagues were justifiably reluctant to invoke the threat of strike action, knowing that this was a risky strategy in even the most favourable circumstances and in time of war would seriously damage the profession's public reputation. As John Marks points out, the strike weapon was impossible to wield effectively without unanimity and with so many doctors absent on active service in the armed forces and given the responsibilities resting on their colleagues' shoulders in their absence, the IAC can perhaps be forgiven for dismissing the idea as impracticable.[70]

Stung by the MPC's accusation that the IAC was still not sufficiently representative of panel GPs, owing to the continued presence on the committee of BMA officials and members of other 'crafts', the IAC asked the BMA's Council to increase the number of the committee's members elected from the LMPC conference by six from England and Wales and one from Scotland.[71] The IAC demanded that the panel GPs' case be referred to arbitration but the LMPCs Conference overruled them, insisting that they return to the Minister backed by a motion authorising mass withdrawal from panel service.[72] When IAC representatives met the new Minister, Ernest Brown, in January 1943 to discuss a war bonus for the panel GPs Gregg put forward arguments, which his colleague Solomon Wand backed with statistics, showing how much GPs workload had increased. Wand mentioned that several 'not small' panel practices he knew of had been relinquished by GPs unable to pay their bills.[73] Brown partially accepted the IAC's arguments but declared himself unable to authorise a war bonus without falling foul of the Treasury's wartime economic restrictions. In response Gregg made a rather surprising admission when he complained that 'Everybody in this country is receiving additional remuneration for additional duties. It is only people who are so weak that they can be ignored who are not getting their dues in this respect'.[74] Another IAC member, Dr J. Hallam added that he had been in touch with a cross section of panel GPs and found them to be 'a disillusioned and very distrustful profession'.[75] The meeting ended with Brown promising to consider their arguments but he subsequently rejected them, including the suggestion of a 'post war credit for work already done'.[76] In February 1943, the Lancashire LMPC declared itself 'disgusted' with the Minister's reply and called on the IAC 'to consider the advisability of recommending panel practitioners give notice on their contracts'.[77] The subsequent LMPC Conference in November 1943 considered a recent letter from Brown offering a war bonus, taking account of wartime increases in the cost of living, equivalent to £25 per annum but payable only to those whose annual income was less than £850 per annum. The Conference rejected the Minister's offer and the scene looked set for a further showdown between the panel GPs and the Government.[78] The whole of the medical profession was by now preoccupied, however, with the issue of health services reform which had been galvanised by the publication in 1942 of the Beveridge report.[79] In considering this, the 1943 LMPC Conference expressed its support for the principle of a comprehensive NHS, but, fearful of the lasting effects of the dislocation of services which would follow demobilisation, urged the government to delay its inception 'until there was sufficient manpower to operate it efficiently'.[80]

The Beveridge report and the search for a negotiating consensus

In searching for the origins of the NHS and the apparent consensus over the 'welfare state' which occurred in post-war Britain, historians differ in the degree of importance they attach to the feelings of solidarity and community spirit which the wartime situation instilled in the public. The regular 'Postscript' broadcasts made on BBC radio in the early years of the war by J.B. Priestley encouraged the idea that everyone was in 'the same boat', and that same boat would serve 'not only as our defence against Nazi aggression but as an ark in which we can finally land in a better world'.[81] Many in government, though not the Prime Minister, Churchill, it seemed, believed that it would increase public morale to set out objectives for improving the social conditions of the masses, and that 'champions of liberty everywhere would take heart when they learned what Britain was fighting for'.[82] This led to the establishment in 1940 of a government 'war aims committee' whose remit required it 'To consider means of perpetuating the national unity achieved in this country during the war through a social and economic structure designed to secure equality of opportunity and service among all classes of the community'.[83] To the astonishment of establishment figures, even Conservative newspapers like *The Times* published leading articles about the need for social justice as a war aim.[84] Charles Hill said that 'the better the life that people saw ahead, the more they were convinced that it was being planned for and worked for during the war, the higher their wartime morale became. There were wartime dividends in plans for peace'.[85] However, Paul Addison feels that the importance of reconstruction plans in raising morale was exaggerated by post-war lobbyists, citing Ministry of Information reports which showed that they were of great interest only to a 'thinking minority' of between 5% and 20% of the population. The rest of the British people, they found, were too preoccupied with immediate dangers and the need for survival to devote much thought to a post-war utopia.[86]

The Beveridge report published in 1942 nevertheless captured the imagination of a great many war-weary Britons of all classes of society and led to enlivened debates about social reconstruction in the press and in air raid shelters, factory canteens, and even among troops in distant battlefield bivouacs. It gave a new impetus to discussions about a future NHS and its importance was immediately recognised by the leaders of the medical profession as much as by officials in the Ministry of Health. Beveridge was an acknowledged expert on unemployment rightly credited with the creation of labour exchanges.[87] As a government official in various ministries during the First World War and afterwards, he had impressed and infuriated his superiors in equal measure. His capacity for hard work, and meticulous attention to administrative detail were matched by an almost evangelical belief in the rightness of his own ideas. During his tenure as the head of the London School of Economics and Master of University College Oxford, he chaired a number of statutory committees through which he honed his ideas about social insurance.[88] He initially embraced, then rejected, before finally returning to, a belief in centralised planning which the outbreak of war served to reinforce.[89]

Dismayed at being denied a senior post in the wartime administration, he was appointed an undersecretary in the Minister of Labour under Bevin who soon proved anxious to be rid of him.[90] Following the failure of a Royal Commission into workmen's compensation, the TUC had sent a delegation in February 1941 to the Health Minister and Secretary of State for Scotland asking for a review of NHI but after consultation with Bevin this was widened into an interdepartmental inquiry into existing schemes of social insurance and allied services.[91] When Beveridge, whom Paul Addison describes as a 'ponderous new broom in Whitehall', was asked to by Arthur Greenwood to chair the inquiry he recognised it as a 'kicking upstairs'[92] But he was soon excited by the prospect, seeing it as an opportunity 'not merely to rationalize the existing insurance system but to lay down long term goals in many other areas of national insurance policy'.[93] The Committee of inquiry Beveridge chaired was unlike the Royal Commissions with which he had previously been associated. It was staffed almost entirely by civil servants from the seven different government departments which at that time were involved in delivering cash benefits to those in need.[94] The majority of the Committee were in sympathy with his stated aims but Government concerns that their conclusions would lead to unrealisable public expectations prompted Greenwood to change the status of the civil service members to 'advisors and assessors'. The Committee's conclusions would therefore be signed by Beveridge alone, which he initially feared would diminish the political weight attached to the report. He soon realised, however, that this gave him unfettered scope to express his ideas for reform of social insurance, developed through more than 30 years of scrupulous analysis and informed debate with economists, social scientists, civil servants, and others, and he seized every opportunity to make the public aware of what he was doing. Through newspaper articles and a series of BBC radio broadcasts he raised public expectation that his proposals would lead to 'radical even utopian social change'.[95] The wording of the report itself served to reinforce that impression, its proposals being 'clothed in an emotive and persuasive vision of Britain after the war'. A vast number of copies of the report were circulated and read and the overwhelmingly positive reception it received from the public benefitted from the fact that its publication coincided with uplifting news of the allied victory at El Alamein. This made Beveridge himself 'a much-feted national hero'.[96]

Central to the report was a belief in comprehensive social planning as the means of combatting 'the five giants' of 'want, ignorance, squalor, idleness and disease'. Progress in this endeavour was predicated on a series of assumptions, perhaps the most memorable of which was 'Assumption B', the establishment of an NHS available to all, offering comprehensive preventative and curative treatment 'from the cradle to the grave'. Despite its obvious propaganda value, Churchill was wary of committing the Government to implementation of Beveridge's proposals, the estimated costs of which made Treasury officials blanche. But the Coalition Government's failure to endorse its provisions led to a revolt by the Labour and Liberal backbenchers and to one of the largest anti-Government commons votes of the war. The Cabinet consequently instructed a group of officials to consider implementation from which it pointedly excluded Beveridge himself.[97] Webster states that, 'The Ministry of Health was shaken by the utopian character of Beveridge's reforms'.[98] But the medical profession was even more disconcerted, fearing that the popularity accorded to Assumption B would result in a headlong rush towards changes in health services which they could neither control, resist, nor modify. Bartrip states that 'existing timetables of reform became obsolete and the work of the MPC irrelevant'.[99]

While there was much in the report with which almost all doctors agreed, such as the replacement of the Approved Societies by a state-controlled insurance fund, it showed Beveridge to be sympathetic to concepts to which the profession had maintained continuous opposition, such as salaried service and local authority control. Beveridge disliked medical commercialism, that is the competition for patients, and felt that the panel system should give way to 'community service' with doctors employed on the same basis as civil servants or university teachers. He also expected the insurance fund 'to make a substantial grant towards the medical service' and therefore that the fund 'as representative of the consumer should have a major voice in the administration of the health service'.[100] Beveridge made no secret of his belief that making doctors salaried employees would make it easier to exercise more rigorous control over the certification of medical benefits which once again raised doctors' fears of an erosion of their clinical autonomy.[101] The IAC's executive committee was asked to consider key aspects of the report.[102] They agreed with BMA Council to support an NHS provided that those who did not wish to avail themselves of the service could still contract with GPs working within the scheme to obtain medical provision on a private basis. While stating that the NHS would offer coverage to 100% of the population, Beveridge had allowed that individuals could opt out and go private if they wished.[103] But this did not reassure the BMA which expressed its fear that in the proposed health service the 'scope of private general practice will be so restricted that it may not appear worthwhile to preserve it'.[104]

Beveridge was not alone in his disdain for the competition for patients which took place under the panel system and his support for a salaried alternative. Sir John Maude, the Permanent Secretary at the Ministry of Health opined that 'commercial competition among doctors is at the root of most of the difficulties of private practice today'.[105] He felt that the panel system encouraged GPs to provide too many drugs and sickness certificates and inhibited teamwork and stated that it was 'notorious' that any doctor could join the panel and remain on it despite failings due to age, infirmity or alcoholism. He also viewed the buying and selling of practices as reprehensible.[106] Honigsbaum's description of Maude's views, closely correlating with those of Beveridge, is strongly suggestive of the professional social ideal and its intellectual origins in Victorian notions of public service:

> In his view, as with others who had been educated at Rugby and Oxford, it was degrading for doctors to act as businessmen; they were members of an honourable profession and should conduct themselves with the same public spirit which motivated civil servants and university teachers.[107]

Maude was apparently 'encouraged' by comments made by the MPC chairman, Henry Souttar and its secretary Charles Hill and even, confidentially, by the redoubtable Alfred Cox, to the effect that a salaried service was perhaps inevitable.[108] However, he and his colleagues recognised that even if the profession could be persuaded to accept the principle of a centrally organised salaried medical service, they would vigorously oppose any idea that GPs be employed by local authorities.[109] Even the MPU which had recently, after considerable argument and soul-searching, decided that the benefits of salary outweighed its disadvantages, could not stomach the idea of local authority control. As the civil servant R.W. Harris put it, 'whereas the medical profession would regard themselves, if under the control of the Approved Societies, as being chastised by whips, they would look upon the control of the local authorities, as they at present exist, as chastisement by scorpions'.[110]

In March 1943, the Coalition Health Minister Ernest Brown invited the BMA to participate in discussions about proposals for a new health service drawn up by his departmental civil servants.[111] A joint meeting between the LMPCs Conference and the BMA's Representative Body subsequently agreed on the appointment of a committee 'representative of the whole profession'. This eventually comprised 40 individuals, including 25 from the BMA plus the Royal College Presidents, and representatives of the MOHs, the MWF, the Society of Apothecaries, and medical teaching staff. GPs nominated by the Conference included Edward Gregg and Frank Gray from London and J.A. Brown and Solomon Wand from Birmingham. The Representative Body nominated doctors Arthur, Cockshutt, Lambie, Miller, Sedgwick, Rogers, and Winstanley, all of whom were also IAC members.[112] The joint meeting rejected, however, a request for representation by the MPU made by their, by now venerable, spokesman, and irritant, Gordon Ward.[113] When discussions began with the representative committee (which refused to call them negotiations and insisted on keeping their own notes of their meetings) Brown tentatively raised the idea of salaried service administered by reformed local authorities but the idea was immediately denounced and rejected. BMA secretary George Anderson warned that salaried service would result in 'stereotyped mediocrity'.[114] And, in explaining the basis of the doctors' dislike of the prospect of being employed by local authorities one Scottish representative stated that 'They did not wish to be controlled in their day-to-day work by the unscientific layman'. Local authority administration was affected by political influence, he said, and doctors had little confidence in the integrity of the average local councillor who 'was inclined to look after his friends'.[115]

The representative committee were similarly unimpressed by Brown's offer of seats for professional representatives on a central advisory body but without voting rights, those giving advice being appointed not elected. Maude then put forward the idea of new regional health authorities to run both the hospitals and GP services based on joint committees of reformed local authorities. However, even the eminent doctors not directly threatened by the prospect of local authority employment expressed doubts that local authorities had the commitment, technical competence or financial resources to run a complete health service. This view was echoed by a member of the Ministry's own medical advisory committee, who, when consulted by Maude, cited the example of Lancashire 'with its seventeen county boroughs, their local jealousies, excess of local patriotism and blighting parochial limitations'.[116] The representative committee was prepared to consider the idea of new regional health authorities but went further in proposing that the new health service be run by an independent, state-financed corporation like the BBC or the NHI Commission on which the medical profession would have nominated representatives.[117] The BMA felt that the Ministry was proceeding too hastily in formulating plans for the health service in order to ensure a swift reorganisation of medical certification and argued for more public consultation through a Royal Commission.[118] For their part, the local authorities made it clear that they were strongly opposed to the idea of professional representation on any joint local authority committees, the LCC objecting that the presence of such outsiders might upset the political balance in the capital.[119] Such views only served reinforce the profession's fears that in a local authority-run service both the needs of the public and professional livelihoods would be subject to party-political concerns. While Hastings and his socialist colleagues accused the BMA of professional self-interest, the idea of an independent corporation free of local or central government influence found favour with Medical Planning Research whose principal, Dr Stephen Taylor, enjoyed the confidence of several of the Coalition cabinet's Labour ministers. Not all the GPs on the negotiating committee viewed the idea of salary with distaste. Dr A. Talbot Rogers, an SMA member on the IAC and a future chairman of the Kent LMC and the BMA's General Medical Services Committee, is described by Honigsbaum as a 'fervent advocate of salaried service' who blamed the failure of negotiation on the fact that the salaries offered by the Ministry were too low.[120]

Before Brown's civil servants could reformulate the arguments for salaried service, the BMA went on the offensive. Charles Hill, who was already something of a media star due to his regular appearances as the BBC's 'radio doctor', established his credentials as the profession's principal spokesman in a rousing speech at BMA House in May 1943.[121] To the consternation of Ministry officials, he accused the Government of seeking to impose salary on GPs as means by which to control social security certification. The *BMJ* took up the cry and a leading article objected that a salaried service would transform 'an independent, learned and liberal profession' into 'a service of technicians controlled by central bureaucrats and by local men and women entirely ignorant of medical matters'.[122] Brown took the hint and at a meeting in May 1943 reluctantly announced that the idea of salaried service had been consigned 'to the discard'.[123] However, the *BMJ*, continuing the card-playing metaphor, warned that this meant that it could reappear following 'a reshuffling of the deck later in the game'.[124] Brown subsequently met with a select group of GP representatives, including Dain, Gregg, and Rogers who suggested that a mixture of salary and capitation fees might be an acceptable way of remunerating GPs. They also acknowledged that achieving the goal of 'family doctoring for all' would require redistribution of GPs but argued that this would result automatically from supply and demand without the need for central 'direction'.[125]

The negotiating committee, the statement of principles, and the 1944 White Paper

At the next meeting between the Minister and the representative committee in June 1943, Hill proposed an alternative to the Ministry's plan based on an extension of NHI with the addition 'of a few health centres tried on an experimental basis'.[126] Maude, however, was concerned to avoid a two-tier system and to quash any suggestion that the GPs themselves be left to run the new centres. A potential breakthrough was reached when Anderson proposed that, as an experiment, GPs could be incentivised to accept salaried service in health centres without direct administrative oversight and operate in parallel with panel practice until a full salaried service could be realised.[127] While local authorities generally continued to object to Maude's joint board plan, those in Scotland, fearing professional interference in their administration, made it known that they were prepared to relinquish involvement in health centres altogether.[128] Meanwhile, the Scottish Secretary of State, Tom Johnson, supported the joint board idea and proposed that in Scotland the whole GP service should be centrally controlled.[129] However, the Labour members of the Cabinet reconstruction committee, urged on by the SMA, made it clear that health centres should remain a central part of any future white paper and, confirmed their support for salaried service, although Bevin disagreed with Morrison about whether GPs should be employed by local authorities or by a central board. The Tory members were opposed to salaried service and insisted that the wealthy remain free to contract for medical services on a private basis.[130]

Opposition to the Ministry's ideas within the profession was hardening and the BMA's Council came under pressure to expatiate its views. They began by publishing in August 1943 a series of 14 principles. These included opposition to the profession becoming 'a salaried branch of central or local government service', a commitment to the patient's right to free choice of doctor, and a belief that Beveridge's Assumption B could be satisfied by an extension of NHI to cover dependants and inclusion of hospital services. This was provided the inclusion of persons above a determined income limit was not compulsory and that they could avail themselves of NHS services, if they wished to, by means of voluntary contributions.[131] In the autumn of 1943 the 'moderate, self-effacing Souttar' responded to the months of personal attacks on him and others on the MPC by declining to seek re-election as chairman of BMA Council and he was replaced, to popular acclaim, by the 73-year-old Guy Dain.[132] A veteran campaigner for the rights of insurance doctors, the diminutive and dapper GP from Birmingham had impressed his opponents when chairman of the IAC and the BMA's Representative Body with his astute grasp of political realities and his mastery of detail. Described by Bartrip as 'pugnacious', he was certainly terrier-like in pursuit of an argument.[133] Bevan's biographer, Michael Foot, who had met him on several occasions referred to him as 'a miniature bundle of energy'.[134] Honigsbaum offers the astute observation that Dain was 'a popular negotiator whose method of appeasing militants was to put forward proposals which he expected the Department to reject. This made him appear aggressive in the eyes of some civil servants'.[135] Hill reports that George Anderson thought Dain 'competent, yes, but not big enough for the job' but Hill, who was to share the burden of leadership with him when he succeeded Anderson as BMA secretary after the latter's death in January 1944, offered a more complimentary, if nuanced, assessment. He described Dain as 'good sense personified' and 'the ordinary general practitioner speaking for ordinary general practitioners' but who yet exhibited 'a serene judgment born of many years of experience in medical organisation'.[136] Dain and Hill were certainly attuned to the profession's mood music and when in November 1943 the National Liberal Ernest Brown was replaced as Minister by the Conservative Henry Willink, they were resolved to articulate, publicly at least, a more determined stance.

The more immediate problem facing Willink was how to avert the threat of a boycott of any proposed new service by GPs angered at repeated denials of their claims for an increase in remuneration to recognise increasing workload and to arrest a decline in living standards. Such was their unhappiness that calls for mass resignation from NHI contracts were once again being discussed.[137] Just as in the First World War, GPs complained that it had fallen to them to provide unaided the care and treatment of thousands of injured service personnel discharged from the forces on medical grounds and that rural practitioners left to cover absent colleagues were incurring additional costs of covering ever larger areas of the country unsupported. Rural practitioners were especially concerned that their particular problems were not overlooked in any future comprehensive medical service.[138] At a meeting in December 1943, presented with evidence which it was impossible to contradict, the reasonable and seemingly guileless Willink agreed to pay panel GPs a war bonus 'analogous to that awarded to civil servants' of 9d, bringing their composite capitation fee to 10s 6d, plus a commensurate increase in the central mileage fund to benefit rural practitioners'.[139] Unlike his predecessors he also agreed to an increased capitation fee, of 16s 6d, in respect of servicemen discharged on medical grounds. Welcome though these concessions were, the GPs' leaders only felt able to accept them when Willink reaffirmed that the whole question of the basic capitation fee would be 'examined from the ground up after the war'.[140] The publication at this time of a Labour party policy document reiterating support for health centres and salary served to convince many Conservative doctors that socialist elements within the wartime administration were bent on removing all the doctors' professional privileges.[141]

When it was finally published in February 1944, however, the White Paper, *A National Health Service* appeared to the SMA and its supporters, as much as to the BMA and the bulk of the profession, as something of a 'curate's egg'. It envisaged a comprehensive health service, including hospital care available to all and free at the point of delivery but neither practitioners nor the public were prevented from contracting privately for health services if they chose to. It was vague about the role of Consultants but expected that the bulk of GPs would receive the most of their remuneration, which would be at an 'adequate and appropriate' level, from the new service. Health centres, owned and run by local authorities, would provide accommodation for group practices whose members would be paid by salary, operating alongside traditional panel practices whose GPs would continue to be paid capitation fees. The issue of whether the buying and selling of practices was to be allowed to continue was left open for discussion but GPs relinquishing practices to work in health centres would receive financial compensation. The service would be overseen by the Minister answerable to parliament who would be advised by an independent professional body, the Central Health Services Council, while a separate Central Medical Board with elected professional representative members would hold the GPs' contracts and exercise powers of direction to ensure an adequate and equitable distribution of GPs was available throughout the country. Local authorities would oversee health centres and other community services and, through joint boards, all hospitals, other than those which opted to decline government incentives and remain independent.[142]

The response to the White Paper from the public and the press was overwhelmingly positive and the medical press generally so, but it was only cautiously welcomed by the profession's leaders who recognised that a significant part of the profession remained deeply suspicious of how a number of its innocuous-sounding intentions were to be developed.[143] In the House of Lords the venerable Lord Dawson gave it a warm welcome but with unconscious irony, given what critics had said of his report in 1920, expressed the fear, shared by many of his colleagues, that, as drafted, the provisions regarding health centres might prove an insidious means of introducing a whole-time service.[144] Echoing Dawson, the *BMJ* warned that the emphasis on local authority-run health centres represented a clear indication of the direction in which the government was heading and that was towards the institution of a whole-time state salaried service.[145] It stated, prophetically, as it turned out in the case of GPs, 'It is difficult to see how... private practice as we know it can survive as much more than a shadow of itself'.[146] Professional fears were fanned by the ominous warnings of right-wing politicians like the MP Guy Lloyd. He wrote to the *BMJ* urging the profession to resist the 'ardent planners of the socialist state' who had insinuated themselves into the coalition government, warning that 'underlying the subtle phrases of the white paper is the mailed fist of bureaucratic control carefully wrapped up in the velvet glove of political diplomacy'.[147]

Fearing a repeat of the debacle which occurred in 1913, the BMA recognised the need to gather more detailed information about what the profession thought about the White Paper and the principles for health services reform previously set out by the Association. They wanted to know what they would and would not tolerate should another showdown with government occur. Their strategy relied on a detailed questionnaire or 'questionary' which was to be circulated on the BMA's behalf by the British Institute of Public Opinion to the entire profession, including non-BMA members and doctors serving in the forces overseas (and even prisoners of war!).[148] A total of 53,728 copies of the questionary, comprising 30 separate questions, were distributed in March 1944. It was accompanied by the Council's analysis of the White Paper provisions. Originally this had been reasonably neutral in tone but following complaints from more vocal opponents it was changed into something much more judgemental.[149] Slightly less than half the forms were returned which reduced the value of the exercise somewhat but just as concerning from the BMA's point view were the inconsistencies it revealed which, Council members admitted, left them in a quandary. Over half the respondents were against the White Paper as a whole, yet 60% favoured the principle of the new health service being available to all and while more than half thought the service would make medicine a less attractive profession, 69% favoured free hospital services and 68% were in favour of GPs working in health centres! Even historians disagree about how the results should be interpreted, with Eckstein calling it a repudiation of the BMA's position while Webster asserts that it showed the profession generally supported it.[150] The BMA delayed an official response pending the resumption of its ARM which was postponed due to the Normandy landings in the summer of 1944.[151]

In the interim, the BMA Council urged the Government to delay any implementation of the White Paper proposals until the war had ended, and the enlisted doctors had been able to return to their practices. The BMA's Council suggested that the government's haste was prompted more than anything by an urgent desire to control the certification of social insurance benefits to the detriment of all other considerations.[152] Willink rejected the accusation as preposterous but it was a notion that was not easy to dispel, given references made to this effect by both Beveridge and Ministry officials at various times.[153] Willink was in any case doing his best to appear conciliatory and sympathetic to the GPs' concerns about wartime workload and remuneration. In June 1944, he wrote to the IAC proposing a general inquiry into GPs' remuneration to be led by a small committee of experts of whom half were to be nominated by the profession.[154] At a subsequent meeting with the CMO, Sir William Jameson, and the Ministry's Deputy Secretary Sir Arthur Rucker, the IAC were informed that if this 'experiment' proved successful it could lead to 'the establishment of a permanent machinery for negotiating remuneration questions'.[155] Equally significantly, the Permanent Secretary, Maude, assured Hill in a letter of August 1944 that the findings of the inquiry 'would apply irrespective of any National Health Service'.[156] The remuneration subcommittee established by the IAC and the BMA's General Practice Committee immediately set to work preparing its evidence to the inquiry as debates continued within the profession about the White Paper and what it foretold.

The BMA's annual meeting which took place in December 1944 was described by the *BMJ* as among the most momentous in its history.[157] It involved four days of debate over 370 motions on the White Paper. At its conclusion, Dain gave a summary of the BMA's position which showed that the results of the questionary had been rendered largely superfluous. The Association was clear, he said, 'that we do not wish to be employed by local authorities; that there should be no civil direction; that there shall be no whole-time salaried service for general practitioners; and that we shall have no clinical control'.[158] The BMA decided that the negotiating committee could resume meetings with the Minister and his officials but there would be no actual negotiation until the question of how the profession was to be represented in all the administrative structures of the new service had been resolved. Realising how popular the Beveridge report still was, the BMA proposed that legislation relating to the health service be entirely separate from that touching social security.[159] Viewing the chorus of critical and frankly alarmist comments on the White Paper and the BMA's subsequent response, *The Times* observed that 'the conference (sic) had willed almost all the ends and rejected almost all the means'. Though it showed what the doctors did not want, it said, 'it has not revealed at all what doctors do want, except to be left alone'.[160] The opposition to the White Paper had been 'cultivated by zealots' the *Lancet* claimed, and demand for professional representation in all the key administrative structures of the new service was unrealistic, it added, and laid the profession open to ridicule.[161]

The meetings between the Minister and the 31-person-strong negotiating committee, which, like the MPC, contained a broad range of interests, including the Royal College Presidents, began in January 1945. Dain chaired the committee with Hill as its secretary. Much of the discussion took place in small groups and the whole process was subject to strict rules of confidentiality.[162] This merely heightened professional anxieties while the press continued its onslaught on what it saw as the hypocritical posturing of professional self-interest. The BMA, the *Daily Mirror* railed, were 'sharpening the surgeon's knife to butcher' the White Paper, and their actions were 'degrading a noble profession'.[163] Hill had meanwhile become 'the darling of the rank of file' with his relentless attacks on salaried service and his stirring defence of professional freedoms.[164] In private, however, he demonstrated a more realistic side in discussions with the Ministry which revealed his sympathy with many of their aims. The committee reiterated their desire to preserve private practice and permit GPs to retain the right to sell their practices but Hill secretly informed his official opposite numbers that the profession could, in time, learn to accept the 100% principle and that 'whatever happened, the present system of buying and selling practices was undesirable and would probably have to go'.[165] In his public-speaking engagements, Hill tried to calm the profession's fears that an experiment with health centres would prove the thin end of the wedge. He urged the profession to remain patient and to put its trust in the negotiating committee but left his audiences in no doubt as to the likely outcome should they prove unsuccessful in their endeavours. 'Trust the people who are doing the talking for you' he counselled, 'and hold your forces until the time comes for a fight'.[166]

Eventually the dove-like Willink, 'too nice a man for the hurly-burly of politics' according to Hill, caved in to the committee's demands.[167] He indicated that he was willing to drop the Central Medical Board's proposed powers of direction and even omit the Board altogether, to abandon local authority employment of doctors in health centres, and to reserve places for professional representatives in both central and municipal structures responsible for health services. 'Medical pressure forced him to retain essential features of the panel system' including, albeit temporarily, the right to sell practices.[168] The concessions were included in a report from the negotiating committee sent under confidential cover to every member of the profession, both BMA members and non-members, as the basis for discussion at a Special Representative Meeting set for May 1945.[169] This greatly angered MPs with whom the Minister had not deigned to share the same information. The SMA bellowed its dissatisfaction in the ears of the Labour ministers and in the commons, Willink was subjected to a withering tirade by the Labour backbencher and by now familiar critic of the Government, Aneurin Bevan. Willink was then roundly criticised, in turn, by the Government's reconstruction committee, the Labour party, the TUC, the local authorities, the press and, privately, by his own civil servants, many of whom, Honigsbaum maintains, continued to advocate greater powers for the local authorities.[170] The BMA's Special Representative Meeting responded bullishly to Willink's compromises: they asked him to drop the Central Medical Board altogether and abandon any thought of part-salaries for GPs in health centres. They did, however, make one apparent concession in line with the findings of the earlier questionary, in agreeing to accept the 100% principle, 'should parliament decide to proceed with it'. This was provided that every citizen, regardless of income, was granted the right to opt out of state health service provision and purchase medical services privately if they wished.[171] The BMA meeting was in congratulatory mood, concluding its deliberations by applauding Dain with a chorus of 'For he's a jolly good fellow'.[172] However, their optimism was short-lived as, when the results of the general election in May were finally revealed in July, a month after VE day, it emerged that the electorate had rejected the party led by 'the man who won the war' and chosen a Labour administration committed to post-war reconstruction on the basis of full implementation of the Beveridge report and wide-ranging social and economic reform.[173]

In 1945, as in 1912, the BMA felt itself under far more pressure from right-wing opponents of reform than from left wingers who wished to embrace it. In 1912, the National Medical Union (NMU) was numerically insignificant but succeeded in making a great deal more noise than their polar opposites, the State Medical Services Association, which had broader appeal but aroused less passionate support within the rank and file of ordinary GPs. In 1945–1948, a group calling itself the Medical Policy Association (MPA) were the successors to the NMU.[174] The structure and membership of this caucus remains obscure, but their conduct and tactics, the effectiveness of their propaganda, and the way they appeared to have infiltrated, invisibly, a number of key BMA divisions, such as Guildford, bear the hallmarks of a fascist organisation. As Honigsbaum has shown, the MPU had already fallen prey to right-wing fifth columnists holding virulently antisemitic views and he identified many of the same individuals behind the MPA's campaigns.[175] Their opponents, the SMA, however, operated in plain sight, making no secret of their views and of their negative opinion of the BMA and the forces of medical reaction. They were, therefore, for mainstream medical politicians, much easier to attack and diffuse.[176] Just how important were the MPA, an organisation of which Honigsbaum was surprised to find almost no mention in the official records? Like sub-atomic particles, we know of their existence largely by the effect they had on those around them.

Honigsbaum sees their influence in a hardening of opinion against the White Paper.[177] But the MPA was almost never mentioned by name by BMA leaders, anxious, no doubt, to deny them the oxygen of publicity. Edward Gregg spoke cryptically of 'a small but active organisation' who had been at work encouraging replies to the questionary from those who shared their views but this could equally have been a reference to the SMA.[178] One *BMJ* editorial in 1943 did identify the MPA leaders and called them out over their antisemitism, and in 1944 Talbot Rogers condemned their attempts to mislead the less politically savvy among the profession with demands for unachievable objectives.[179] When pressed, however, the BMA's leaders denied that they exercised any influence on the Association's thinking. It is possible that Honigsbaum has credited them with rather more influence than they actually enjoyed. The SMA, however, concentrated on influencing the Government more than the profession and in that regard were much less successful than they would have hoped.[180] Nor was their influence within the Labour movement itself as great as might have been expected. The lukewarm response of the Labour leadership, especially Bevin, may have owed something to the fact that the SMA insisted on maintaining a broad membership which included communists, and also to their constant championing of the LCC, which seemed to alienate and annoy provincial colleagues.[181] Their relations with the TUC had been continually strained since the latter established their amicable relationship with the BMA in the late 1930s.[182] The TUC's canny leaders, Bevin and Citrine, recognised that the real power in the medical profession lay in the BMA. They consequently had little time for the SMA and even less for the seemingly crypto-fascist MPU.[183]

In all the political manoeuvring of the various interest groups vying to win over the doctors to their views, propaganda was a key weapon and the opinions voiced in national newspapers mattered as much as anything that was said in parliament or in ministers' conferences with their officials. While helping the nation prepare for the eventuality of international conflict in the mid-1930s, the BMA had been preparing for a propaganda war of its own. In 1912, their leaders had learned to their cost the dangers of not getting their message across to the public and their successors were determined not to make the same mistake. While mass circulation newspapers occasionally supported the profession's point of view, they were more often than not more eager to publish the views of those who opposed them. Even as the influence of their traditional antagonists, the Approved Societies, waned, the profession found it had many other enemies willing to seize the opportunity to accuse them of all manner of misdemeanours, from enriching themselves at the state's or the public's expense, of callous indifference to the suffering of their patients, or of having an inflated view of their ability to cure and relieve illness and consequently of their true value to society. 'In those days' Charles Hill intoned, 'the newspapers showed few signs of love for the BMA'.[184] The BMA sought to remind the public of its many campaigns in support of public health and in the 1930s renewed this with a committee on nutrition whose pamphlet on 'Family meals and catering' gave the public 'a new and warmer view of a professional body it had often feared and sometimes scorned'.[185]

The BMA soon recognised the need to develop a public relations function in order to counter the negative propaganda directed at them. It established a publicity committee in the 1920s which was re-established in 1932 and a separate propaganda committee was created in 1938.[186] According to Bartrip, neither was particularly successful until the urgent need to influence the public's perception of the debates over the nature of the proposed NHS gave provided a focus for their activities.[187] The central committees distributed to local affiliates a succession of posters, pamphlets and outlines for letters to local press on subjects of interest and concern. In 1943, the Association engaged the services of a PR adviser, a journalist named Colin Hurry, who penned regular letters for them to the national press while a list of speakers was drawn up to offer themselves as professional spokesmen or experts on medical matters.[188] The BMA's medical secretary, Charles Hill, led by example, becoming widely known to the public through regular broadcasts on the BBC as 'the radio doctor', and he and Hurry wined and dined national newspaper editors in an effort to win their support. The Association even commissioned documentary films to be shown alongside newsreels in public cinema presentations. Their efforts were only partially successful.[189]

Handicapped by insufficient resources and, on occasion, the lack of a coherent message, they found it hard to counter the lobbying of politicians and government officials, and the Association even found itself having to resort to libel action to obtain retraction of some of the most heinous falsehoods to which it fell victim.[190] There is no doubt, however, that when it sought to oppose and water down the most popular elements of the 1944 NHS White Paper, and even more so when it declared its opposition to the NHS Act of 1946, the medical profession had absolutely no chance of winning the battle for public opinion. The professional social ideal was not readily appreciated or understood by the public and all talk of professional freedom being ultimately to the public's benefit had a hollow ring in the ears of a cynical and war-weary public eager to avail itself of the free and comprehensive new service Beveridge and others had promised them. The problem for the BMA leadership was that too many doctors failed to appreciate this and advocated continuation of an increasingly bitter battle that they could not hope to win and for which there was actually little necessity, since the concessions granted to them were in reality more than they had any right or reason to expect.

Conclusion

It may be trite to talk of history repeating itself, but the profession's response to the Second World War emergency bore remarkable similarity to its response to that of the First World War. As in that conflict, the BMA made its services available to the Government and managed the supply of doctors to the armed forces with quiet efficiency. Meanwhile, the diminished workforce of practitioners left at home was overstretched, if not overwhelmed, by the health needs of the civilian population, and did all that was required of them while continuing to vent their pre-war complaints. The wartime Coalition Government remained as deaf to their entreaties as their predecessors had been until the threat of mass withdrawal from NHI contracts was discussed with more immediacy and purpose. A modest increase in the capitation fee, a limited war bonus and financial recognition of the extra work caused by invalided service personnel put these fears to rest only when accompanied by the promise of an independent review of the panel GPs' remuneration 'from the ground floor up'.[191]

There was widespread surprise, not least among Ministry officials, when the report of the MPC was published, revealing a consensus in favour of a range of measures which, given the profession's well-rehearsed fears and obsessions, would previously have seemed unthinkable. They proposed a unified and comprehensive health service available to all, based on a centrally controlled network of regionally grouped hospitals together with primary healthcare centres housing groups of partially salaried GPs, in which distribution of medical manpower would be regulated and the sale of goodwill in state-funded practices eventually prohibited. The optimistic spirit with which this report was imbued began to evaporate when the Beveridge report was published and had all but disappeared when its plan became, for a reluctant wartime Government, a seemingly mandatory prescription for a radical overhaul of the health and social security benefit system. Even before the Government had announced its response to the Beveridge report, the forces of medical reaction had begun to muster, as they had in 1911–1912, leaving the Government and the public perplexed at the doctors' rejection of policies they had only recently appeared supportive of. The outbreak of peace in Europe, it turned out, was to signal the resumption of hostilities between government and the medical profession over the shape of health services in Britain.

Notes

1 David Edgerton, *Warfare State: Britain, 1920–1970* (Cambridge, 2006). ch.1, passim.
2 See, for example, the 2021 film *Munich: The Edge of War* starring Jeremy Irons as Chamberlain, based on the 2017 Novel, *Munich*, by Robert Harris, for a critique of which see www.historymatters.group.shef.ac.uk/netflixs-munich-the-edge-war-film-time/ 'Guilty Men' was the title of a polemical book written by Michael Foot, Frank Owen, and Peter Howard under the pseudonym 'Cato' and published in London in July 1940.
3 Peter Bartrip, *Themselves Writ Large: The British Medical Association, 1832–1966* (London, 1996). p. 220.
4 John Stewart, *The Battle for Health: A Political History of the Socialist Medical Association, 1930–1951* (Abingdon, 1999). pp. 118–119.
5 Bartrip, *Themselves Writ Large*, p. 220.
6 *Ibid.*

7 Elston Grey-Turner and Frederick M. Sutherland, *History of the British Medical Association, 1932–1972* (London, 1982). p. 16.
8 Bartrip, *Themselves Writ Large*, pp. 220–221.
9 Grey-Turner and Sutherland, *History of the British Medical Association*, pp. 16–17.
10 Bartrip, *Themselves Writ Large*, p. 221.
11 Grey-Turner and Sutherland, *History of the British Medical Association*, p. 17.
12 *Ibid*, p. 18.
13 *BMJ*, 9 September 1939, pp. 571–572.
14 Geoffrey Barber, *Country Doctor* (Woodbridge, Suffolk, 1974). pp. 70, 80, 87.
15 Bartrip, *Themselves Writ Large*, p. 224.
16 Charles Webster, *The National Health Service: A Political History* (2nd ed., Oxford, 2002). p. 6.
17 Grey-Turner and Sutherland, *History of the British Medical Association*, p. 19.
18 Barber, *Country Doctor*, pp. 95–96.
19 Bartrip, *Themselves Writ Large*, p. 225.
20 *Ibid*, p. 226.
21 *BMA Archive*, B/203/1/ 34, minutes of IAC meeting on 26 March 1943, min. 29.
22 *Ibid*, B/203/1/35, Agenda of IAC meeting on 1 February 1945, item 44.
23 *BMJ*, 17 November 1945, Supplement, p. 105.
24 Grey-Turner and Sutherland, *History of the British Medical Association*, p. 21.
25 Barber, *Country Doctor*, p. 78.
26 Paul Addison, *The Road to 1945* (London, 1975). p. 130.
27 Helen Jones, *Health and Society in Twentieth Century Britain* (London, 1994). pp. 93–94 and 98.
28 Barber, *Country Doctor*, p. 94.
29 Harry Eckstein, *The English Health Service: Its Origins, Structures and Achievements* (Cambridge, MA, 1958). p. 93.
30 Barber, *Country Doctor*, p. 83.
31 Jones, *Health and Society in Twentieth-Century Britain*, p. 99.
32 Frank Honigsbaum, *The Division in British Medicine: A History of the Separation of General Practice from Hospital Care* (London, 1979). p. 244.
33 Paul Vaughan, *Doctors' Commons: A Short History of the British Medical Association*, (London, 1959). p. 217.
34 Charles Webster, *The Health Services Since the War, Volume 1, Problems of Healthcare: The National Health Service Before 1957* (London, 1988). p. 25.
35 Bartrip, *Themselves Writ Large*, p. 228.
36 John Pater, *The Making of the National Health Service* (London, 1981). p. 31.
37 Bartrip, *Themselves Writ Large*, p. 228.
38 Eckstein, *The English Health Service*, p. 119.
39 Pater, *The Making of the National Health Service*, p. 35.
40 *Ibid.*
41 *BMJ*, 20 June 1942, 'Medical Planning Commission: Draft Interim Report', pp. 743–753.
42 Webster, *The Health Services Since the War*, p. 25.
43 Charles Hill, *Both Sides of the Hill: The Memoirs of Charles Hill (Lord Hill of Luton)* (London, 1964). p. 82.
44 Bartrip, *Themselves Writ Large*, p. 23.
45 Grey-Turner and Sutherland, *History of the British Medical Association*, p. 38.
46 Eckstein, *The English Health Service*, p. 118.
47 Stewart, *The Battle for Health*, pp. 132–133.
48 *Ibid*, pp. 136–137 and 139.

49 Hill, *Both Sides of the Hill*, p. 83.
50 Honigsbaum, *The Division in British Medicine*, pp. 184–186. Compare Hill, *Both Sides of the Hill*, pp. 81–84.
51 Frank Honigsbaum, *Health, Happiness and Security: The Creation of the National Health Service* (London, 1989). p. 47.
52 *Ibid.*, p. 41.
53 Pater, *The Making of the National Health Service*, p. 63. See also *BMJ*, 4 September 1943, G.C. Anderson, 'Evolution not revolution', Supplement, pp. 30–31.
54 Pater, *The Making of the National Health Service*, p. 22.
55 *BMJ*, 15 March 1941, Supplement, 'Scheme for State Medical Service', p. 29.
56 Pater, *The Making of the National Health Service*, p. 36.
57 *BMJ*, 20 June 1942, pp. 764–765 and 26 September 1942, Supplement, p. 33.
58 Pater, *The Making of the National Health Service*, p. 28.
59 *Ibid.*, p. 40.
60 *BMA Archive*, B/203/1/34, Agenda for the IAC meeting of 24 September 1942, LMPC responses to draft report of MPC, pp. 1–6.
61 Eckstein, *The English Health Service*, p. 121. *BMJ*, 5 December 1942, Supplement, p. 70.
62 Bartrip, *Themselves Writ Large*, p. 238.
63 John H. Marks, *The History and Development of Local Medical Committees, Their Conference, and Its Executive.* (Edinburgh University MD Thesis, 1974). p. 148.
64 *Ibid.*
65 *BMJ*, 7 March 1942, Supplement, p. 43.
66 Marks, *The History and Development of Local Medical Committees*, p. 149.
67 *Ibid*.
68 *Ibid*, p. 150.
69 *Ibid.*
70 *Ibid*, p. 151.
71 *BMJ*, 7 March 1942, Supplement, p. 42.
72 *Ibid.*, 21 November 1942, Supplement, p. 62.
73 *BMA Archive*, B/203/1/34, Agenda for IAC meeting on 4 January 1943, pp. 2–4.
74 *Ibid.*, pp. 4–6.
75 *Ibid.*, p. 8.
76 *Ibid.*, Supplementary agenda.
77 *Ibid.*, Supplementary agenda for IAC meeting of 25 February 1943, item 17.
78 *BMJ*, 13 November 1943, Supplement, p. 83.
79 *Report on Social Insurance and Allied Services.* Cmd. 6404 (London, 1942).
80 *BMJ*, 13 November 1943, Supplement, p. 84.
81 Addison, *The Road to 1945*, p. 118.
82 *Ibid.*, p. 121.
83 *Ibid.*, p. 122.
84 Peter Clarke, *Hope and Glory: Britain 1900 – 2000* (2nd ed., London, 2004). p. 208.
85 Hill, *Both Sides of the Hill*, p. 79.
86 Addison, *The Road to 1945*, pp. 215–216.
87 Jose Harris, *William Beveridge: A Biography* (2nd ed., Oxford, 2003). pp. 148–198.
88 *Ibid.*, pp. 326 and 346.
89 *Ibid.*, p. 353.
90 *Ibid.*, p. 362.
91 *Ibid.*, pp. 368–370. Eckstein, *The English Health Service*, pp. 168–169.
92 Harris, *William Beveridge*, p. 363.
93 *Ibid.*, p. 374.

94 *Ibid.*, pp. 365 and 371.
95 *Ibid.*, p. 406.
96 *Ibid.*, pp. 417 and 424; Clarke, *Hope and Glory*, p. 213.
97 Harris, *William Beveridge*, p. 426.
98 Webster, *The Health Services Since the War*, p. 36.
99 Bartrip, *Themselves Writ Large*, p. 231.
100 Webster, *The Health Services Since the War*, p. 36.
101 Honigsbaum, *Health, Happiness and Security*, p. 37. Pater, *The Making of the National Health Service*, p. 63.
102 Marks, *The History and Development of Local Medical Committees*, p. 153.
103 Bartrip, *Themselves Writ Large*, p. 232.
104 Grey-Turner and Sutherland, *History of the British Medical Association*, p. 40.
105 Honigsbaum, *Health, Happiness and Security*, pp. 48–49.
106 *Ibid.*, p. 39.
107 *Ibid.*, p. 49.
108 *Ibid.*, p. 50.
109 *Ibid.*, pp. 40–41.
110 R.W. Harris, *National Health Insurance* (London, 1946). pp. 174–175.
111 Bartrip, *Themselves Writ Large*, p. 234; Grey-Turner, *History of the British Medical Association*, p. 41.
112 *BMJ*, 20 March 1943, p. 359.
113 *Ibid.*, 10 April 1943, Supplement, p. 45.
114 Webster, *The Health Services Since the War*, p. 48.
115 Honigsbaum, *Health, Happiness and Security*, p. 54.
116 Webster, *The Health Services Since the War*, p. 48.
117 *Ibid.*, p. 55; Pater, *The Making of the National Health Service*, p. 61.
118 Pater, *The Making of the National Health Service*, p. 63.
119 Webster, *The Health Services Since the War*, p. 55.
120 Honigsbaum, *Health, Happiness and Security*, p. 62.
121 Bartrip, *Themselves Writ Large*, p. 236.
122 *BMJ*, 29 May 1943, pp. 670–671.
123 Bartrip, *Themselves Writ Large*, p. 237. Honigsbaum, *Health, Happiness and Security*, p. 57.
124 Grey-Turner and Sutherland, *History of the British Medical Association*, p. 42.
125 Pater, *The Making of the National Health Service*, p. 66.
126 Honigsbaum, *Health, Happiness and Security*, p. 58.
127 *Ibid.*
128 *Ibid*, p. 65.
129 *Ibid*, p. 62; Webster, *The Health Services Since the War*, pp. 53, 65; Pater, *The Making of the National Health Service*, p. 70.
130 Honigsbaum, *Health, Happiness and Security*, pp. 67–68; Pater, *The Making of the National Health Service*, p. 72.
131 Grey-Turner and Sutherland, *History of the British Medical Association*, p. 43. *BMJ*, 7 August 1943, Supplement, 'Supplementary Annual Report of Council, 1942–43', pp. 19–20.
132 Bartrip, *Themselves Writ Large*, p. 238.
133 *Ibid.*
134 Michael Foot, *Aneurin Bevan, 1897–1960* (abridged edn, London, 1977). p. 20.
135 Honigsbaum, *Health, Happiness and Security*, p. 74.
136 Hill, *Both Sides of the Hill*, p. 90.
137 *BMJ*, 13 November 1943, 'Report of Annual Panel Conference', Supplement, p. 83.
138 *BMA Archive*, B/203/1/ 35, minutes of meeting of the IAC's Rural practices sub-committee on 13 May 1943, min. 3, 'The position of the rural practitioners under a comprehensive post war medical service.'

139 *Ibid,* minutes of IAC meeting with Minister on 30 December 1943, min. 67.
140 *BMJ,* 8 January 1944, 'War Bonus for Insurance Practitioners', Supplement, p. 6.
141 Stewart, *The Battle for Health*, pp. 153–155.
142 Bartrip, *Themselves Writ Large,* p. 239. *BMJ,* 26 February 1944, Supplement, pp. 31–36 and editorial pp. 293–295.
143 Bartrip, *Themselves Writ Large*, pp. 239–240.
144 Pater, *The Making of the National Health Service*, p. 82.
145 Bartrip, *Themselves Writ Large*, p. 240.
146 *BMJ,* 26 February 1944, 'The White Paper', p. 295.
147 *Ibid.*, 1 April 1944, Supplement, p. 67.
148 Grey-Turner and Sutherland, *History of the British Medical Association*, p. 45.
149 Bartrip, *Themselves Writ Large*, p. 241.
150 Eckstein, *The English Health Service*, p. 147. Webster, *The Health Services Since the War*, p. 61.
151 Bartrip, *Themselves Writ Large*, p. 242.
152 Pater, *The Making of the National Health Service*, p. 84.
153 *Ibid*, p. 85
154 *BMA Archive*, B/203/1/36, Agenda for meeting of IAC on 26 June 1944.
155 *Ibid.*, minutes of IAC meeting on 26 June 1944, min. 122.
156 *Ibid.*, minutes of joint meeting of IAC and BMA General Practice Committee's subcommittee on GP remuneration on 29 August 1944.
157 *BMJ,* 16 December 1944, editorial, p. 794.
158 *Ibid.*, Supplement, p. 165.
159 Grey-Turner and Sutherland, *History of the British Medical Association*, p. 47.
160 *The Times*, 9 December 1944, 'The Doctor's Programme', p. 5.
161 *Lancet*, 16 December 1944, pp. 789–790.
162 Bartrip, *Themselves Writ Large*, p. 244.
163 *Daily Mirror*, 7 May 1945.
164 Honigsbaum, *Health, Happiness and Security*, p. 76.
165 *Ibid.*, p. 73.
166 Hill, *Both Sides of the Hill*, p. 85.
167 *Ibid.*
168 Honigsbaum, *Health, Happiness and Security*, p. 89.
169 Grey-Turner, *History of the British Medical Association*, p. 48.
170 Honigsbaum, *Health, Happiness and Security*, pp. 80–81.
171 Grey-Turner and Sutherland, *History of the British Medical Association*, p. 48.
172 *Ibid.*, p. 49.
173 Bartrip, *Themselves Writ Large*, p. 248.
174 Honigsbaum, *The Division in British Medicine*, pp. 276–283.
175 *Ibid.* and pp. 169–170.
176 Stewart, *The Battle for Health*, pp. 161–162 and 164.
177 Honigsbaum, *The Division in British Medicine*, p. 280. Honigsbaum, *Health, Happiness and Security*, p. 81.
178 *BMJ,* 4 August 1944, Supplement, p. 30.
179 *Ibid.*, 30 October 1943, 'The Opponents of the Medical Profession', p. 552; *BMJ,* 2 September 1944, letter from A. Talbot Rogers on MPA 'The Apostasy of the BMA.' Supplement, pp. 49–50.
180 Stewart, *The Battle for Health*, pp. 144–145.
181 *Ibid.*, pp. 123–124, 170–172 and 217.
182 Ray Earwicker, 'A Study of the BMA/TUC Joint Committee on Medical Questions 1935–1939.' *The Journal of Social Policy*, 8 (3) (1979). pp. 335–356.
183 Stewart, *The Battle for Health*, pp. 72–73 and 104–110.
184 Hill, *Both Sides of the Hill*, p. 55.
185 *Ibid.*, p. 60.

186 Bartrip, *Themselves Writ Large*, p. 196.
187 *Ibid.*, p. 233.
188 Grey-Turner and Sutherland, *History of the British Medical Association*, p. 310. Bartrip, *Themselves Writ Large*, p. 233.
189 Bartrip, *Themselves Writ Large*, pp. 233–234.
190 *Ibid.*, p. 227.
191 *BMJ,* 8 January 1944, Supplement, p. 5.

12 Facing the future?

Bevan, the BMA, and the ghost of conflicts past, 1945–1948

There were some ironic cheers when news was announced at the BMA's Annual Representative Meeting in July 1945 that Beveridge had failed in his bid to become the (Liberal) MP for Berwick on Tweed.[1] The Conservative-minded representatives found little else to cheer about, however, when the full results of the general election that year were made known. The 'Labour landslide' raised fears that the hard-won concessions wrung from Willink might soon be repudiated. According to Kenneth Morgan, the new Labour administration had appropriated the Beveridge report 'as its own' but was vague on key social issues, including the idea of a state medical service.[2] It was initially committed to implementation of the Coalition Government's White Paper and a resolution to that effect was passed at the Labour Party annual conference in 1945.[3] However, a change to this situation was inevitable when the new Prime Minister, Attlee, made the daring and entirely unexpected decision to appoint as his Health Minister the Welsh firebrand and most vocal critic of Coalition health policy, Aneurin Bevan. The sphinx-like Attlee realised that the man whom Churchill dismissed as 'a squalid nuisance' was in fact highly capable. He reasoned that if Bevan's considerable energy and talent were directed towards the difficult but essential objectives of delivering the much-anticipated National Health Service (NHS), and overseeing an ambitious post-war house-rebuilding programme, his indomitable personality could prove an asset rather than a liability. In his biography of Bevan, John Campbell writes that 'Attlee recognised the subtlety, the thoughtfulness, the essential seriousness beneath the crude and provocative irresponsibility of Bevan's public conduct'. He was supported by Bevan's sometime antagonist Bevin, who opined that Bevan had 'sense as well as blarney' and that 'he will not let our people down'.[4]

Bevan was not bound to implement Willink's plan which some of Labour's coalition ministers had already repudiated, but nor did he feel bound by the SMA's policy obsessions. Bevan was among many in the Labour movement who felt that Beveridge's proposals had been 'emasculated by the negotiators at Tavistock square'.[5] However, he recognised that he could not easily row back on Willink's concessions to the BMA without the risk of reigniting a conflict with

DOI: 10.4324/9781003438274-12

the largely conservative doctors without whom no plans for an NHS would be viable. He therefore proceeded cautiously at first in his dealings with the profession while clarifying his thoughts about the best way of achieving the objective which had all but defeated his predecessors. His relations with the SMA 'were not particularly close' according to Webster.[6] He dismissed them collectively as 'pure but impotent' and when, later, they attacked elements of his plans, expressed private annoyance at 'SMA hotheads'.[7] The BMA was initially horrified at the thought of having to deal with a Minister who was working-class, an ex-miner, and a trade unionist demagogue to boot. Remembering their clash with Lloyd George, they noted that he was 'another Welshman' who, to make matters worse, had once played an active role in one of the hated miners' Medical Aid Societies in South Wales.[8]

Bevan was initially less concerned with the GPs than he was to reform the hospital service and his main focus was to embrace the challenge which his predecessors had shied away from by nationalising the voluntary and municipal hospitals. Regionalisation of hospital services was a concept which had gained wide support during the course of the war, aided by the success of the Emergency Medical Services (EMS) and was in Eckstein's words now accepted as 'orthodox doctrine'.[9] He was therefore, according to Webster, 'aligning himself with a distinct body of expert opinion'.[10] The boldness of his plan, however, was a shock for many of his officials whom Honigsbaum and Webster agree were still captivated by the notion of a pluralistic health service under local authority control. The LCC was for them an essential exemplar, 'a state within the medical state... strategically well placed to influence the Ministry of Health during the evolution of its thinking'.[11] But advocates of the reform of local government singled out health services as an illustration of their deficiencies, stating that the creation of a modern integrated hospital system was beyond their administrative and financial capabilities.[12] Bevan shared this view of local government which soon put him at odds with Morrison and other cabinet colleagues whom he had to work hard to win over with irrefutable logic and his characteristic rhetorical flair.[13]

For Bevan, a nationalised and regionalised scheme was an essential prerequisite for social and geographical equality, something 'which would achieve a uniform standard of service for all', and would be available to everyone everywhere.[14] Much of Bevan's approach involved permutations of previously agreed proposals but his hospital plan was unique and daring.[15] He was able to capitalise on growing support for the idea of a unified hospital service among Consultants, whom he managed to appease by offering to maintain their private practice privileges, by means of part-time contracts and the transfer of pay beds into the NHS. This he termed, memorably, as 'stuffing their mouths with gold'.[16] While doing so, he fought off attacks from the voluntary hospital lobby, strongly supported by the Conservative opposition, and the elements within his party, including the SMA, who resented the proposed loss of local authority power.[17] Bevan reassured his cabinet colleagues that while the local authorities would lose control over the hospitals 'many other avenues were being opened where their responsibilities would be expanded'.[18] Apart from Sir John Hawton, whom Pater credits with encouraging Bevan to adopt the nationalisation idea, his senior officials were initially less than enthusiastic, but soon realised that he was not a Minister to be deflected by civil service obduracy or obscurantism.[19] They, like his opponents, soon appreciated that the strength of Bevan's convictions was matched by the sharpness and subtlety of his mind. His prodigious memory and grasp of administrative detail were such that he could argue with opponents without the need for notes. He carefully weighed the advice his officials gave him and was not dominated by them and when he had made up his mind, he was clear and decisive in his instructions. He was accordingly adjudged by many of those who served him to have been the most outstanding Minister of Health the country had ever had as well as 'on his day, the most outstanding parliamentary speaker of his generation'.[20]

Initial encounters and professional frustration

Bevan was determined not to make the mistake which Willink had made of allowing himself to become mired in complex negotiations with the BMA. In his first official speech as Minister at a dinner in September 1945, Bevan assured the profession's leaders that he would not use 'bullying methods' in his dealings with them and that doctors could expect full involvement 'in the management of their work and the policies that govern it'.[21] Nevertheless in a letter to Charles Hill in November, he dismissed any notion of there being 'a long series of protracted negotiations' while still expressing his readiness to listen to the profession's views. In his initial encounters with the profession's leaders Bevan impressed them with his intelligence, wit, and charm. One of the GP members of the BMA's negotiating team, Roland W. Cockshutt, judged Bevan 'the finest intellect I ever met. From the outset we were startled by the calibre of his mind'.[22] Comparisons with that other Welsh politician were obvious when, in reporting his address to the Society of Physiotherapists in January 1946, the *BMJ* noted, disapprovingly, that Bevan was someone who 'could say infuriating things in such a way that his audience, after a gasp of indignation ends by laughing and applauding'.[23] While Bevan set about demolishing the arguments of the voluntary hospital lobby the BMA, frustrated by Bevan's prevarication over meeting with the profession's negotiators, decided to set out a new series of principles deemed essential to secure doctors' participation in the new NHS. The 'seven principles' announced by the negotiating committee in December 1945 were:

1 no full-time salaried medical service;
2 doctors to retain complete clinical autonomy;
3 patients to have free choice of doctor, hospital, or of any medical service they wish to avail themselves of, whether public or private;

4 doctors to be free to choose the form, type, and place of work they prefer without governmental or other direction;
5 every patient to be free to avail themselves of the NHS services;
6 hospital services to be regionally organised around university teaching hospital areas;
7 doctors to be adequately represented on all administrative bodies associated with the NHS.[24]

However, when Bevan met the negotiating committee in January 1946, it was with the sole purpose of explaining the structure and content of his forthcoming NHS Bill and they were dismayed to find that he considered its contents non-negotiable.[25] They subsequently concluded that the Minister's proposals were potentially in conflict with principles 1, 4, and 7 and sought to persuade him to institute appropriate modifications. Bevan, however, pressed ahead with the Bill, which was introduced in March 1946 with an accompanying White Paper. The response from the press and the public was overwhelmingly positive. The *Lancet* observed that it was in many respects little different from what Brown and Willink had agreed with the profession, but the BMA was fearful of 'the devil in the detail'.[26] While reaffirming Council's approval of the principle of an NHS, Dain and his colleagues emphasised the threat which the Bill in its present form posed to what they described as 'professional freedom'. They were not altogether dissatisfied with the proposed nationalisation of the hospitals, and certainly preferred Bevan's plan to the confused plan concocted by Willink which Pater described as being of 'almost unworkable complexity'.[27] Nor were they unhappy with how doctors working in the hospitals were to be accommodated as regards their status and their right to undertake private practice. Publicly though, they lamented that the voluntary hospitals were to be 'disinherited' and were disquieted to find ultimate control over the whole hospital system vested in the Minister.[28]

   Their first stated objection was that the tri-partite system, which Bevan had pragmatically proposed to ensure that the service could be introduced speedily with minimum administrative dislocation, solidified the separation of GPs from the hospital service and threatened to create a health service based on separate and mutually distinctive parts rather than an integrated whole.[29] In this, their criticism was not without justification, as it proved to be a complaint which in later years many observers, particularly within the Labour party itself, were to level at Bevan when discussing the effectiveness of his 'legacy'.[30] Bevan seems to have assumed that the profession's leaders would be reassured by the continuity of the separate administrative structures governing independent contractors, as indeed they should have been.[31] The BMA's main concern, however, was with the status and work of GPs within the new service. They objected to the fact that GPs in the new NHS could only practice in areas where a new central government-appointed body, the Medical Practices Committee, had determined that there was a need for them, and that new doctors would be expected to practise in local authority-owned and managed health centres and to receive part of their remuneration as salary. Given the Labour Party's declared policy, it was not unreasonable to assume, the *BMJ* claimed, that this was the first step towards a whole-time salaried service.[32]

The other aspect of the plan of considerable concern to a number of GPs was the proposed abolition of the buying and selling of practices, which Bevan had resurrected from among ideas consigned by Willink to the 'back burner'. In this, Bevan was at one with the SMA in regarding the custom as morally repugnant. How could it be right, he asked in a later debate in the Commons, for a doctor to be allowed to succeed to a practice 'not on account of his professional qualifications but on the size of his purse?'[33] Bevan also felt that it was 'improper' for doctors to benefit from the sale of practices almost wholly built up out of public money. Nevertheless, he concluded that it would be 'inhuman and most unjust' not to compensate doctors for the loss of their practices.[34] He set aside a sum of £66 million for the purpose, to be distributed to doctors on their retirement from the service or on death, to their next of kin, the value of each award being based on one and a half years' income, while the owners of those practices were to receive interim interest payments.[35] He tried to placate MPs speaking on the profession's behalf by stating that the Bill 'would strengthen democracy by giving doctors full participation in the administration of their own profession'.[36] Although little attention was given to this assertion at the time, his statement speaks to a deeply held belief on Bevan's part in democracy, among whose manifestations he counted not just the parliamentary system but the guild socialists' idea of workers' participation.[37] He was therefore sympathetically inclined towards professional representation in the new administrative structures and when left-wingers, including the SMA, criticised his decision to allow doctors the right of appeal against dismissal from their contracts to an independent tribunal, he justified the decision by invoking the principle of workers' control. The party could hardly deny to the medical profession, he argued, the privileges they had been demanding for other public sector workers.[38]

At the BMA's Special Representative Meeting in May 1946, however, a string of resolutions condemned the principal measures in the Bill, including state ownership of hospitals, and, worked up by what they perceived to be an implicit attack on their 'professional freedoms', the meeting pledged to inform the public that Bevan's proposals were against the public interest. Typical of the dire warnings uttered from the platform on that occasion was that of Dr Cockshutt who thundered that the NHS Act 'would reduce the status of doctors to that of West Indian slaves'.[39] Taking his cue from the tone of the debate, Dain himself condemned the Act as a vehicle for 'socialist ideals' which would render the Minister a 'complete and uncontrolled dictator'.[40] In this, he was echoing the views of Alfred Cox who had denounced Bevan in the *BMJ* as a would-be medical 'Fuehrer'.[41] The representatives, 'drunk on their own rhetoric', according to Bartrip, convinced themselves that the profession was, aside from a minority of SMA 'cranks', solidly behind them and against the Government's proposals.[42] They demanded a series of amendments which would have succeeded in making the Act unworkable.[43] Bevan and his supporters were not impressed, concluding, as Lloyd George had once done, that the profession's leaders were out of touch with the needs and wishes of the rank and file and, more importantly, that they were out to frustrate the declared will of parliament. Bevan explained to the medical MP Sir Henry Morris Jones that he had consulted rather than negotiated with the profession because parliament alone was responsible for approving legislation and was not answerable to outside bodies.[44]

Attempts by the Conservative opposition to throw up obstacles in the path of the Bill using arguments supplied from BMA House proved entirely ineffective.[45] In the Lords meanwhile, the medical grandees, Lords Horder and Dawson, sounded ominous warnings, echoing the fears expressed by the Association. However, the effect of these pronouncements was muted by the more balanced but always sightly ambiguous comments of the President of the Royal College of Physicians, Lord Moran.[46] It was during the second reading of the Bill in the Commons, however, that Bevan made a 'seriously maladroit' remark which was to come back to haunt him. In response to a Conservative MP's questioning of his comment that the time was not right for the profession to become salaried, he responded with the ill-judged remark that 'there was all the difference in the world between plucking fruit when it was ripe and plucking it when it was green'.[47] Professional leaders immediately seized on this as evidence of a nefarious intention to dragoon the profession into salaried service at some not too distant date. Bevan's protests that he had no plans to introduce a full-time salaried service were negated by his admission that 'he could not prophesy what might be done by future governments'.[48] This one comment served to undo what little trust the profession had in the new administration and encouraged the diehards in their opposition to the Bill in all its particulars. Campbell suggests that the doctors' fears were supported by comments Bevan had made to cabinet colleagues the previous year, but points out that Bevan was at that time under pressure to convince Attlee, Morrison, and others that he had not completely abandoned the idea of salaried service which, after all, had been a central plank of Labour's policy pamphlet, *A National Service for Health*, published in April 1943.[49] Although Bevan had committed himself in the Bill to retaining capitation as the basis for independent contractors' remuneration, resistance to the threat of salaried service, and its implied subordination of doctors to local authority or central bureaucratic control, was to become the rallying cry of the BMA during all its subsequent campaigns and negotiations prior to the 'appointed day' on which the service began in 1948.

The Spens report and the questionary

The amount of capitation the GPs were to receive before and after that date was to prove another important factor in determining the profession's relations with the Minister and the Government at this time. Given the fact that unhappiness with remuneration had been the single biggest grievance of the panel GPs throughout the history of NHI, it is surprising how little attention has been shown by historians to the fate of the Spens report in descriptions of this period. Only Charles Webster seems to have acknowledged its importance.[50] The Interdepartmental Committee of Inquiry into GPs' Remuneration in the Public Service was established by the Coalition Government in February 1945 under the chairmanship of the respected academic Sir Will Spens. The committee comprised equal numbers of medical and lay experts, including four GPs nominated by the BMA.[51] The inquiry succeeded in confirming what the profession had been saying for some years, namely that, for substantial numbers of GPs, incomes had fallen steadily in real terms over successive years prior to and during the war. In its report, published in May 1946, the inquiry consequently recommended a substantial increase in remuneration equivalent to a rise in the capitation fee from 10s 6d to 15s per patient, an amount Webster adjudges 'fair to the profession'.[52] Importantly, the committee sought to redress the decline in GPs' incomes not only in terms of economic reciprocity but with reference to 'the social and economic status of general medical practice and its power to attract a suitable type of recruit to the profession'.[53]

The Spens committee assumed that the remuneration of GPs working in the public service would continue to be based on capitation which, they argued, 'allowed the highest incomes to accrue to the best, or at least the most popular doctors'.[54] Further, capitation did in their opinion 'at least reward practitioners in proportion to the number of their patients and thus preserves the competition for patients which existed under the old medical system'.[55] In that sense, the Spens report, according to Webster, placed a 'formidable obstacle' in the path of the salaried alternative and helped deflect the Government from that course.[56] The profession's negotiations with Ernest Brown had raised expectations that a settlement based on the Spens report would 'clear up past injustices' and that 'establishing accord over remuneration was…a necessary precondition to gaining support for the new health service'.[57] The BMA's Annual Representative Meeting (ARM) welcomed the Spens report enthusiastically and, had Bevan agreed to implement it immediately, it would have dampened the ardour of the some of the professional opponents of his Bill and 'undermined professional solidarity'.[58] Bevan, however, prevaricated. He threatened to impose an interim award of 12s 6d, hinting that his agreement to full implementation of the Spens recommendations could be dependent on the profession's acceptance of the NHS Bill.[59] This was a tactical error on his part. It flew in the face of assurances given by previous ministers and civil servants and so was seen as an act of bad faith. The IAC made it clear in correspondence with officials that they saw this as a potential resignation issue.[60] At a subsequent meeting with Ministry officials the impasse was only broken after Charles Hill and the Ministry's permanent secretary, Sir William Douglas, retired from the meeting to thrash out a form of words which allowed for an acceptable compromise. Essentially the Government agreed to fully implement the Spens recommendations 'on account' from January 1946 on the understanding that the profession would enter into meaningful discussions about the NHS. Both sides glossed over the fact that the BMA was committed to hold another plebiscite which might vitiate that undertaking.[61]

This agreement came too late, however, to counter the negative effect it had produced in the profession and relations between the two sides were soured still further when 'hotheads' like Cockshutt exulted in the Minister's apparent climb-down.[62] The BMA's leaders now talked openly of conflict with the government being inevitable and, regardless of the Government's claims that it had already conceded much that was of concern to the profession, that it would only be re-solved by the Government meeting all of the profession's remaining demands.[63] For many impartial observers, this sounded very much like the position which the BMA had taken over the National Insurance Act in 1912. But, despite their bellicose language, the BMA's leaders were anxious not to fall into the same er-ror as their predecessors did on that occasion. They felt confident that they knew the minds of the silent majority of the profession but needed to be sure that, when the anticipated battle commenced, that majority would follow them to the barricades. Charles Hill had endured repeated 'history lessons' by his 'predeces-sor but one', Alfred Cox, on the mistakes made by the Association in its battle with Lloyd George. 'There had been confusion, frustration and bitterness', he noted, 'not so much because of a lack of leadership but more because the lead-ership failed to refresh its authority from the rank and file'. He summed up the challenge faced by him and his colleagues:

> It is not enough for the leadership to be bloody, bold and resolute: it must be continually in touch with the rank and file…it is the duty of leaders to remind their followers of what has already been gained as well as what has not, and of what is possible and what is not.[64]

This was the philosophy on which in the summer of 1946 the ARM based its de-cision to undertake a plebiscite of the entire profession to ascertain its views on how they should respond to the Bill, which became law when it received Royal assent in November 1946. Once the NHS Act was passed, the profession's fate seemed to many to have been sealed. The BMA was anxious, however, to try to mitigate, by means of political pressure, the elements of Bevan's plans to which they took the greatest exception. They could attempt this by seeking to negotiate modifications via the explanatory regulations following the Act; or they might force the Government to abandon key elements of those proposals altogether through the threat of orchestrated non-participation. The plebiscite was meant to guide the profession's leaders as to how to proceed. The key question was 'Do you desire the negotiating committee to enter into discussions with the Minister on the regulations authorised by the National Health Act?' The *Lancet* argued that the answer needed to be 'yes' in order to see 'the whole structure shaped and completed under the most favourable conditions'.[65] The BMA leadership was, however, hoping for a decisive 'no' as strongly implied by the comments in its accompanying explanation of the Act which stated that 'the independence of medicine is at stake'. Such comments led some newspapers to accuse the BMA of trying to manipulate the result.[66]

Like the questionary, the plebiscite was sent to every member of the profession for whom an address could be found. Unfortunately, the results failed to deliver an unequivocal message. Bartrip claims that 46% of those who voted favoured negotiations while 54% disapproved, whereas Grey-Turner prefers to quote the percentage of the total issued being against negotiations as 55% and those voting for them as only 37%.[67] Both agree, however, that the result was indecisive and showed that the profession was divided, though as Grey-Turner puts it, 'the results were sufficient to inform the Minister that his cherished scheme was in danger'. The *Lancet* discerned a host of coincidental reasons to explain the unhappiness of the profession as represented in the plebiscite results. These were:

1 misrepresentation by the BMA;
2 GPs' indignation over the capitation fee dispute;
3 a feeling that there had not been adequate consultation with the profession;
4 the Minister's insistence on new GPs being paid a basic salary;
5 the effect of the recent incident in Willesden (where a Labour-led local authority had tried to compel hospital staff to join a trade union);
6 general middle-class irritation at Government controls and fears of the loss of privileges.[68]

The BMA informed Bevan that following the plebiscite it could not enter into negotiations with his officials due to the 'divergence' between the profession's principles and those of the NHS Act.[69] Just how true was this assertion and, if the Act was not as intrinsically inimical to the principles the BMA had set out, what was the BMA's motivation for opposing it?

Principles, politics, and the medical lords' intervention

The aspiration to develop health centres as the future locus of NHS primary care had attained a symbolic significance for the GPs as a harbinger of a whole-time salaried service. The offer of a state salary for new doctors working in them was likewise viewed as insidious even though it would, as Bevan said, free those doctors from the necessity of enduring exploitative assistantships or 'borrowing from a usurer' to support themselves when starting out in practice.[70] The arguments in favour of the buying and selling of practices hardly stood up to scrutiny. It was suggested that a practitioner who owned the goodwill of a practice had an incentive to develop it but as *The Times* pointed out, 'the right of the doctor to sell his place in the public service to the highest bidder' could hardly be admitted to be one of the 'essential freedoms of medicine'.[71] The effects of the ban would mainly be felt by older doctors, and they and their dependants were to be adequately compensated. The criticisms levelled by the BMA at Bevan's plans to control the distribution of GPs via the actions of a Medical Practices Committee, of which half the membership would be professional representatives, also seem to lack real substance. After all, the profession's own MPC had come up with the idea of trying to solve the problem of maldistribution of GPs by this means. Moreover, Bevan's proposals only relied on 'negative direction', that is by requiring those wanting to open new practices to apply for permission to the Medical Practices Committee. Permission would only be granted if the area in question was one not deemed 'over-doctored'. No attempt was made to prevent the continuation of practices in those areas already well served with GPs or to force GPs to practise in 'under-doctored' areas.

The BMA characterised this, however, as a gross infringement of doctors' traditional freedom to set up practice wherever they wished, even though it could be argued that it helped preserve the practices in those over-stocked areas from the threat of further competition.[72] They continued to invoke the old battle cry of 'free choice of doctor' but the patient's choice was not in any way restricted by the Act, and, as many in parliament and press were keen to point out, this was in practice a right which patients rarely exercised with any assiduousness. Patients generally stayed with the same doctor and with the same practice when ownership changed hands and, in the absence of any objective measures of quality or medical knowledge, were not in any position to judge how competent or up to date their doctor was compared with the generality of practitioners.[73] John Campbell claims that the BMA's hostility towards Bevan and the Act was due partly to 'pique at his refusal to treat them with the deference they thought they deserved' and partly because it served as a means of 'throwing up a smokescreen of simulated outrage from behind which to chip away a few concessions'.[74] Once the Act had become law, the chances of wringing major concessions from the government seemed to have diminished, but the arguments used by professional spokesmen portrayed this as an existential struggle for the soul of the medical profession and the future of medicine in Britain.

Webster states, 'When devising means for translating the national health service legislation into practice the government was entering a house haunted by the ghosts from 1911'.[75] He and others allege that the BMA leadership was determined to use this occasion to reverse the humiliation they had suffered at the hands of Lloyd George. Certainly, they were, as already noted, anxious not to make the same mistakes as their predecessors but the circumstances were arguably less propitious than they had been in 1912–1913, given the absence of support from an effective parliamentary opposition or any significant portion of the press or public opinion. The BMA leaders hoped to ensure that the profession knew its mind and was united behind their leadership, but the key lesson history should have taught them was that no interest group, no matter how powerful and united, could hope to win in a fight against an elected government regardless of the size of its parliamentary majority. The outcome of the general strike by trade unions in 1926 offered ample evidence of this but the BMA's leadership seemed undeterred. In the increasingly bitter war of words that followed between the Minister and the profession's leaders in late 1946 Bevan condemned them as politically reactionary.[76] They were likewise demonised by an increasingly hostile press and mercilessly lampooned by political cartoonists as self-righteous hypocrites motivated by self-interest and hubris.[77] Yet, Bevan's most hagiographic biographer, Michael Foot, who witnessed these events first-hand, offers a more magnanimous assessment of the profession's motives. Their opposition was compounded of many elements, he writes, but chiefly by 'fear that the doctor/patient relationship would be damaged by state interference'. Some doctors 'may have been actuated by political hostility' he says, but many 'felt they were fighting a noble battle in defence of the Hippocratic oath'. Foot discerns in them a 'non-political conservatism' based on 'a revulsion against all change, a habit of intellectual isolation which enabled them to magnify any proposals for reform into a totalitarian nightmare'.[78] This attitude is observable in many of the letters written to the press and professional journals at this time, fuelled by inflammatory comments by the BMA leadership.

By the close of 1946, an impasse had been reached and seems likely not have been broken but for the intercession of the Presidents of the three London Royal Colleges, Lord Moran, Sir Alfred Webb-Johnson, and Mr William Gilliatt. On 2 January 1947, they wrote to the Minister seeking clarification on certain matters of concern to the profession and requesting his assurance that he would endeavour to satisfy professional objections.[79] Lord Moran enjoyed an unusually positive relationship with Bevan and may have primed him of the Presidents' intentions beforehand.[80] In any event, Bevan was poised to respond in a conciliatory manner. The BMA leaders expressed outrage at the Presidents' action, of which they had had no prior warning, and had not been properly sanctioned by their respective institutions, but it did allow the BMA to recommence negotiations with government without seeming to lose face. Moran later justified his actions stating that once 'the extremists' were in control of the BMA 'the brakes were taken off, the machine got out of control. Those at the wheel shut their eyes and waited for the collision'. The three Presidents, he suggested, succeeded in slamming on the brakes and steering the profession's 'machine' round the corner.[81] In fact, the BMA was not entirely unaware of what was being proposed. Webb-Johnson had met with Charles Hill a week beforehand and 'mysteriously' asked him what form of words an intermediary might use in approaching the

Minister and, in effect, what the Minister might say to enable negotiations to recommence. Hill says, rather unconvincingly, that he thought the discussion was entirely hypothetical and was taken aback by what then transpired. He said he was relieved that the Minister had shifted his position but the 'presidential letter was the wrong way to go about it'.[82] His opinion of Moran, or 'Corkscrew Charlie' as he was known to medical colleagues, can be judged by the cryptic comment in his autobiography that 'In those days I had some difficulty in understanding the workings of Lord Moran's subtlety, though not in appreciating his devotion to the interests of his college, the Royal College of Physicians, and to Consultants generally'.[83] Pater states that 'Moran rightly regarded (the BMA) as dominated by the general practitioners and their particular concerns'.[84] He was anxious not to lose the benefits which Consultants stood to gain from concessions Bevan had already made.[85] Hill agrees that many Consultants regarded the Association as a GP body and were disdainful of the BMA's concern with remuneration and other 'bread and butter' issues. [86]

The BMA's Council was not convinced by Bevan's emollient words but, fearful of what the press would say if they refused, felt that they had no choice but to accept the olive branch. They accepted the offer of further negotiations on the proviso that they were 'comprehensive in scope and that the possibility that they may lead to further legislation is not excluded'.[87] They also insisted that when these further negotiations were concluded acceptance would be subject to a second plebiscite. Bevan responded graciously and explicitly did not rule out the possibility of amending legislation. Negotiations with Ministry officials took place throughout 1947 but they operated in an atmosphere of mutual suspicion and barely concealed hostility. Much of the discussion took place in subcommittees established to tackle contentious matters of detail rather than principle.[88] However, the profession's representatives would not agree to anything which they deemed to be in conflict with their previously stated 'principles' and it was Bevan's turn to feel frustrated by the lack of constructive dialogue and agreement. According to Campbell, Bevan was obliged to make 'concession after concession... while the BMA boasted that it had not conceded an inch'.[89] For example, the profession's negotiators won an agreement to obtain clarification of the legal status of medical partnerships, and the right of all GPs, whether obstetrically qualified or not, to attend their own midwifery cases in hospital. They demanded that GPs be allowed a right of appeal against dismissal (or rather, the cancellation of their contracts) to the high court which Bevan denied, stating that they would in any case enjoy greater protection than accorded any comparable workers in the public service.[90] Besides, he said, the Minister's powers only extended to restoring practitioners removed from the list, not removing them. However, there would, he agreed, be medical representatives in administrative bodies at every level of the service: the Central Health Services Council, Regional Health Boards, Boards of Governors of Teaching Hospitals, General Hospital Management Committees, and Executive Councils, and there would be a state administered NHS pension scheme in which the GPs could participate along with employed doctors.[91] On the subject of Health Centres, the Ministry conceded, importantly, that practice from them would be entirely voluntary.[92] Despite these concessions, the BMA's Council remained firmly of the opinion that the Act was deeply flawed and were angered that, while hinting at the possibility of amending legislation, Bevan had conceded nothing that would allay their greatest fear. Hill summed up their position by stating: 'There is one criterion by which, as a profession, we can measure these matters…it is whether these proposals do or do not bring us closer to a whole-time salaried service of the state'.[93]

When the negotiations had run their course there was nothing left to do but to seek the verdict of the profession via the promised second plebiscite. At a Special Representative Meeting in January 1948, six months before the 'appointed day', the details of the plebiscite were agreed after heated debate. The meeting insisted that the profession be given 'a strong lead' on how to vote and issued a 'solemn declaration' that the NHS Act was 'so grossly at variance with the essential principles of our profession that it should be rejected absolutely by all practitioners'.[94] The Council wrote separately to every member of the profession urging them 'not to accept service under the Act in its present form'.[95] The aim of the plebiscite, Pater says, was not to seek approval for detailed amendments to the Act but 'to sabotage it completely'.[96] This view was shared by newspapers like the *Daily Mirror* and by Bevan himself. Bevan had informed his cabinet colleagues in January that he had no wish to enter into a war of words with the BMA. He anticipated that the plebiscite might support the BMA position but was confident that as the appointed day approached the majority of practitioners would sign up for service.[97] The Cabinet was however, not convinced, and it was this that led to the Commons debate in February in which Bevan condemned the BMA leadership as 'a small body of politically poisoned' and 'raucous voiced' people engaged in 'a squalid political conspiracy' and 'organised sabotage'. He appealed for cross-party support when commenting that the House had not yet 'made BMA House into another revising chamber'.[98] These comments were condemned by the normally conciliatory *Lancet* which complained that such intemperate language would only inflame the situation.[99]

Bevan further damaged relations with the BMA by impugning the integrity of the referendum process. He suggested that the requirement for participants in the plebiscite to state their names and addresses, which had been introduced to negate any chance of numbers being inflated fraudulently was, 'a long way from the secret ballot and the working of democracy in this country'.[100] The BMA invited Bevan to come and inspect the count for himself which he declined to do. The press took up the offer and concluded that the process, managed by auditors Price Waterhouse and co, was conducted with due propriety.[101] However, several SMA members unwisely accused the BMA of trying to manipulate the result in a letter to the press. The BMA reacted swiftly by suing them and *The Daily*

Mirror and the defendants were eventually forced to apologise in open court, meet the BMA's costs and make a donation to the Red Cross by way of reparations.[102] Bevan's indignation at the behaviour of his medical opponents provided plenty of material for the leader writers in the national press and for the political cartoonists who found it easy to caricature the distinctive features of Bevan and Hill, often depicted arguing over the recumbent body of a hapless patient.[103]

Of roughly the same age but from vastly different backgrounds, the two men shared a number of similarities. Both were highly intelligent and skilled communicators. Each was described as 'cherubic' in appearance, though Bevan was imposing physically, whereas Hill was, by his own admission, corpulent. In fact, Hill looked surprisingly like Frank Richards' popular schoolboy anti-hero Billy Bunter, who featured in the early twentieth-century boys comic *Magnet* which Hill read avidly as a boy and which was also, according to Bevan's biographer, Michael Foot, among the favoured reading material of the miner's son from Tredegar.[104] Hill dismissed any notion of a personal conflict between himself and Bevan, whom he clearly admired, despite the differences of their political affiliations.[105] But his prominence as the profession's spokesman made him the obvious target of MPs and left-wing doctors who jeered at news that he was standing as a Conservative candidate in a forthcoming byelection in Luton. Hill admitted that the responsibility of his office and the personal attacks on him caused 'physical strain' but claimed that he accepted, philosophically, that it came with the job he was required to do and that, like a good civil servant, he merely responded to his BMA masters' bidding.[106]

If Bevan hoped to drive a wedge between the BMA's leaders and the rank of file, the results of the plebiscite showed how far he had failed in that objective. Around 90% of the doctors who voted, some 75% of those on the medical register, declared their opposition to accepting service under the Act.[107] Even the doctors already in whole-time service voted against it.[108] Though the views of the profession appeared to have been expressed quite clearly, the BMA's policy could only be decided by a meeting of its Representative Body of which a special meeting was hastily convened in March 1948. The meeting resolved to demand, in the public interest, an amendment to the Act 'to prevent doctors being turned into civil servants' and to preserve the 'integrity' of medicine.[109] They further resolved that the Association be ready to recommence negotiations with government on the understanding that the profession was not prepared to participate in the new service unless and until the necessary amendments to the Act had been guaranteed.

The final showdown

Like Lloyd George, when faced with the prospect of a mass medical boycott, Bevan did not entertain any idea that his scheme might not begin on the appointed day. He was confident that in this high-stakes poker game, it was he who held the winning hand.[110] By Act of parliament, the scheme under which the majority of doctors, the GPs, were currently paid by the state to attend their patients was to be abolished in July 1948. Those who did not sign up for the new service would forfeit any income in respect of those patients and lose the right to a share in the compensation being offered in return for relinquishing the right to sell the goodwill in their practices. Without the patients in any case there was no goodwill to sell. The remuneration for those who accepted service had also been much improved. In response to the profession's claim that the betterment factor indicated that the appropriate rate at which the GPs should be paid in the new service was 20s per patient, Bevan had managed to persuade the Chancellor of the Exchequer, Sir Stafford Cripps, to raise the Government's offer to a final, non-negotiable ceiling of 18s per patient.[111] This was significantly more than GPs had previously been paid, with the prospect of a great many more patients than before and no risk of unpaid bills for treatment. The Consultants meanwhile would lose any right to have any private patient in any pay bed in any hospital if they declined to participate, and the separate Spens committee report into their remuneration offered them a more than sufficient personal incentive to sign up for the new service.[112]

The principal weakness in the profession's case was the lack of an alternative once NHI had effectively been wound up. The BMA's GP leaders had been aware of this for some time. In March 1943, the LMPCs' conference had resolved that

> in the event of negotiations failing to secure conditions satisfactory to the profession, the Council of the BMA should have a plan ready to carry on the treatment of the sick by the profession without its participation in the government's plan.[113]

By the end of 1945, the plan, based on the existing PMS schemes, had been drawn up but, aside from the practical difficulties of implementing it at scale across the country, a significant number of LMPCs surveyed (62 out of 109) rejected the scheme on principle.[114] Now that the profession was bent on not participating in Labour's NHS, the need for an alternative was paramount. A report on the feasibility of administering the national PMS scheme by a specially appointed committee chaired by Dr Frank Gray had been circulated to LMPCs.[115] At a special LMPCs conference at BMA House in March 1948, the IAC chairman Edward Gregg was asked to provide assurance that the plan was ready to be implemented should it prove necessary, as now seemed likely. Gregg reported that the responses to Dr Gray's report suggested that LMPCs did not favour a uniform alternative scheme but felt that each area should determine what sort of scheme it wished to introduce and how it was to be administered.[116] There was, therefore, 'no clear-cut plan as to how doctors were to carry on their practices, and earn their incomes, if they refused to join the National Health Service'. Gregg reluctantly concluded that 'Our alternative is the National Health

Service Scheme with the changes in it for which we have asked'.[117] The importance of this devastating admission seems to have escaped the attention of most historians.

The BMA's Special Representative Meeting the same month was characterised by a great public show of support for the leadership, and the negotiating committee. They applauded Dain, and decried the attacks made by Government spokesmen on the representativeness of the Association and what they considered the deliberate misrepresentation of the reasons for their opposition to the Act.[118] Lord Horder, who now put himself forward as the darling of the diehards, claimed these unjustified attacks had only served to make the profession more determined to resist the 'tyranny' of government service. The meeting resolved to set up an independence fund as a means of financing the campaign of resistance that was to come.[119] This was made possible by an initial donation of £400,000 from the GPs' National Insurance Defence Trust which Gregg justified as providing 'the sinews of war for the conduct of the campaign'.[120] The scene was set for an evitable showdown, yet within a few months that eventuality had evaporated. How did this happen? The first steps towards preventing the collision were made, as they had been the year before, via the intercession of Lord Moran. In a private meeting with Bevan the week before the Special Representative Meeting Moran explained that GPs' fears about salaried service would not be assuaged without some form of legislative guarantee.[121] While it was true that Bevan could not bind his successors to not entertaining the idea of a whole-time salaried service in future, an amending Act which ensured that such a policy could not be executed by regulation or executive order might be all that was needed to break the deadlock. There was insufficient time to bring in an amending Act before the approved day, but Bevan was persuaded to give an official undertaking to introduce such an Act if expressly asked to do so by his lordship on behalf of his College. Unlike the BMA, the Royal of College of Physicians was not a representative body, and its president did not need the backing of all its members to undertake such an action, provided it had the support of its comitia, or executive council. Only one thing stood in the way of Moran being able to execute his plan: he had to win the forthcoming presidential election in which he was opposed by the diehard-in-chief, Lord Horder. This he managed to do, albeit by a narrow majority, and with the tacit approval of the other college presidents whom he had informed beforehand, Moran duly wrote to the Minister on 4 April 1948.[122] Three days later Bevan made an announcement in the commons agreeing to Moran's suggestion of amending legislation.

His announcement included further concessions designed to address other longstanding concerns. First and foremost, he agreed that the initial salary of £300 per annum available to new GPs would only be paid in cases of proven need determined by Executive Councils in consultation with LMCs, and would last for a maximum of three years after which it would be replaced by patient capitation payments.[123] He said that an expert committee would be appointed to look into the disputed effect of the Act on doctors' partnership agreements which, if necessary, would also be dealt with by means of amending legislation. He accorded statutory recognition to LMCs and granted them the right to a statutory levy of GPs' remuneration to defray their expenses and agreed to increase the GPs' maternity fee, though it was to be set at a higher rate for those on the obstetric list.[124] He clarified that the chairman of the Health Services Tribunal which would adjudicate on disciplinary matters affecting the GPs' rights to hold NHS contracts would be a senior lawyer appointed by the Lord Chancellor. Finally, he conceded, there would be no interference with a doctor's medical practice or their freedom of speech.[125] According to Foot, Moran's intervention was not only critical it was, for Bevan, very timely. It allowed him to appear conciliatory at just the right moment. 'Made too soon, the move would have been interpreted as weakness...Delayed too long, the benefits would be squandered'.[126] This comprehensive attempt to address the profession's concerns put the BMA leadership in a quandary. Dain responded publicly that the Minister's announcement offered insufficient reassurance, but the BMA's NHS Executive Committee welcomed the apparent olive branch and without consulting Council sent Bevan a list of 14 questions which it agreed to send a deputation to discuss with him. 'As a result', Grey-Turner says, 'many doctors gained an impression that their leaders, having taken their followers to the brink, were now beginning to waver'.[127]

Cracks were beginning to appear in the facade of professional unity, moreover, signalled by a conciliatory editorial in the *BMJ* penned by its editor Hugh Clegg.[128] In the article, titled 'Mr Bevan's gesture', Clegg, who privately congratulated Moran on his efforts to break the deadlock, described Bevan's announcement as 'a big concession' which he argued should be met by the Association in the same spirit. This created for perhaps the only time in its history a major rift between the 'organ of the association' and its parent body.[129] Angry correspondents denounced Clegg's 'treachery' and he narrowly avoided being sacked. Conscious that they were losing the battle for public opinion, the BMA's Council decided there was no other option than to call for another plebiscite. Hill was undoubtedly influential in this decision, given his views on the absolute necessity of regularly 'taking the temperature' of the profession. In keeping with Hill's mantra of being open with the profession about what had been gained and what had not, the BMA's Council justified this decision in the *BMJ*. With regard to the new proposals, it stated:

> We have succeeded on some points, such as the bar on the introduction of a whole-time salaried service by regulation, and the universal basic salary. We have failed on others, such as the ownership of goodwill and the right of appeal.

It went on to say that the Council considered that the freedoms of the profession were 'not sufficiently safeguarded' and urged doctors to attend one of the many local meetings taking place across the country and to express their views clearly in the forthcoming plebiscite.[130] The *BMJ* editorial of 24 April 1948 continued to aver that the Minister had made significant concessions on the issues of most concern to the profession.[131]

Bartrip says the *BMJ* made no secret of its views that the profession should give its approval to the NHS and agree to work in it.[132] But would that be enough to end the conflict? On 19 April 1948, forms were dispatched to 54,667 practitioners for return by 28 April. The BMA agreed to refrain from adverse publicity and had already dropped its objections to the sale of goodwill and the Medical Practices Committee.[133] The respondents were once again asked if they approved of the NHS Act, whether they were in favour of accepting service under it, and whether, if a majority opposed such acceptance, they would refuse to participate themselves. As in the previous plebiscite there was, however, an important caveat. The GPs were not the only doctors whose future was to be determined by the proposed NHS, but they were absolutely critical to the success of any proposed boycott. Based on their experience in 1913, the BMA was aware that the number of GPs refusing to serve under the new arrangements had to be sufficiently large to ensure that the Government could not operate at least a skeleton service as this would, over time, lead to an inevitable haemorrhaging of support for any boycott. The BMA's Council had determined therefore that, regardless of the level of support for its campaign among other branches of the profession, the boycott had to be supported by at least 13,000 GPs out of a total of approximately 20,500.[134] The first plebiscite had secured the support of well in excess of that number of GPs. But as the appointed day approached would the number, given the Minister's recent reassurances, still be sufficient? The answer to that question was clear. Out of a reduced turnout of 74%, 64% expressed disapproval of the Act despite the concessions and only 36% approved. But on the question of accepting service the difference was narrower, with 52% not in favour and 48% in favour and the majority against accepting service included only 9,588 GPs, well short of the stipulated minimum. As Grey-Turner puts it: 'The great and natural fear of many general practitioners was that enough of their colleagues might join the Service on the appointed day to make it workable and so take away the bulk of the patients'.[135]

The *BMJ* declared that the Association had lost the mandate to organise collective opposition but, given that most doctors still had grave misgivings, was not at all optimistic about the chances of the new service being an immediate success.[136] However the knowledge that there were sufficient GPs willing to accept service to make it workable persuaded many others that it was time to accept the inevitable. By the end of May 1948, 26% of English and 36% of Scottish and Welsh GPs had joined the service.[137] The undignified stampede to join the NHI panels in 1913 looked like being repeated. On 5 May, the BMA's Council met to discuss the plebiscite results. After a long, difficult, and fractious session, they decided to recommend to the Representative Body that the

profession should cooperate in the new service on the understanding that negotiations with the Minister would continue on outstanding matters relating to the
doctors' terms and conditions of service and on the wording of the amending
Act.[138] The war was 'all over bar the recriminations'.[139] A *BMJ* article entitled
'What we have gained' listed ten gains apparently secured by the Association's
tenacious campaign. It denounced those of its correspondents who, it said, had
no desire to see a comprehensive medical service for the nation, pointing out
that this was a view which was both untenable and at variance with the oft-
stated policy of the Association.[140] It then hailed Bevan's recent concessions as
a worthy compromise stating, in words which echoed those of other great BMA
peacemakers of the past like Lauriston Shaw and E. Rowland Fothergill, that
'compromises are the traditional English way of settling disputes'. There were
still many doctors, BMA members and non-members, who did not subscribe to
that view, however, and at the meeting of the Representative Body on 28 May,
there were accusations of treachery and defeatism.[141] A motion questioning the
decision to opt for a second plebiscite so soon after the first was actually carried
but others challenging the Council's recommendation to cooperate, and one put
forward by the MPA-dominated Guildford division expressing no confidence in
the leadership, and criticising the editor of the *BMJ*, were soundly defeated.[142]

The diehards made their presence felt and made it clear that they as individuals would not accept the decision to support the new service. Contrasting
views were expressed about what had happened. One of the GP negotiators, the
redoubtable Solomon Wand, said that the army was so satisfied with the gener-
als' achievements that they had decided to go home. A Dr Breach of Bromley
responded that the truth was that the army thought that its leaders had gone
home.[143] It was pointed out that many in the press were congratulating the BMA
on having won a great victory in defence of professional freedom. *The Economist* for example opined that 'the doctors have won a big victory, for Mr Bevan
does not easily climb down to the extent that he has'.[144] Many others declined
to see it as such. Alfred Cox urged the Council to recognise defeat and not persist in enduring the humiliation which had accompanied the climb-down in
1913. He acknowledged the gains but expressed astonishment that GPs had not
thought retaining the right to sell the goodwill in their practices, which he saw as
a guarantee of their professional independence, an object worth fighting for.[145]
Among the loudest critics of that policy and of the BMA's decision to cooperate
generally was Lord Horder. Horder, Hill says cryptically, 'pursued an uncertain
course'. He seemed to be motivated as much by the desire to oppose anything
which his rival for the Royal College of Physicians presidency, Lord Moran,
supported, as by any ideological conviction. Horder and fellow diehards made
one final forlorn and unsuccessful effort to deflect the course of history at the
BMA's Annual Representative Meeting in June while writing to the press claiming that there was insufficient time to launch the service properly and calling for
the appointed day to be postponed.[146]

Bevan dismissed such talk as nonsense and he confidently toured the country inspiring administrators, professional groups and the public alike with excitement at the transformative prospect which the new service offered the British people.[147] Having failed to unseat Moran or to turn the BMA towards continued opposition to the Act, Horder eventually led his 'fellow Adullamites' off into the political wilderness to form a right-wing caucus called 'The Fellowship for Freedom in Medicine', a body which, despite its longevity, proved to have no real purpose or credibility.[148] Hill himself was, as has been noted, no real fan of the sale of goodwill but fell short of admitting it. In his autobiography he merely says 'Whether the abolition of the ownership of medical practices has, in fact, reduced the clinical independence of general practitioners in the Service, I find difficult to say. My guess is that it has not'.[149] At the ARM, the BMA acknowledged the futility of trying to resist the implementation of the Act and resolved to allow practitioners to sign up as they wished. Dain wrote to *The Times* stating, 'This decision reached, the profession will do its utmost to make the new service a resounding success... Only the best is good enough for the public service and we shall do our best to provide it'.[150] Bevan meanwhile sent a goodwill message to all doctors wishing them success and an end to all their professional anxieties.[151] By the appointed day around 20,000 GPs, some 90% of the total, had signed up and 75% of eligible patients, a figure rising to 97% by the end of the year.[152]

After defeat, the reckoning

In their condemnation of the BMA's capitulation, Horder and his fellow die-hards had denounced the Council's 'defeatism'.[153] But wiser heads had taken their cue from the feeble response to the call for contributions to the profession's campaign war-chest, the 'independence fund'. When it was launched one doctor wrote to the *BMJ* about immediately contributing £100 while expressing fears of 'surrendering our liberty to the State'.[154] But in the end the number of doctors contributing totalled no more than 6000.[155] According to Hill, this was very discouraging and a 'chastening reminder that some hands are more active in applause than in signing cheques'.[156] As another example of history seeming to repeat itself, a small number of commentators felt the BMA had, as in 1913, secured a victory of sorts. Hill argued that it had secured five of its stated seven principles.[157] However, most historians interpret the outcome of the conflict as a defeat for the BMA. Bartrip states that 'it is hard to point to the extraction of many concessions of true value during the period 1944–1948'.[158] According to Foot, all the concessions Bevan incorporated into both the Act and the amending Act merely 'gave legislative form to pledges he had given of his own volition on the second reading and the committee stage... It gave nothing it had not always intended to give'. He says that Bevan regarded the Amending Act as no more than a move which could help save the face of the BMA leaders.[159] Webster agrees that the concessions were in that sense 'insignificant' but says that their 'embodiment in the amending legislation was of great symbolic importance to the BMA ... it was presented as a belated token of reparation by a penitent government'.[160] Campbell describes it more simply: the BMA had effectively been 'crying wolf' when there was no wolf, so it was consistent now for them to state that 'the wolf had been seen off'.[161]

Many doctors sought to argue that in preventing the establishment of a salaried service the BMA's campaign had done a great service to the public. Although he states that he was confident 'from the outset' that the NHS would not be built on a whole-time salaried GP service, Hill claimed 'This was a victory for the public as well as for the doctors'.[162] This was because, he said, the right of free choice on which the soundness of the relationship between doctor and patient was based could not remain safe if the doctor was a salaried subordinate of the state.[163] However, Foot maintains that Bevan himself strongly supported the principle that the patient should have free choice of doctor which he saw as the 'the best safeguard against poor service'.[164] The SMA profoundly disagreed with this view and the longer the NHS continued the greater was their regret that salaried service had not been introduced.[165] They were even more gravely disappointed at what had become of their grand plans for the reorganisation of general practice on a grouped basis in local authority-run health centres.[166] Despite all the expectations, fears and arguments, the expected network of health centres failed to materialise. As the Minister of Housing faced with a shortage of materials and skilled labour, Bevan prioritised house building over support for public building projects, even hospitals, but Campbell contends that by 1948 Bevan and his officials, recognising that the majority of GPs would not accept them, had 'gone cold' on the health centre idea.[167] Eckstein records Bevan telling him in an interview that 'while he had always been in favour of group practice, he had never really believed health centres to be required'.[168]

Several historians have made the point that in one sense the vehemence with which the BMA opposed Bevan's plans did him one great favour. It provided the excuse he needed to ditch those aspects of Labour's, or rather the SMA's, health policies of which he was not especially enamoured and allowed him to concentrate on those he considered absolutely essential. As one of his critics put it: 'His outstanding success was the way he applied the anaesthetic to supporters on his own side, making them believe in things they had opposed almost all their lives'. To do this, Campbell says, 'he needed the public row with the BMA'.[169] For it was not in general practice that the greatness of Bevan's achievement lay. It was the creation of a nationalised and comprehensive hospital service for which he is chiefly remembered and justifiably feted. Even his opponents agreed. Henry Willink openly acknowledged that Bevan had succeeded where he and others had failed, and Charles Hill stated in his autobiography 'Whatever the flaws in the service today, nothing can detract from the greatness of the unified hospital plan'.[170] Once he had taken the decision to 'cut the Gordian knot' and had succeeded in pushing his plans through cabinet he settled the shape of the future health service and 'the other parts of the jigsaw fell relatively easily into place'. After this, Campbell says, 'the long-drawn-out tussle with the BMA was an unseemly irrelevance'.[171]

With the benefit of hindsight, it seems the profession really had little to fear from Bevan's proposals. Why then did the BMA persist in its fight with government and why were they not prepared to take Bevan's repeated reassurances at face value? One reason acknowledged by several historians, is the deep distrust of government itself which lay behind some of the most vehement outbursts from the rank and file during this period. As already noted, the 'repeated setbacks' over capitation payments in the interwar period changed the BMA's view of the Ministry of Health and left it fearful of its expanding bureaucracy.[172] In 1942, the Ministry's permanent secretary, Sir John Maude, acknowledged an attitude of hostility towards the department and that relations had deteriorated since the arbitration of 1937.[173] Two years later the Chief Medical Officer, Sir William Jameson, informed the BMA negotiators of Willink's hopes that the Spens inquiry would end 'the atmosphere of suspicion'.[174] In the words of John Pater, himself a Ministry official in the 1940s, 'to general practitioners…the Ministry was the unsympathetic skinflint which had fought them over the level of the NHI capitation fee no less than seven times since 1920'. Moreover, it had ignored advice given by the profession and was guilty of 'subordinating its medical and professional staff to a dominant lay administration'.[175] When the coalition government published its White Paper in 1944 the *BMJ* had commented 'Of the emotional cross-currents in the life of the profession today, the strongest is suspicion'.[176] Frank Honigsbaum's study of the Ministry of Health prior to 1948 confirms that the support of many officials for the idea of local authority control proves that the GPs in particular had much to be suspicious about.[177] The wartime health ministers, MacDonald, Brown, and Willink had each succumbed eventually to professional pressure, but as the doctors soon found, Bevan was an altogether different animal. Wily, charismatic, and capable, his working-class affiliations and reputation as a socialist firebrand aroused in the largely conservative medical body politic an irrational fear – that the doctors were to become the first victims of a class war soon to be fought by socialist politicians across all sections of the economy.[178] He was a bogeyman to the right wing of the profession as the frankly hysterical comments describing him as a would-be Nazi dictator attest.[179] As Grey Turner puts it, 'There was an emotional, even political, undercurrent to the dispute'.[180] Bartrip goes further and says, 'it is hard to avoid the conclusion that BMA leaders were, as Bevan believed them to be, motivated by hostility towards the Labour government'.[181]

The origins of this are not hard to fathom. The doctors had fought and worked hard for over a century to achieve the status of respectable middle-class professionals. Like other members of the middle classes they were unnerved by the utterances of their new socialist political masters who in the words of one prominent class warrior, the Labour MP and cabinet member Manny Shinwell, 'did not care a tinker's cuss for the middle classes'.[182] Some came to view themselves therefore as standard bearers for democracy, freedom, and independence, engaged in resisting, not just on their own behalf, but for the greater good of society, a centralising socialist bureaucracy. Some sections of the press agreed. *The Daily Sketch* described their actions as 'the first effective revolt of the professional classes against socialist tyranny'.[183] Harry Eckstein observed, however, that the BMA's opposition to many of the proposed reform measures rested less on political ideology than on a general distrust of organisation. Acceptance of this, he said, renders the BMA's conservatism 'at once more comprehensible and less offensive'.[184] But, however strongly they believed themselves to be representing the public interest, the BMA signally failed to win the battle for public opinion. As E.S. Turner puts it, 'Masses of the public felt, rightly or wrongly, that progress was being impeded for reasons which, if not selfish, were unimportant and even unintelligible'.[185]

And it was not just the working classes who lost patience with what was often seen as the profession's political posturing. As Harry Eckstein observed, the middle classes had as much to gain as anyone else from the new NHS and, as the profession found somewhat to its surprise, demonstrated this with the alacrity with which they signed up for NHS services on the appointed day. While the poor had previously been able to obtain medical care free of charge or at nominal rates, the middle classes had had to endure often ruinous bills both for GP and for hospital treatment and therefore welcomed the levelling out of entitlement which the NHS promised.[186] Bevan himself was well aware of this. In the debate in the Commons in February 1948, he had stated: 'There is nothing that destroys the family budget of the professional worker more than heavy hospital bills or doctors' bills'.[187] In their continued defence of private practice the doctors had utterly failed to appreciate this point. Another factor worth bearing in mind is that non-panel doctors, amounting perhaps to no more than 10% of the nation's GPs, were more vehemently opposed to Bevan's plans than the rest because those plans threatened to destroy the middle-class market for private general practice. It would thus leave them with no alternative but to participate in a state service which they had shown themselves to be against on principle by remaining aloof from NHI.

Why, in the end did GPs, the group which had complained longest and loudest about the threat, real or imagined, which Bevan's plans posed to their well-being, set aside their objections and sign for the service in huge numbers before the appointed day? The answer is simple. As Bevan had pointed out to the Cabinet, once the NHS began the alternative of NHI disappeared and with it not just the GPs' working-class patients but most of their private practice since the middle classes were now able to avail themselves at last of state-funded medical services. Moreover, the right to compensation for the loss of the right to sell their practices expired on the appointed day. As Dain observed, 'The General

Practitioner is in a cleft stick, that is if the Act starts and he has not come in, then he loses the right to compensation'.[188] This was not something GPs could readily forego, especially as there was a risk that sizeable debts might be called in, since practice loans were often made on condition that the GP maintained contract work like that provided by NHI and, from now on, by the new NHS.[189] As one Nottinghamshire GP put it more prosaically,

> In the event- and let us not forget this- the GPs were whipped into line by Aneurin's promise that our Practice Purchase Money would never be repaid if we waited until after 5th July to sign a contract. Not surprisingly, with over two years' income at stake the vast majority committed themselves in early July.[190]

Conclusion

As events were to show, GPs in the new NHS were, initially at least, far from happy with their lot and it was not long before dissatisfaction with workload, remuneration and the absence of investment in their services brought their dissatisfaction once more to a head. As David Widgery put it, 'The Consultants ruled the new health service... general practice and public health were neglected grievously, cast out into the fields of worthy neglect as hospital medicine flourished'.[191] But, all things considered, it has to be acknowledged that their leaders, backed by a determined, if fleeting, show of professional unity, had succeeded in preserving many of the features of contract practice which most of them professed to value. GPs were to remain independent contractors accountable to local Executive Councils which looked and acted much like the Insurance Committees with which they were intimately acquainted, except that GPs now constituted half the membership and no longer had to deal with the Approved Societies. The Executive Councils were, moreover, obliged to consult the GPs' democratically elected and statutorily recognised representative bodies, now called simply Local Medical committees (LMCs), on all matters touching the local interpretation of their contracts and terms of service. GPs remained the strongest voice in the disciplinary procedure and although, at Bevan's insistence, patients were no longer subject to sanctions for misuse of medical services, GPs were still free to accept or decline to accept patients on to their lists subject to maximum list sizes prescribed in regulations. There was effectively no interference in, and no greater budgetary control over, their clinical decision-making – that is in terms of treatment, prescribing, or certification allowed under the NHS regulations, or in referral to other NHS services. Nor was there any inhibition of their freedom of speech. Doctors were, as Bevan promised, represented at every level of NHS administration, and therefore enjoyed a degree of involvement in the running of health services far greater than they could honestly have expected when the tortuous process of negotiations began in 1943. They were therefore in a position to shape the new health service and make it their own, and within a fairly short time the profession did just that.

Before long doctors counted themselves among the most enthusiastic advocates of the NHS and many GPs began to wonder why they had ever troubled to question the wisdom of Bevan's plan, as even the Conservatives acknowledged its benefits and sought to expunge their opposition to it from the public memory. Passing quickly over the events of 1947–1948, professional commentators sought to rescue their leaders' reputations by pointing out that from the early days of NHI the BMA had called for a more comprehensive health service and that most of the controversial measures which Bevan incorporated in the NHS Act had actually been suggested in 1943 by the non-partisan professional forum that was the Medical Planning Commission. In that sense, they attempted to claim much of the credit for the new service for themselves and were entitled to do so, Campbell claims, asserting that the profession was 'arguably more responsible than any other body for the final shape and limitations of the NHS'.[192] John Pater says that 'There is a very real sense in which the story of the making of the NHS is the story of the long-delayed implementation of the Dawson Report'.[193] In his biography of Bevan, Michael Foot generously endorsed the words of a *BMJ* editorial that stated, 'The historian who will be able to view these events dispassionately in the future may come to the conclusion that after 1911 the principal architect of the National Health Service was the medical profession itself'.[194]

Notes

1 Peter Bartrip, *Themselves Writ Large: The British Medical Association, 1832–1966* (London, 1996). p. 248.
2 Kenneth O. Morgan, *Labour in Power, 1945–1951* (2nd ed., Oxford, 1987). p. 143.
3 Bartrip, *Themselves Writ Large*, p. 248.
4 John Campbell, *Nye Bevan: A Biography* (London, 1987). p. 151.
5 Harry Eckstein, *The English Health Service: Its Origins, Structures and Achievements* (Cambridge, MA, 1958). p. 156. Charles Webster, *The National Health Service: A Political History* (2nd ed., Oxford, 2002). p. 12.
6 Charles Webster, *The Health Services Since the War, Volume 1, Problems of Healthcare: The National Health Service Before 1957* (London, 1988). p. 76.
7 John Stewart, *The Battle for Health: A Political History of the Socialist Medical Association, 1930–1951* (Abingdon, 1999). p. 182.
8 Charles Hill, *Both Sides of the Hill: The Memoirs of Charles Hill (Lord Hill of Luton)* (London, 1964). p. 86. Morgan, *Labour in Power*, p. 151.
9 Eckstein, *The English Health Service*, p. 113.
10 Webster, *The National Health Service*, p. 18.
11 Webster, *The Health Services Since the War*, p. 78.
12 Webster, *The National Health Service*, p. 17. Frank Honigsbaum, *Health, Happiness and Security: The Creation of the National Health Service* (London, 1989). p. 177.
13 Campbell, *Nye Bevan*, p. 177.

14 Webster, *The National Health Service*, p. 18.
15 Webster, *The Health Services Since the War*, p. 80.
16 Campbell, *Nye Bevan*, p. 168.
17 Webster, *The Health Services Since the War*, p. 85.
18 Michael Foot, *Aneurin Bevan, 1897–1960* (abridged ed., London, 1977). p. 301.
19 John Pater, *The Making of the National Health Service* (London, 1981). p. 178. Honigsbaum, *Health, Happiness and Security*, pp. 217–218.
20 *BMJ*, 16 July 1960. 'Aneurin Bevan' p. 203. Hill, *Both Sides of the Hill*, pp. 93–94.
21 Bartrip, *Themselves Writ Large*, p. 250.
22 Foot, *Aneurin Bevan*, p. 293.
23 *BMJ*, 12 January 1946, Supplement, p. 5.
24 *BMJ*, 15 December 1945, p. 833.
25 Bartrip, *Themselves Writ Large*, p. 251.
26 *Ibid.*, p. 252.
27 Pater, *The Making of the National Health Service*, p. 104. Campbell, *Nye Bevan*, p. 167.
28 *BMJ*, 20 April 1946, 'The Press, the Minister and the Bill', pp. 612–613.
29 Elston Grey-Turner and Frederick M. Sutherland, *History of the British Medical Association, 1932–1972* (London, 1982). p. 53.
30 Stewart, *The Battle for Health*, p. 223.
31 Webster, *The National Health Service*, p. 15.
32 *BMJ*, 20 April 1946, 'The Press, the Minister and the Bill', p. 613.
33 Hansard, HC, 9 February 1948, col. 40.
34 E. S. (Ernest Sackville) Turner, *Call the Doctor: A Social History of Medical Men* (London, 1958). p. 300.
35 Pater, *The Making of the National Health Service*, p. 121.
36 Grey-Turner and Sutherland, *History of the British Medical Association*, p. 55.
37 Campbell, *Nye Bevan*, p. 173.
38 Honigsbaum, *Health, Happiness and Security*, p. 97.
39 *BMJ*, 11 May 1946, Supplement, 'Report of the Special Representative Meeting', p. 124.
40 Pater, *The Making of the National Health Service*, p. 132.
41 Honigsbaum, *Health, Happiness and Security*, p. 98.
42 Bartrip, *Themselves Writ Large*, p. 253.
43 Pater, *The Making of the National Health Service*, p. 130.
44 Foot, *Aneurin Bevan*, p. 307.
45 Campbell, *Nye Bevan*, p. 172.
46 Grey-Turner and Sutherland, *History of the British Medical Association*, pp. 54–55.
47 *Hansard*, HC, 2 May 1946, 422, col. 392.
48 Bartrip, *Themselves Writ Large*, p. 254.
49 Campbell, *Nye Bevan*, p. 173. Grey-Turner and Sutherland, *History of the British Medical Association*, p. 56.
50 Webster, *The Health Services Since the War*, p. 93.
51 Grey-Turner and Sutherland, *History of the British Medical Association*, p. 59; Bartrip, *Themselves Writ Large*, p. 254.
52 Webster, *The Health Services Since the War*, p. 92.
53 *Ibid.*
54 Eckstein, *The English Health Service*, p. 197.
55 *Ibid.*, p. 198.
56 Webster, *The Health Services Since the War*, p. 93.
57 *Ibid.*, pp. 91–92.

58 Bartrip, *Themselves Writ Large*, p. 255.
59 Webster, *The Health Services Since the War*, p. 109.
60 *BMA Archive*, B/203/1/38, minutes of meeting of IAC on 5 September 1946, minute 29.
61 *Ibid.*, Minutes of meeting on 17 October 1946, minute 45.
62 Foot, *Aneurin Bevan*, pp. 317–318. Webster, *The Health Services Since the War*, pp. 107–108.
63 *Ibid.*, p. 108.
64 Hill, *Both Sides of the Hill*, pp. 96–97.
65 Bartrip, *Themselves Writ Large*, p. 255.
66 See, for example, *The Times*, 15 November 1946, p. 5.
67 Bartrip, *Themselves Writ Large*, p.255; Grey-Turner and Sutherland, *History of the British Medical Association*, p. 60.
68 *Lancet*, 21 December 1946, 'Risk or Opportunity', p. 909.
69 *BMJ*, 21 December 1946, Supplement, p. 161.
70 Foot, *Aneurin Bevan*, p. 316.
71 *The Times*, 11 April 1946, p. 5.
72 Turner, *Call the Doctor*, pp. 300–301.
73 *Ibid.*, p. 301. For the questioning of this by the SMA, see Stewart, *The Battle for Health*, p. 41.
74 Campbell, *Nye Bevan*, p. 172.
75 Webster, *The Health Services Since the War*, p. 107.
76 Foot, *Aneurin Bevan*, p. 316.
77 Bartrip, *Themselves Writ Large*, p. 260.
78 Foot, *Aneurin Bevan*, p. 287.
79 *Ibid.*, p. 320. Grey-Turner and Sutherland, *History of the British Medical Association*, p. 60. Bartrip, *Themselves Writ Large*, p. 256.
80 Honigsbaum, *Health, Happiness and Security*, p. 136.
81 Pater, *The Making of the National Health Service*, p. 143.
82 Hill, *Both Sides of the Hill*, pp. 89–90.
83 *Ibid.*, p. 91.
84 Pater, *The Making of the National Health Service*, p. 140.
85 Honigsbaum, *Health, Happiness and Security*, pp. 143–145.
86 Hill, *Both Sides of the Hill*, p. 88.
87 Bartrip, *Themselves Writ Large*, p. 256.
88 *Ibid.*, p. 257.
89 Campbell, *Nye Bevan*, p. 174.
90 *Ibid.*, Bartrip, *Themselves Writ Large*, p. 257.
91 Pater, *The Making of the National Health Service*, p. 151.
92 Campbell, *Nye Bevan*, p. 174.
93 Pater, *The Making of the National Health Service*, p. 153.
94 Grey-Turner and Sutherland, *History of the British Medical Association*, p. 63.
95 Bartrip, *Themselves Writ Large*, p. 258.
96 Pater, *The Making of the National Health Service*, p. 155.
97 Campbell, *Nye Bevan*, pp. 174–175.
98 Pater, *The Making of the National Health Service*, p. 156.
99 *Ibid.*, p. 157.
100 Bartrip, *Themselves Writ Large*, p. 259.
101 Hill, *Both Sides of the Hill*, p. 101.
102 Bartrip, *Themselves Writ Large*, pp. 259–260.
103 *Ibid.*, p. 260. Hill, *Both Sides of the Hill*, p. 76.

104 Hill, *Both Sides of the Hill*, p. 21. Foot, *Aneurin Bevan*, p. 23.
105 Hill, *Both Sides of the Hill*, pp. 93–96.
106 *Ibid.*, pp. 100 and 103.
107 Bartrip, *Themselves Writ Large*, p. 260.
108 Grey-Turner and Sutherland, *History of the British Medical Association*, p. 64.
109 Bartrip, *Themselves Writ Large*, p. 261.
110 Campbell, *Nye Bevan*, pp. 175–176.
111 Webster, *The Health Services Since the War*, p. 114.
112 Pater, *The Making of the National Health Service*, p. 161.
113 Bartrip, *Themselves Writ Large*, p. 254.
114 *BMA Archive*, B/203/1/37, minutes of IAC meeting on 7 March 1946, min. 99.
115 Grey-Turner and Sutherland, *History of the British Medical Association*, p. 64.
116 *BMJ*, 17 March 1948, 'Report of Special Panel Conference', Supplement, p. 58.
117 Grey-Turner and Sutherland, *History of the British Medical Association*, p. 65.
118 *Ibid.*
119 Bartrip, *Themselves Writ Large*, p. 261.
120 Grey-Turner and Sutherland, *History of the British Medical Association*, p. 66. Foot, *Aneurin Bevan*, p. 345.
121 Pater, *The Making of the National Health Service*, p. 158.
122 Bartrip, *Themselves Writ Large*, p. 261.
123 *Ibid.*, p. 262. Webster, *The Health Services Since the War*, p. 116.
124 Webster, *The Health Services Since the War*, pp. 117–118.
125 Paul Vaughan, *Doctors' Commons: A Short History of the British Medical Association* (London, 1959). p. 231.
126 Foot, *Aneurin Bevan*, p. 347.
127 Grey-Turner and Sutherland, *History of the British Medical Association*, p. 68.
128 *BMJ*, 17 April 1948, 'Mr Bevan's Gesture', pp. 737–738.
129 Bartrip, *Themselves Writ Large*, p. 262.
130 *BMJ*, 24 April 1948, 'Statement by Council', Supplement, pp. 105–106.
131 *Ibid.*, 'The Plebiscite', pp. 791–793.
132 Bartrip, *Themselves Writ Large*, p. 263.
133 Webster, *The Health Services Since the War*, p. 118.
134 Grey-Turner and Sutherland, *History of the British Medical Association*, p. 69.
135 *Ibid.*, p. 70.
136 Bartrip, *Themselves Writ Large*, p. 263.
137 Webster, *The Health Services Since the War*, p. 124.
138 Grey-Turner and Sutherland, *History of the British Medical Association*, p. 70.
139 Turner, *Call the Doctor*, p. 306.
140 *BMJ*, 15 May 1948, 'What We Have Gained', pp. 936–937.
141 *Ibid.*, 5 June 1948, 'Special Representative Meeting', Supplement, pp. 147–155.
142 *Ibid.*, pp. 149 and 154.
143 *Ibid.*, p. 153.
144 *The Economist*, 24 April 1948, 'The BMA Replies', pp. 664–665.
145 *Ibid.*, Foot, *Aneurin Bevan*, p. 353.
146 Foot, *Aneurin Bevan*, p. 536.
147 *Ibid.*, pp. 356–537.
148 Webster, *The Health Services Since the War*, p. 119. See also Andrew Seaton, 'Against the "Sacred Cow": NHS Opposition and the Fellowship for Freedom in Medicine,1948–1972.' *Twentieth Century British History*, 26 (3) (2015). pp. 424–449.
149 Hill, *Both Sides of the Hill*, p. 99.

150 Vaughan, *Doctors' Commons*, p. 324.
151 *Ibid.*
152 Foot, *Aneurin Bevan*, p. 357.
153 Grey-Turner and Sutherland, *History of the British Medical Association*, p. 72.
154 *Ibid*, p. 66.
155 Eckstein, *The English Health Service*, p. 162.
156 Hill, *Both Sides of the Hill*, pp. 97 and 102.
157 *Ibid.*, p. 100.
158 Bartrip, *Themselves Writ Large*, p. 264.
159 Foot, *Aneurin Bevan*, p. 353.
160 Webster, *The Health Services Since the War*, p. 129.
161 Campbell, *Nye Bevan*, p. 177.
162 Hill, *Both Sides of the Hill*, p. 87.
163 *Ibid.*, p. 98.
164 Foot, *Aneurin Bevan*, p. 300.
165 Stewart, *The Battle for Health*, pp. 192–194.
166 *Ibid.*, p. 197.
167 Campbell, *Nye Bevan*, p. 179.
168 Eckstein, *The English Health Service*, p. 252, n. 69.
169 Campbell, *Nye Bevan*, p. 178.
170 Honigsbaum, *Health, Happiness and Security*, p. 217. Hill, *Both Sides of the Hill*, p. 99.
171 Campbell, *Nye Bevan*, pp. 167 and 169.
172 Bartrip, *Themselves Writ Large*, p. 265.
173 *BMA Archive*, minutes of IAC meeting on 24 September 1942, min. 3.
174 *Ibid.*, minutes of meeting on 29 June 1944, min. 122.
175 Pater, *The Making of the National Health Service*, p. 61.
176 *BMJ*, 13 May 1944, Editorial 'Before Negotiations Begin', p. 663.
177 Honigsbaum, *Health, Happiness and Security*, pp. 37–41.
178 Webster, *The Health Services Since the War*, p. 110.
179 *Ibid.*, p. 98.
180 Grey-Turner and Sutherland, *History of the British Medical Association*, p. 75.
181 Bartrip, *Themselves Writ Large*, p. 265.
182 Grey-Turner and Sutherland, *History of the British Medical Association*, p. 75.
183 Foot, *Aneurin Bevan*, p. 342.
184 Eckstein, *The English Health Service*, pp. 129–130.
185 Turner, *Call the Doctor*, p. 306.
186 Eckstein, *The English Health Service*, p. 9.
187 Foot, *Aneurin Bevan*, pp. 339–340.
188 *BMJ*, 10 January 1948, pp. 59–60.
189 Webster, *The Health Services Since the War*, pp. 100–103.
190 Atholl MacLaren, 'Fifty Years On: How a Fledgling Health Service Proved its Worth,' in Chris Locke (ed) *GPs in Nottinghamshire 1948–1998: A Health Service Record* (Nottingham, 1999). p. 16.
191 David Widgery, *Health in Danger: The Crisis in the National Health Service* (London, 1979). pp. 31–32.
192 Campbell, *Nye Bevan*, p. 177.
193 Pater, *The Making of the National Health Service*, p. 8.
194 Foot, *Aneurin Bevan*, p. 360.

Conclusion

*Assessing GPs' political activities
and their context*

The Introduction to this book suggested that prior to the advent of the NHS, British GPs were an important but misunderstood minority. Though never at any time numbering, during the period studied, more than around 25,000 individuals, GPs played a central part in the social administration of the country and in maintaining the health and well-being of its citizens. But they were frequently maligned by opponents, politicians, and the press and their reasonable complaints were more often than not disregarded. One of the objectives of this study was to throw some light on the factors motivating their emergent collective political ideology and its effects. The book has also attempted to show how GPs' desire for self-determination impacted the development of organised healthcare services in early twentieth-century Britain. Additionally, it has sought to explain how new representative structures came into being following the introduction of NHI that reflected and embodied GPs' aspirations and professional 'articles of faith'. As has been shown, these structures sought to protect GPs' professional interests but were not always successful in doing so. Personal interest was not, however, their sole motivation. Among the common misconceptions about GPs' conflicts with governments which this analysis has sought to dispel is the idea that GPs were consistently opposed to state coordination of healthcare services, and that there was no higher purpose to their leaders' actions than their own material benefit. As has, hopefully, been demonstrated, the profession was, in general, consistently supportive of efforts to extend the range and improve the quality of the services GPs offered, provided they were adequately funded, but they were always fearful of the consequences of ceding more control over their activities to lay authorities. This study has sought to encourage a greater appreciation of the individual and collective sacrifices of GPs in this period. It has also made clear why collective opinions formed during this period continued to exercise an influence on the thinking of the GPs of subsequent generations, extending even to the present.

Considering the political ideology of GPs during the period studied and how the principles it encompassed became so engrained in their collective culture,

DOI: 10.4324/9781003438274-13

the survival of such an ideology to the present day, as testified by the actions of their representatives in 2016 described in the Introduction, is, therefore, not altogether surprising. This study has demonstrated how GPs' limited ability to self-regulate encouraged a desire to resist governmental interference, fostered a distrust of politicians, and engendered a belief in the profession's unique ability to identify and meet the public's need for healthcare. This formed the basis of a professional narrative which GPs of more recent times have found no less compelling. This study has been structured around an accumulation of interlocking themes which are considered sequentially in this Conclusion as a means of drawing together the central points of its analysis. It is hoped that a coherent picture emerges from this synthesis which makes sense of the disparate elements of which the preceding narrative is composed, and the occasionally beguiling complexities it has sought to explain.

Individualism, contractor status, and professional autonomy

Throughout the period studied, general practice remained very much an individualistic undertaking. Sir George Newman believed that individualism was a determining characteristic of the medical profession and central to the doctor's success as a clinician, stating that their 'resourcefulness, adaptability, common sense and imagination' were individual virtues, and that 'the medical practitioner is individualistic in upbringing and in purpose'.[1] Partnerships between GPs thus often proved difficult to sustain, given the inevitable personality clashes which occurred when strong-minded individuals disagreed. Single-handed practice remained predominant therefore throughout this period.[2] The GP's practice was, essentially, a personal enterprise in which individual doctors invested much of their waking lives.[3] The advent of NHI did not put an end to commercial rivalry and competition between practitioners. Even without the divisions which resulted from the bitter intra-professional disputes which accompanied NHI, many doctors found it hard to cooperate with their local competitors, even though they were occasionally compelled to seek assistance from other doctors, whether for a second opinion, the administration of an anaesthetic during an operation, or treatment for themselves or their families when sick. A layman, Mr Atherton Moore, writing in *Medical World* in 1914, offered the following astute observation:

> Accustomed throughout their professional lives to act alone, to come to decisions in a moment, guided by the needs of the moment, without opportunity for consultation with others, they develop a moral temper which unfits them to act with others. The very quality of being self-contained, adequate to the task of the moment which is so invaluable a part of the mental equipment of a country Doctor, this quality itself makes it difficult for him to sink his individuality and cooperate with other men.[4]

Many regretted the isolationism which single-handed practice led to and believed that primary health centres, as recommended by the Dawson report, would provide the antidote. They hoped that GPs operating in shared premises or in group practices would also share new ideas and opportunities for postgraduate training and engage more frequently and productively with specialist colleagues. Cottage hospitals and professionally run PMS schemes brought some GPs together in collective endeavours but these could never amount to more than a partial realisation of Dawson's suggested regimen. In no real sense was it possible for GPs to work in teams without a fundamental reorientation of the medical mindset coupled with root and branch reorganisation of state-commissioned healthcare. A representative of the trade unions' Approved Societies, Mr F. Jordan, complained in a press article in 1931:

> There is too much individualism in the medical profession. It would be highly beneficial if ... local practitioners (spent) time in the hospitals and other medical centres, away from their practices at stated periods, so that they can be thoroughly posted in up-to-date practice.[5]

The IAC hoped that their proposals in *A General Medical Service for the Nation* would bring some of the benefits of team working without GPs forfeiting any of their independence or autonomy. However, the separation of general practice and hospital medical care which they hoped to prevent, though never as complete as Honigsbaum postulated, was already becoming a reality by the late 1930s and was solidified in Bevan's tri-partite NHS structure. For most GPs, independent contractor status, as the embodiment of their individualistic spirit, was an article of faith which they expected LMPCs and their national executive, the IAC, to defend at all costs. Steve Watkins observes that independent contractor status has 'a deep emotional appeal' to GPs and that the MPU 'suffered very heavily when it declared its support for a salaried service'.[6] As noted in the Introduction, the desire for autonomy is common to all branches of the medical profession internationally. It was their ability as independent contractors to undertake their clinical work unsupervised, and without being monitored by those to whom they were contractually responsible, which made British GPs feel superior to salaried doctors. So too with any of their continental counterparts, who may have been less free to determine who to accept as a patient, when and where to deliver treatment, or determine how many patients they could safely be responsible for. These freedoms exercised a powerful attraction for which the fringe benefits of a salaried service, such as nominally fixed hours and employer-sponsored pensions, never succeeded in outweighing.

Watkins believes that the freedom of action which doctors believed independent contractor status accorded them is largely illusory in that doctors have always had an overwhelming tendency to conform to accepted norms of practice and behaviour.[7] But whenever individual GPs were singled out for criticism by the Ministry of Health in the 1930s, the doctors' representative bodies closed ranks, and rose to defend to the utmost their constituents' right to exercise their clinical and professional freedom without lay interference. They did so even where their constituents' behaviour exceeded the bounds of what they believed to be good practice.[8] The preservation of independent contractor status gave rise to what Watkins describes as the 'laager mentality' which resulted from the profession's sense of 'being embattled, being powerless, pushed around by hostile and powerful forces against which it must maintain relentless hostility in order to have some slight influence on events'.[9] The GPs' original antagonists – non-qualified quacks, interloping professional rivals, self-enlarging local authorities, and power-hungry friendly societies – were soon supplanted in the GPs' imagination by manipulative politicians hell-bent on reducing the doctors' autonomy, and by a hostile press reflecting the political preferences and prejudices of the political elite. This feeling was accelerated by the events of the 1920s and 1930s when the panel GPs' patience and reserves of goodwill and public-spiritedness were tested by the persistent undermining of the profession's claim for just reward by ministers, civil servants, and a hostile press dismissive of their claim to be acting in the public interest. Out of this process emerged a collective feeling, which survived into the era of the NHS, which Watkins describes as 'a fierce libertarianism'. This was manifested in an indiscriminate distrust of politicians, administrators, and any groups representing the public who might question their professional autonomy or the extent of their authority in medical matters.[10]

Free choice of doctor, private practice, and 'the professional social ideal'

Hand in hand with independent contractor status was the principle which became in itself a separate article of faith for the profession, that is, free choice of doctor. This was something which was calculated to appeal to the man in the street as much as it did to Lloyd George but it was not, as W. J. Braithwaite maintained, a specious claim.[11] GPs genuinely believed in the patient's right to choose their medical attendant because the effectiveness of the confidential relationship between doctor and patient was based on trust, even if, judging by many contemporary accounts, there was often a good deal of suspicion on both sides. The BMA strongly believed that the patient's free choice of doctor would be vitiated if GPs were forced to become salaried employees of the state. It was a principle the public could readily appreciate even if, in practice, they rarely exercised this freedom. As E.S. Turner, writing in the 1950s, rather cynically put it, 'The average person spends more care in choosing a car or a television set than in choosing a doctor. In any event he has neither the means nor the ability to check on a doctor's professional skill or knowledge'.[12]

Many people in Britain today are unable to equate the ideals of medicine with the idea of competition for patients and making a profit. But, in an era when as many patients were treated under private arrangements as through national insurance or other forms of contract practice, few doctors saw in this any ethical dilemma. In a debate in the House of Lords in 1947 about the profession's fears of becoming salaried, the revered Lord Dawson commented that a state-salaried doctor could not be expected to show the same responsibility for a patient as 'a doctor whose good work brings reputation and later, maybe, material reward'. He stated his belief that 'a healthy thought of self is a spur that consorts well with a desire and an endeavour to help others'.[13] That is not to say that there were not any doctors whose desire to make money sometime overrode their professional and ethical responsibilities. There was always a small minority who were motivated by what Harry Roberts referred to as 'The cad's code', that is, 'Get all that you can, and give as little as you must'.[14] Frank Layton's fictional character McFadd offers a rather two-dimensional example of this archetype.[15] However, Francis Brett Young's Jacob Medhurst offers a more interesting character study. Medhurst has acquired a level of competence and knowledge of his craft which is put to good use in treating patients; yet, he is an unabashed hedonist who lives only to please himself. His personal philosophy represents a challenge to the accepted professional wisdom about the noble profession and its ethics but is, however, compelling in its honesty.[16] Professional leaders would have been embarrassed to admit to such views although they represented an attitude which critics within the Approved Societies claimed to encounter all too frequently. It would be unwise, however, to take the Societies' criticisms at face value. They were seldom free of malice and were fuelled by resentment at their loss of authority. David B. Green's argument that the friendly societies were the unheralded champions of consumer choice falls down when he accuses the GPs of being anti-competitive.[17] Their adherence to the principle of free choice of doctor proved that GPs were in favour of competition, provided it was 'fair' competition, that is, competition based on quality of service or the doctor's reputation rather than price, and this is effectively what they got under NHI. Their collective experience of the excesses of the free market had led them to believe that undercutting by impoverished and unscrupulous doctors would, by lowering the market rate for their services, result in an increasingly lower quality of service being delivered by an increasingly inferior brand of doctor.

NHI brought a halt to that process but when the refusal of successive governments to increase the panel GPs' remuneration was followed by actual reductions in what they were paid, the consequent lowering of standards should have come as no surprise, as many panel GPs gave up insurance practice or sought to maximise their income from private practice. In many cases, this enabled them to maintain the standard of living they believed they deserved, and which guaranteed their proper place in society. They believed very strongly, as has been shown, that an adequate lifestyle was necessary for them to maintain proper standards of practice and to do their best for patients. As contemporary commentators noted, patients' respect for their doctors and the advice they gave was often influenced by the outward appearance of 'respectability'. Thus, James Smith Whitaker asked, when commenting on the GPs' pay claim in 1919 if the amount the doctors were asking for was no more than sufficient 'to remunerate a doctor working at the maximum of his single-handed capacity *taking into account the social position it is desirable that he should occupy?'* (added emphasis).[18] In the BMA's evidence to the Court of Inquiry into GPs' pay in 1923, their statistician Professor Bowley offered a perfect description of the 'professional social ideal' when he said that the doctors' 'professional success, from the financial point of view, is to some extent dependent on their maintaining a social position in proper relationship to those among whom they work'.[19] Harry Eckstein agrees that 'external traits of success have a great deal to do with the public's assessment of professional abilities'. Thus, he concludes, 'The young doctor who valued his "goodwill" was well advised not to economise even on the most inconsequential trappings of successful practice'.[20] Accompanying this view is the belief that to be effective in all aspects of their work, GPs needed to be cultured individuals, a view endorsed by the League of Nations' report quoted by Brackenbury in his book, *Patient and Doctor*, which said that, 'The Doctor should, in the best sense of the words, belong to the elite. His professional knowledge should be enhanced by his general culture'.[21] According to one authority, 'For much of the nineteenth and twentieth century, culture was understood to be a significant – if not indispensable – part of what it meant to be middle class'.[22] Class, culture, and financial reward were thus inextricably bound together in the GPs' professional philosophy and the political ideology which arose from it. Rightly or wrongly, GPs believed that they could not achieve that level of 'culture' without an adequate standard of living.

The mixed economy of care and the threat of salaried service

Independent contractor status was the foundation of the mixed public and private practice model and essential to GPs' autonomy. It allowed them to maintain a list of panel patients as large as they felt able to manage while still allowing them time to treat dependants of the insured and fee-paying middle-class patients and undertake other remunerative medical work. It was acknowledged by the GPs themselves that fee-paying patients generally enjoyed greater courtesies and convenience than panel patients, but GPs devoted no less attention to panel patients' medical needs. As this study has demonstrated, GPs, other than the minority who favoured a salaried service, wanted a comprehensive national medical service available, though not free, to all, and expected those able to afford to pay for a GP's services privately to continue to do so. From the perspective of historians writing in the late twentieth century, this attitude seemed reactionary and inconsistent with the altruistic outlook which doctors professed, and the public had come to expect of them, under the NHS. There is more than a hint of determinism in this, influenced by the views of a generation of historians and social scientists whose reverence for the NHS inclined them to see the 'welfare state' as the inevitable culmination of a century of social reform and state expansion.[23] Now that such path-dependant views no longer go unchallenged, the motives of the profession's leaders warrant a more open re-examination. If those who accuse the doctors of these times of being interested only in their own well-being are correct, then the public pronouncements of their leaders were a cynical façade, of which one would expect to find evidence in their confidential documents and communications. The absence of any such evidence supports the contention that they were sincere in their adherence to the ideals of public service, albeit in their own terms, and that they genuinely wanted to establish the best possible health service the country could afford, based on a mix of private and public funding.

It should be remembered that many panel GPs had almost no private patients other than the families of the insured, whom they endeavoured to cater for through PMS schemes in the expectation that they would eventually be included in any future state-organised health service. The level of bad debts incurred by many 'slum doctors' is, moreover, consistent with the continued element of charity which they were forced to adopt towards their poorest patients. The GP Francis Maylett Smith, for example, observed that 'receipts from the Clubs, for looking after their families (who gave twice as much trouble) scarcely covered the cost of drugs and dressings'.[24] As has been shown, private practice among the fee-paying middle classes remained an area in which GPs enjoyed greater freedom to experiment with new treatments, pursue special interests, and acquire new skills which could prove to be of benefit to their panel patients. For those GPs able to grasp its opportunities, private practice offered the prospect of greater financial rewards. It also offered freedom from the increasing effects of 'red tape' and officialdom which the panel GPs found irksome. It was therefore viewed as a potential bolthole into which GPs could retreat if their experience as reluctant agents of the state proved unpalatable or unsustainable.[25] This was an essential weapon in their conflicts with the government and proved to be one of the sticking points on which their subsequent opposition to Bevan's proposals for the NHS was based. The other factor animating professional opposition to Bevan's plans was the fear that they would inevitably lead to GPs being forced to become salaried employees of the state.

In the debates about the Dawson report, Guy Dain warned of the consequences of GPs not embracing the health centre idea.[26] His warning was only partially borne out, however, as the profession successfully resisted any attempt to expand the role of local authority clinics or replace GPs with other healthcare professionals. The overtly socialist ambitions of some local authorities, notably in London in the 1930s, alarmed conservative-minded GPs and convinced many that they would eventually be forced to become salaried employees of those authorities. When this became official Labour Party policy, it was inevitable that it would become a central point of contention between the profession and any future Labour Government, and it completely coloured the profession's view of the Beveridge report and successive government proposals for the NHS. GPs could consider themselves fortunate that Bevan's faith in local authorities was not sufficient for him to allow them a greater role in the provision of curative treatment in the new NHS than they had enjoyed under the interwar regime. The profession's fears always blinded them to the benefits which greater integration of medical services offered and left them in a state of glorious isolation as, within a few years, politicians and the public focused most of their attention on the new hospital system and its merits and deficiencies. The GPs' leaders were soon complaining that they were the 'Cinderellas' of the NHS.[27] But on this occasion, Cinderella had only herself to blame at being left out of everyone's considerations. She had declined to wear the apparel she had been offered and subsequently ruled herself out of contention for the prince's hand by not turning up to the ball.

Self-regulation and 'bounded pluralism' vs bureaucratisation and state control

For doctors, autonomy demanded professional control over the setting of standards for competence and behaviour. This control was not at any time surrendered by the profession during the period studied. The GMC, as the ultimate arbiter of professional conduct and standards and of who could be and could remain a qualified medical practitioner, continued to be dominated by clinicians and its power and decision-making was seldom questioned by government. When it came to NHI, the state had every right to expect a role in determining if those it contracted with to deliver medical services were complying with their contracts but accepted the need to defer to the profession's expertise in clinical matters. The doctors generally exercised the decisive voice in medical service subcommittee investigations and successfully fought off attempts by the Approved Societies to carve out a role for themselves in the initiation of patient complaints. Politicians were also content, as was shown, to grant the profession the responsibility to police disputes between practitioners and share ground-rules for professional etiquette through LMPCs. The deference shown towards the profession by Lloyd George, Addison, Morant, and their key officials in the early days of NHI did not sit well with the Approved Societies or their allies in parliament and the press but was consistent with Liberal party views of how the expanding state should operate, that is, by means of 'bounded pluralism'.[28] The nature of the relationship between the state and the medical profession in this regard is also consistent with the previously mentioned concept of 'regulated self-regulation'.[29] For the BMA and their critics in the MPU, 'there were no severer critics of delinquent doctors than a body of their own colleagues invested with the control of purely professional affairs'.[30] But while excessive prescribing, inappropriate charging of fees, or failure to offer treatment required might be punished, service subcommittees found it difficult to agree on matters of competence or negligence. The Local Medical Committees (LMCs) also found it difficult to censure doctors of whom other constituents complained, for fear of being sued and being without funds, they were never fully able, in the absence of state indemnity, to realise their potential as professional 'courts of honour'.

The advent of the RMO Service signified a change in the dynamics of the relationship between panel GPs and the state. Relations between the GPs, LMPCs, and Insurance Committees remained cordial but, being directly accountable to the Ministry, the plenipotentiary RMOs soon merited, in many panel doctors' eyes, the same degree of opprobrium they accorded to the local authorities' MOHs. While rigorously exercising their inquisitorial functions in inspecting GPs' records and prescribing, and questioning their judgement in issuing certificates, the RMOs came to represent for some panel GPs an unwelcome, intrusive, and in some cases feared emissary of the state. As a commentator in *Medical World* put it in 1926, 'the panel doctor is being brought more and more under the stultifying influence of authority'.[31] In 1923, the Walsall GP Frank Layton had welcomed the changes wrought by the advent of NHI in his novel *The Old Doctor* whose publication the BMA had helped sponsor as propaganda supportive of their claim for increased remuneration. Layton had dedicated his novel to Morant. Ten years later in his novel *The Little Doctor*, Layton complains that the Ministry has 'ruined' the scheme of which GPs like him had such high hopes. He concludes his fulminations with regret at Morant's passing: 'Why did the big man die…? His death was a catastrophe…He would never have consented to panel doctors being treated as untrustworthy clerks'.[32] For Layton, it would seem that the relationship between panel GPs and the state was scarcely one of partnership. Moreover, the behaviour of Ministers and officials like Robinson hardly merited the degree of confidence and trust which Cox had expressed in his paean to the 'incorruptible' civil service.[33] Though it would be considered distinctly 'light touch' by modern standards, the degree of monitoring of contractual noncompliance by Insurance Committees and RMOs was seen by many GP as a constraint on their professional freedom and unwelcome evidence of increasing state control, fuelling concerns about the possibility of a future state medical service. It was to their representative bodies that the GPs looked to counter this and other existential threats.

Class consciousness, party political affiliations, and the nature of representative authority

In describing the changing fortunes of GPs, this study has shown how middle-class insecurities were manifested politically and otherwise during a period of massive social and economic upheaval which saw the sweeping away of the old Liberal order. As has been shown, the nineteenth-century GP was motivated by a desire for social acceptance and respectability. Professionalisation helped improve the status of GPs, but its effects were offset by an increase in the number of doctors which served to depress wage levels and lower standards of practice. Insecurity fuelled protectionism. The increasing cost of medical education in the early twentieth century had the effect of making the profession less socially diverse but, while new entrants were increasingly middle class, the level of debt most of them were obliged to incur jeopardised their social status as they struggled to keep up appearances. As self-employed businessmen and women, GPs were instinctually conservative and shared the political establishment's fears of Bolshevist revolution and regret at the breakdown of the values by which the, now ailing, British Empire had been held together. They compared the apparently improving fortunes of their working-class clientele with their own diminishing prospects, considering themselves part of the 'new poor'. They felt aggrieved that their sacrifices had not been acknowledged and they were not accorded a greater share of the social product. Most doctors thought of medicine as a 'liberal' profession. But it comprised a broad spectrum of political opinion, including some distinctly reactionary elements. In 1896, the *Lancet* opined that country doctors were solidly Tory, arguing that similarities between medicine and the priesthood meant that 'naturally a medical man bears the interior instinct of Toryism'.[34] Isolation breeds suspicion of change, so rural GPs were perhaps less open to new ideas than their urban or suburban counterparts who enjoyed a wider cultural experience and had more opportunity of testing their ideas in informed debate. But what this book has demonstrated more than once is that GPs were unquestionably a heterogeneous group and as their individual and collective circumstances changed, so, often, did their outlook and political affiliations. GPs could be liberal in some respects and conservative in others, or open to change one minute and fiercely resistant to it the next. At times, the herd instinct, or the 'mob complex' as Alfred Cox described it, made it relatively easy to steer the profession in a particular direction, whereas for the majority of the time, the experience of those trying to lead GPs was, to employ a much-overused metaphor, like 'herding cats'.

Unity was the profession's main weapon in its battle against a hostile world.[35] But unity was, as has been shown, elusive. While it was the desire for an effective political response which led the profession back to the IAC leadership in moments of crisis, the BMA's inability to speak forcefully and monolithically for a united profession was a constant constraint on its effectiveness. The dilemma faced by those who sought to organise the profession for political objectives was how to bring these individuals together in a common cause. Doctors, as Woodcock had observed, were not by nature rebels, so it took a lot to move them to the point where they felt compelled to collaborate in mutual self-defence.[36] The 'battle of the clubs' was really a succession of local skirmishes taking place over several decades with an enemy which an astute minority of doctors recognised as representing a serious and long-term threat to their well-being. The effect of the agitation following the Manchester conference in 1900 was to force the BMA to recognise its political role and, to become, for the benefit of its largely GP membership at that time, though it hotly denied it, a trade union in all but name. Its structures, the divisions and new central committees, were not fully developed when the first great opportunity came for the BMA to flex its political muscles as it galvanised the profession in opposition to the National Insurance Act. However, their collective judgement of what this legislation offered the profession was off target, as was readily admitted by later generations of its leaders. Their inexperience was their undoing. As Lloyd George, in forgiving mood, informed a dinner organised in his honour by veterans of the conflict in 1933, 'It was the first time the profession as a body had come into politics, and politics is a very heady wine if you are not used to it, and they were not'.[37]

As was shown, the conflict over NHI divided the profession and the very wide spectrum of political opinions it encompassed included extreme wings which those who aspired to lead the profession at times found difficult to ignore. Yet, while every GP had an opinion, the number who were sufficiently motivated or had the time and energy to become actively involved in professional politics remained small. In 1912, Woodcock opined that the local branches of the BMA 'were too much in the hands of correct and starchy men, dry, longwinded, antisocial', confessing to being one such man himself.[38] He observed, however, that 'the political doctor' was 'now born' and there were among those who emerged as local and national leaders of the GPs after 1912 a group of capable individuals who took a pragmatic approach built on painstaking efforts to build relationships with those at the centre of power in the state. While many medical luminaries found it hard to disguise their distaste for the squabbling over financial reward which much of their political activity necessarily involved, the reaction of a good proportion of the profession, other than at times of greatest agitation, was one of resignation and apathy. Even when great political questions affecting the work and future of panel practices were at issue, few GPs could rouse themselves to attend meetings. Writing to the *BMJ* in 1916, a Dr J. MacBeth-Elliot reported that when enquiring as to why BMA division meetings were poorly attended, one colleague had informed him that, 'These medico political matters do not interest me in the least'.[39] When collecting evidence to present to the Royal Commission in 1926, one regional committee of LMPCs noted that 198 meetings had taken place across the country at which not more than 21% of panel GPs had attended.[40] Even when the profession was apparently convulsed by concerns about the prospects offered by the NHS White Paper in 1944 and doctors were urged to attend local meetings to make their views known, the GP negotiator Roland Cockshutt declared himself 'rather depressed by the smallness of attendance at some division meetings'.[41] Eckstein shrewdly observes, 'There is power which rests on sympathy and power which rests on apathy; that of the BMA's leaders rests on apathy. It is therefore easily turned into weakness under circumstances requiring strong corporate cohesion'.[42]

The local structures on which the profession's power rested remained peopled by representatives nominally elected by their peers but who were, in reality, largely self-selected, as the numbers of uncontested elections and vacant seats on LMPCs during this period attest. The political allegiances of these institutions were sometimes determined by the personalities of their local leaders and battles for control are evident in the minutes of LMPCs and the debates at their annual conference. In Kent, the LMPC's adherence to the MPU effectively came to an end in a showdown in the late 1920s between the Union's local spokesman, Gordon Ward, and the LMPC officers, and by 1938, the accommodation between the London Panel Committee and the IAC was complete when E.A. Gregg became the chairman of both, as well as the chairman of the London Insurance Committee and the London Public Medical Service.[43] LMPC representatives were meant to reflect the views of their constituents, which was why elections were conducted on the basis of geographical districts, but in the face of widely diverging views among those constituents, it was the representatives' own views which usually emerged more strongly. They might have justified their actions by quoting one of Edmund Burke's sayings of which Harry Roberts was fond: 'Your representative owes you not his industry only but his judgement; and he betrays, instead of serving you, if he sacrifices it to your opinion'.[44]

Critics of the BMA both within government and the profession itself liked to portray the Association as unrepresentative. Just how fair is this criticism? Eckstein sees the medico-politician, whether GP or Consultant, as stereotypically among the more established and wealthy practitioners, and concludes, with some justification, that medical 'representative' bodies were 'inevitably weighted in favour of age, affluence, private practice and the suburb'.[45] He might have added that women, ethnic or religious minorities, and the full-time salaried were among those excluded by implication from this assessment. In their battles with Bevan, Bartrip argues that it was largely Consultants and GPs from the home counties who led the BMA in a fight for principles which GPs and other doctors in the regions and other nations of the UK had little appetite.[46] Participation in 'associative affairs' was, however, extraordinarily low, Eckstein notes, due to the sheer pressure of the doctor's work.[47] Beyond this, it is a feature of politics in whatever form it takes for those with the most extreme opinions to express themselves with the greatest conviction and in so doing influence, albeit momentarily, a great many others whose natural inclinations are more moderate. The MPA and the SMA not only added a great deal of noise and colour to the debates about the NHS, but they also succeeded in muddying the waters, making it harder on occasion for ordinary practitioners to determine which matters they should be most concerned about. 'Moderation is never easy or popular when tempers and temperatures are high', Charles Hill complained, accusing those on the right wing of the profession especially of forgetting that it was the profession itself that had initially called for a comprehensive NHS, and advocated many of the things they now condemned as inimical to professional interests.[48]

But, as Hill was also at pains to point out, the BMA was committed to democratic principles to a far greater extent than most representative bodies or trade unions. He described it, proudly and not unjustifiably, as 'the most democratic professional organisation in the world'.[49] This was why the Association went to such enormous lengths to ascertain the views of its members, and non-members, through independently conducted and expensive plebiscites, frequent special meetings of its Representative Body and through local meetings and roadshows. The views of all sides of the political spectrum were allowed to be aired in the *BMJ* and the BMA's leaders made themselves available to answer the questions of, and engage with, practitioners, the public and other interested parties at every turn. It is true that they did try to influence the outcome of the plebiscites, but the Association was committed to abide by the decisions of not just its membership, but of the whole profession, when those views were clearly expressed and understood. But when it came to complex and controversial issues of policy or principle, the preferences of the rank and file were not always easy to discern and were apt to change rapidly in response to outside pressures. Looking back, Hill felt that the 'questions they ask and the cash contributions they make are a useful guide to what men and women are really thinking' and 'The fact that a body of members does not vote as their leaders advise does not prove that they are wrong'.[50] Comparing the situation of Hill and Lord Moran, Honigsbaum notes that, 'The very nature of Moran's oligarchic rule had its advantages; it gave him freedom to take initiatives which were denied to Hill. Hill was more sensitive to the medical mood, but he was also imprisoned by it'.[51] Bartrip concludes that the accusation that the BMA was unrepresentative therefore is both inaccurate and unfair. The problem it faced was the gap between active and passive participation in political matters and the fact that those interested in political concerns and who took the trouble to vote, committed the non-political and apathetic to policies which they were ultimately reluctant or disinclined to support. This, he says, 'was not lack of democracy, it was the product of it'.[52]

The limitations of 'bargained corporatism' and the battle for public approval

Views are divided about the success of the BMA's attempts at bargained corporatism. Norman Eder is guilty, perhaps, of exaggerating the extent of the consensus between the profession and officials through which the administration of NHI was conducted during the interwar period. Eckstein argues that the BMA and the Ministry worked constructively together most of the time and that while GP leaders did not succeed in major confrontations, they made up for this with less well-publicised successes in more minor matters.[53] Digby questions Eckstein's assessment of this 'meso-corporatist' approach pointing to the

BMA's failure to secure an increase in state payments to panel doctors in the interwar period.[54] She accords this failure to the difficulty of bringing the profession together in a united effort. As has been seen, the profession's leaders in the 1920s and 1930s generally sought to give ministers and officials the benefit of the doubt as to their motives for wanting to reduce expenditure and increase regulation. However, the effects of government actions were to depress panel GPs' income and morale, which fomented dissatisfaction both with government and with GPs' professional leaders, whom many GPs, like the MPU, deemed too conciliatory. A frequent critic of the IAC, Dr Genge, a representative of Croydon LMPC, typified this view when he said in 1931 that the IAC contained too many 'perfect little gentlemen' and that the GPs should instead be represented 'by someone who was not quite a gentleman'.[55] His comments might, of course, be interpreted as a personal dig at the chairman of the IAC, Guy Dain, who was of diminutive stature and known for his courteous and respectful manner. In any event, the government's deference to professional expertise was tempered by its ability to put forward its own medical experts, namely the Ministry's senior medical advisers and the network of RMOs, who came to be despised by many rank and file GPs as the proverbial 'poachers turned gamekeepers'.

Yet, as has been shown, the principal bulwark against government control and chief weapon in GPs' battle for self-determination was the collective might of the professional representative institutions to which NHI had given birth, the LMPCs. Although their individual effectiveness and influence over Insurance Committees was often dependent on the personalities of the committees' membership, collectively they represented a powerful lobby group bolstered by a nominally democratic mandate, able to articulate (what they believed were) the opinions of grassroots GPs. They were certainly capable of mobilising their constituents in support of political objectives. Over time, the local relationships between the LMPCs and the Insurance Committees became close to the point of being almost incestuous, especially when, as in a few cases, the LMPC chairman became the chairman of the Insurance Committee, or their secretary was the Insurance Committee Clerk! In 1926, a *Medical World* editorial lamented the fact that only about 6 out of 126 Insurance Committees in England were chaired by Panel GPs, dismissing newspaper claims that this was a new development.[56] To remain free of government control, however, it was essential that LMPCs remained self-funded, but this represented a fundamental weakness. The amount of statutory levy payments they could collect to support their activities was circumscribed by regulations and the level of voluntary contributions constrained by their constituents' ability, or willingness, to pay. Without the resources necessary to pay for much beyond the honorarium of a secretary and members' travelling expenses, the LMPCs could not fulfil the active leadership role which Addison and others had hoped they would, and the policing of professional behaviour was, as we have seen, fraught with legal difficulties. Those LMPCs who produced formularies and professional guidance for their constituents did so at their own expense and on their own initiative, but such actions show how much more effective they could have been had they been funded adequately.

From a political perspective, the importance of the LMPCs' Conference as a policy-making body has been overlooked by historians who in general have tended to see it as less important than the BMA's Annual Representative Meeting. This was certainly true when it came to the negotiations about the NHS in the 1940s, when the Conference and its executive consciously deferred to the BMA as representative of the wider profession. But during the interwar period, the IAC and its leaders were in no doubt that their power, though bolstered by the resources of the BMA, rested squarely on the democratic mandate which the Conference of LMPCs had bestowed on them. The increasing proportion of IAC members elected by the LMPCs Conference, regardless of whether they were BMA members, is, moreover, testament to the overriding political necessity of keeping the Conference loyal and 'on side'. Failure to do so, the IAC's leaders believed, would result in attempts to establish a rival organisation. As has been seen, this was no idle threat, but it was one which the IAC and its supporters just about managed to suppress. The fortunes of the MPU waxed and waned depending on general levels of dissatisfaction within the profession. They never looked like supplanting the IAC and their activities sometimes seemed only to increase the latter's bargaining power, not by forcing them to take a more extreme stand, but by providing the Ministry with a less palatable alternative if an accommodation with the IAC proved unattainable.

What is not disputed is the fact that dissatisfaction with their lot encouraged successive generations of GPs to continue to create lobby groups and new organisations threatening the BMA's political hegemony. For those on the extreme wings of political opinion, the BMA's business-like relationship with the Ministry smacked of collusion and the LMPCs' equally cordial relationship with Insurance Committees was deemed just as reprehensible.[57] Political extremists are always difficult to accommodate and often made use of the political platform offered them by the Conference of LMPCs. As a *BMJ* editorial in 1919 stated: 'In every body of ardent reformers there have always been doctrinaires who will make more noise and thus exerted more influence than their numbers or the weight of the arguments warranted'.[58] In many cases, the strategy adopted by those playing to the gallery at the LMPCs Conference involved advocating extreme forms of action to which the word 'strike', whether justified or not, was widely applied. The fact that the IAC backed away from such extreme measures was characterised as weakness, but the profession's leaders' reluctance was due to an abiding wish to avoid harm to patients, and fear of losing the moral high ground in arguments about the public interest. It was also due to the recognition that even a temporary reduction in panel income could prove fatal to many doctors' businesses. The BMA had flexed its muscles successfully in disputes over Medical Aid Institutes, even if it had got its knuckles rapped during the Coventry case, but implementing industrial action on a national scale was fraught with risk to doctors' livelihoods and reputations and the IAC's reluctance was therefore understandable.

The IAC's leaders recognised that the threat of mass resignation was not only a measure of last resort should purposeful negotiations fail, but was, as Eder described it, 'a gun with a single bullet'.[59] For this threat to be effective, the profession had to be determined to carry it through and be fully prepared for the consequences. It required proof of support from an overwhelming majority of the profession and a viable alternative through which the existing panel GPs could sustain themselves financially. Both these conditions were met in 1923, but in the 1930s, the profession was noticeably less willing to engage in political brinkmanship as both their leaders and their Government antagonists knew only too well. Between 1945 and 1948, the profession was galvanised by the ongoing debate about the future NHS and the perceived threat to their professional freedom which many felt it represented. In 1948, however, the GPs' leaders reluctantly concluded that there was no viable alternative, so the prospects of a mass boycott were largely illusory. The memory of GPs' collective and not wholly unsuccessful determination to achieve political ends through direct action was nevertheless to survive that conflict and the idea of mass resignation continued to exert a powerful appeal to the more politically astute among subsequent generations of dissatisfied GPs. Only once in the history of the NHS did desperation take GPs to the point where the threat of mass resignation proved real enough to secure the government's capitulation. That was in 1965. Thereafter, periodic ballots for mass resignation, such as those preceding the imposed new contract of 1990 and the negotiated new contract of 2004, proved increasingly unconvincing. GPs brought up with the NHS and working their entire professional lives within it identified themselves too much with the new system to want to abandon it. They felt that it was *their* NHS which they were defending when defying the wishes of government and, knowing how much their patients relied on it, found it difficult to contemplate industrial action, given the inevitable damage to patient care that would result. The 'professional social ideal' notwithstanding, the paradox of how to equate the ostensibly selfish need for material reward with the selfless calling of a noble profession was perplexing to many doctors, as their opponents recognised only too well. John Marks, the GP chairman of BMA Council in the 1990s and sometime historian of LMCs, stated in his autobiography that, when studying the origins of LMCs, he had concluded that civil servants and politicians had 'ruthlessly exploited doctors' vocational spirit' knowing that 'doctors were unwilling to take any action that would jeopardise their patients and that, under pressure, they would blame the BMA for their troubles and form splinter groups'.[60] It is clear from the account of discussions between the profession and the ministry that this somewhat jaundiced view contains much truth.

The other factor which the profession's representatives had to contend with was the battle for public opinion. Professional leaders, nationally within the IAC and the BMA's Council, and locally, within the LMPCs and BMA divisions, recognised the importance of public support for their political campaigns, and devoted considerable energy to developing a public relations function. The main obstacle to success was the hostility of the mainstream national press for whom doctors were always an easy target. The antagonistic and one-sided comments about doctors in the interwar press drew on a deep well of anti-medicalism and lay resentment of the soft power which profession enjoyed in its dealings with patients. The newspaper barons, moreover, had an ulterior motive in seeking to weaken the scientific authority of the medical establishment. They feared the effect which the profession's repeated attacks on unlicenced and alternative medicines might have on their advertising revenue, given the extent of it made up of purveyors of homely remedies and questionable medicaments, and fiercely resisted attempts to outlaw or restrict their unjustified claims.[61] The humble, hardworking family doctor could do nothing to withstand the orchestrated character assassination to which the profession was periodically subjected by the press, especially as their legal and ethical responsibilities to keep the contents of their consultations with patients confidential forbade them from offering comments on even the most outlandish claims of disgruntled patients. Indignant letters to the press from professional spokesmen were seldom sufficient to correct the damage done by journalistic misrepresentation or selective use of facts.

Nor did the charm offensive launched by sophisticated leaders like Brackenbury, Dain and Hill prove sufficient in preventing journalistic excess. Ultimately, the profession's attempts to win public support were undone by the lack of a coherent message, or at least one that the public could readily understand and sympathise with. It is a challenge with which they struggle to the present day. Doctors, and GPs especially, have always come out well in public opinion surveys of those most trusted by the public, and certainly much higher than journalists and politicians.[62] But this made little difference when major political decisions were at issue. As E.S. Turner noted sagely, 'patients who generally had no quarrel with, and indeed had every admiration for, their own doctor, were apt to grow impatient with the behaviour of doctors in the mass, especially when they group themselves under political labels'.[63] When Bevan and the BMA traded insults, neither party emerged with much credit. Webster makes the surprising comment that in their campaign against Labour's NHS proposals, the BMA 'employed techniques of megaphone diplomacy imitative of totalitarian regimes'.[64] The packed meeting of doctors which Charles Hill addressed at Wimbledon Town Hall in 1947 hardly merits comparison with the Nuremberg rallies but for many of the public, the spectacle was as disconcerting as any similar gathering of militant trade unionists.

The profession tried hard to cultivate the good opinion of the public by popularising the idea that medicine was a noble calling and promoting the image of the family doctor as a saintly, selfless, and often put-upon public servant. All this goodwill rapidly evaporated whenever doctors revealed themselves to be like ordinary men and women in wanting pay increases to maintain their standard of living. The public has proved unforgiving when doctors declined to regard a good public reputation as sufficient reward for their labours. This often proved, and was to prove on many subsequent occasions, a major weakness in the profession's political campaigns and contributed to the doctors' repeated defeats in their disputes with government. For GPs, the events of 1948 were merely the latest of a series of bruising encounters with lay authorities stretching back into the nineteenth century. They served to reinforce the 'laager mentality' mentioned earlier, if not the mythology of noble sacrifice many of them had maintained after their defeat in 1913. Following the profession's defeat over the introduction of the NHS, their apologists argued, with some justification it must be said, that the movement which led to its creation had begun with the profession itself. Since the inception of NHI, the BMA and the LMPCs Conference had been consistent advocates of more comprehensive and integrated health services. But when it came to how those services would be organised and paid for, the doctors' instinct for self-preservation and distrust of government control served to dissipate their radicalism and combined to drive them into alliance with the forces of political reaction. If subsequent generations of doctors, when valuing and defending the NHS, were puzzled, bemused, and, to some extent, embarrassed by the profession's condemnation of its principal architect and the Act which brought it into being, their distrust of central government and its officials remained undiminished. Clashes between GPs and government over their pay and terms and conditions of service were to occur regularly throughout the remainder of the twentieth century, the GPs' sense of grievance being compounded by consistent misrepresentation of their motives by politicians and the popular press. If suspicion of government had had been the strongest of the 'emotional cross currents' of the life of the profession in the 1940s, it was to become a permanent feature of GPs' professional mindset and one that has persisted throughout the long history of the NHS.

Notes

1 Quoted by Sir Henry B. Brackenbury in *Patient and Doctor* (London, 1935). p. 134.
2 Elliot Friedson, *Profession of Medicine: A Study of the Sociology of Applied Knowledge* (New York, 1970). p. 91.
3 Charles Webster, 'General Practice Under the Panel: The Last Phase.' *Bulletin of the Society for the Social History of Medicine*, 32 (1983). p. 23. Anne Digby, *The Evolution of British General Practice, 1850–1948* (Oxford, 1999). p. 136.
4 *Medical World*, 8 January 1914 'Doctor's Disunion', pp. 57–58.
5 Quoted by 'AGP', *This Panel Business* (London, 1933). pp. 106–107.
6 Steve Watkins, *Medicine and Labour: The Politics of a Profession* (London, 1987). p. 96.
7 *Ibid.*, pp. 21–24.
8 See above, pp. 199–200, for example, the defence of the anti-vaccinationist, Harvey.
9 Watkins, *Medicine and Labour,* pp. 22 and 18.
10 *Ibid.*, p.22.

11 See Chapter 4, Sir Henry Bunbury (ed.) *Lloyd George's Ambulance Wagon: The Memoirs of W.J. Braithwaite* (London, 1957). p. 198.

12 E.S. (Ernest Sackville) Turner, *Call the Doctor: A Social History of Medical Men* (London, 1958). p. 301.

13 *Ibid.*, p. 297.

14 Winifred Stamp, *Doctor Himself: An Unorthodox Biography of Harry Roberts MD, 1871–1946* (London, 1949). p. 80.

15 Frank G. Layton, *The Old Doctor* (Birmingham, 1923). pp. 162–164.

16 Francis Brett Young, *Doctor Bradley Remembers* (London, 1938). p. 239.

17 David B. Green, *Working-Class Patients and the Medical Establishment: Self-Help in Britain from the Mid-Nineteenth Century to 1948* (Aldershot, 1985). p. 132.

18 *National Archives* MH 62/118, Memorandum from Whitaker to Morant dated 24 July 1919, part 4, point 10.

19 *BMJ*, 5 January 1924 'Court of Inquiry into the Insurance Capitation fee' Appendix D, Memorandum by Professor Bowley dated 21 December 1923, Supplement, p. 11.

20 Harry Eckstein, *The English Health Service: Its Origins, Structures and Achievements* (Cambridge, MA, 1958). pp. 76–77.

21 Brackenbury, *Patient and Doctor*, p. 261.

22 Simon Gunn, 'Translating Bourdieu: Cultural Capital and the English Middle Class in Historical Perspective.' *British Journal of Sociology*, 56 (2005). p. 54.

23 Richard Titmuss, for example. For a comprehensive analysis of this issue, see Martin Gorsky, 'The British National Health Service, 1948–2008: A Review of the Historiography.' *Social History of Medicine*, 21 (3) (2008). pp. 437–460.

24 Francis Maylett Smith, *A G.P.'s Progress to the Black Country* (Hythe, Kent, 1984). p. 86.

25 Frank Honigsbaum, *Health, Happiness and Security: The Creation of the National Health Service* (London, 1989). p. 58.

26 *BMJ*, 3 July 1920, 'Report of Annual Representative Meeting', Supplement, p. 21.

27 Stephen Taylor, *Good General Practice* (Oxford, 1954). p. 446.

28 As noted in the Introduction and Chapter 4, the phrase coined by Pat Thane, *Foundations of the Welfare State* (2nd ed., London, 1996). p. 291.

29 See Peter Collin, Sabine Rudischhauser, and Pascale Gonod "Autorégulation régulée. Analyses historiques de structures de régulation hybrides = Regulierte Selbstregulierung. Historische Analysen hybrider Regelungsstrukturen." *Trivium. Revue franco-allemande de sciences humaines et sociales*, 21 (2016), available at http//journals. openedition.org/trivium/5245.

30 *BMA Archive*, B/177/2/1, BMA, *A General Medical Service for the Nation* (London, 1930). para. 30.

31 *Medical World,* 1 October 1926, G. Rome Hall, 'Improving the Medical Service.' p. 37.

32 Frank G. Layton, *The Little Doctor* (Edinburgh, 1933). p. 200.

33 *BMJ*, 7 April 1923 Supplement, p. 106.

34 *Lancet*, 4 July 1896, p. 40.

35 Watkins, *Medicine and Labour,* p. 19.

36 Herbert de Carle Woodcock, *The Doctor and the People* (London, 1912). p. 100.

37 Alfred Cox, *Among the Doctors* (London, c.1949). p. 197.

38 Woodcock, *The Doctor and the People*, p. 94.

39 *BMJ*, 30 September 1916, p. 477.

40 *YORLMC Archive,* minutes of meeting of Group C Regional committee of LMPCs on 10 March 1925.

41 *BMJ*, 5 August 1944, Supplement, p. 30.

42 Harry Eckstein, *Pressure Group Politics: The Case of the British Medical Association* (London, 1960). p. 72.
43 *Kent LMC Archive*, minutes of Kent LMPC meetings on 9 October and 6 November 1924 and 22 December 1927; John H. Marks, *The History and Development of Local Medical Committees, Their Conference, and Its Executive* (Edinburgh MD Thesis, 1974). pp. 139–140. Douglass W. Orr and Jean Walker Orr, *Health Insurance with Medical Care: The British Experience* (New York, 1938). p. 175.
44 Winifred Stamp, *Doctor Himself,* p. 110. Believed to have been said during one of Burke's Speeches on arrival at Bristol (1774), *Oxford Concise Dictionary of* Quotations (4th ed., Oxford, 2001). pp. 74, 17.
45 Eckstein, *The English Health Service*, p. 154.
46 Peter Bartrip, *Themselves Writ Large: The British Medical Association, 1832–1966* (London, 1996). p. 265.
47 Eckstein, *The English Health Service*, p. 155.
48 Charles Hill, *Both Sides of the Hill: The Memoirs of Charles Hill (Lord Hill of Luton)* (London, 1964). p. 98.
49 *Ibid.*, p. 60.
50 *Ibid.*, pp. 102–103.
51 Honigsbaum, *Health, Happiness and Security*, p. 216.
52 Bartrip, *Themselves Writ Large,* p. 266.
53 Eckstein, *Pressure Group Politics*, p. 96.
54 Anne Digby, 'Medicine and the English State 1901–1948,' in S. J. Green and R.C. Whiting (eds) *Boundaries of the State in Modern Britain, 1851–1951* (Cambridge, 1996). p. 217.
55 *BMJ,* 31 October 1931, 'Report of Annual Panel Conference', Supplement, p. 248.
56 *Medical World,* 26 November 1926, p. 224.
57 *Ibid.,* 8 October 1926, 'Grettir', p. 80.
58 *BMJ,* Editorial 22 March 1919, p. 349.
59 Norman R. Eder, *National Health Insurance and the Medical Profession in Britain, 1913–1939* (New York, 1982). p. 211.
60 John Marks, *The NHS: Beginning, Middle and End? The Autobiography of John Marks* (Oxford, 2008). p. 101.
61 See Paul Vaughan, *Doctors Commons: A Short History of the British Medical Association* (London, 1959). pp. 91–105.
62 Ipsos Mori, as quoted in John Eversley, *Continuity in a Changing World: 100 Years of GP Representative Bodies,* BMA (London, 2012). p. 18 (available at http//:www.gpdf.org.uk).
63 Turner, *Call the Doctor*, p. 311.
64 Charles Webster, *The National Health Service: A Political History* (2nd ed., Oxford, 2002). p. 27.

Epilogue

NHS GPs and the legacy
of medical professional protest

On the 'appointed day' in July 1948, family doctors across the UK found their surgeries full of new and existing patients anxious to avail themselves of whatever the new NHS had to offer. The first few weeks and months were frantically busy as the volume of demand for medical services was matched only by the volume of paperwork necessary to facilitate it.[1] One thing which became patently obvious from the start was that the fears expressed in the professional journals about the fate of private practice had proved justified. The middle classes might come to miss the genteel courtesies they had previously enjoyed as fee-paying clients, but they were quite prepared to forego these in order to escape ruinous bills for treatment.[2] GPs remained independent contractors, free, within contractual limits, to manage their time and workload as they saw fit and to take on other remunerative work outside general practice, but their contracts forbade them from charging their NHS patients for any treatment. The market for private general practice was dead and was never to be resuscitated. Moreover, as the NHS Chief Medical Officer, Sir George Godber, noted, most GPs were glad to be free at last of the necessity to chase up unpaid bills.[3] GPs now had effectively only one client and that was the NHS itself. The patient's free choice of doctor was guaranteed in the new system and never again became an issue, and fears that GPs might yet be forced into salaried employment never materialised. Neither, to the great regret of socialist doctors and others in the Labour movement, did the expected health centres. A handful were opened in the 1950s, but it was not until the late 1960s and 1970s that they were constructed in any significant numbers, and then somewhat shoddily. But by then, the availability of finance under the new cost rent scheme saw a great many more GP practices undertake their own successful surgery-building projects.[4]

GPs soon proved their worth as gatekeepers to secondary care and other services but the problem of resourcing the family doctor service itself adequately had not been solved by Spens and within two years of the appointed day, the threat of mass resignation by a demoralised GP workforce loomed once again. It was mitigated by the result of another independent pay inquiry, the Dankwaerts Award, in 1952, and the establishment in 1962 of a permanent independent pay

DOI: 10.4324/9781003438274-14

review mechanism (the Doctors and Dentists Pay Review Body).[5] But, as successive governments wrestled with the increasing costs of the NHS, costs which were not as great or as unjustified as critics averred, according to the Guillebaud report, GPs complained that their pay and status had declined in comparison with their Consultant colleagues and with other comparable professions.[6] It was not purely about how much income GPs took home after expenses, their leaders argued, but about the need for investment in ancillary staff, facilities, equipment, and postgraduate education. All of this was needed to arrest the decline in general practice observed in the studies by Collings, and Hadfield, in the 1950s.[7] This decline was still felt to be very much in evidence when the profession, threatening in earnest once again to resign en masse in 1965, set out their demands of the government in the *Family Doctors Charter*.[8] This proved the high water mark of negotiating success for GPs in the early history of the NHS and the resultant investment provided a spur to much needed improvements in the standard of service.[9]

While the 'professional social ideal' was not talked about explicitly, most GPs have continued to believe that what is good for the profession is good for patients. And they are not necessarily incorrect. Politicians have always been reluctant to concede that recognition and reward are intricately bound up with the quality of medical services. Maintaining standards has always depended to a considerable extent on having a sufficient number of motivated practitioners and a cadre of willing trainees ready to replace them. In periods when GPs felt demoralised, underpaid, and unsupported, increasing numbers left the profession, leaving those remaining even more overworked. This led to a downward spiral of lowered standards and declining morale as GPs were forced to cut corners in order to cope with unrelenting demand, and the newly trained opted for seemingly more lucrative careers in hospital medicine or the rewards of a less pressurised environment in other English-speaking countries.[10] The recruitment crisis accentuated the continuing problems of maldistribution of GPs which the best efforts of the Medical Practices Committee failed to eradicate, resulting in the persistence of what the respected socialist GP Julian Tudor Hart called 'the inverse care law'.[11] The void was filled to some extent by an influx of doctors from the Indian subcontinent and other commonwealth countries from the 1950s to the 1970s.[12] But, as successive governments failed to adopt constructive proposals from the BMA and the newly established Royal College of General Practitioners, the profession continued to be beset by cyclical recruitment crises. Eventually, the continuity of care which patients came to value most about the NHS GP service proved impossible to sustain. By the turn of the twenty-first century, the shortage of GPs led to increased substitution by nurses and other primary care workers and after several decades in which out of hours cover provided by deputising services and GP cooperatives had become the norm, professional leaders negotiated an end to the GPs' 24-hour commitment in the New Contract settlement of 2004.[13]

It no doubt seemed curious to historians and others that so soon after the profession's leaders had denounced Labour's plans for the NHS as being against the public interest and inimical to the 'essential freedoms' of the medical profession, doctors should have become its most passionate supporters and GPs the most vocal in defending it against its political opponents. It had been just the same with NHI. GPs complained long and hard about their situation within the service but never again questioned the values on which it was based. They also relished and made the most of the degree of involvement in administration of the family health services which Bevan had guaranteed them. With half the membership of the Executive Councils and their successors, the Family Practitioner Committees, GPs dominated the local administration of NHS primary care for the first 30 years of the NHS.[14] The Local Medical Committees continued the traditions established by their predecessors in the interwar period of ensuring that local administration of GP services operated without rancour or disruption while they simultaneously mobilised the profession in national pay campaigns involving repeated threats of mass resignation. In the 1980s, the successors to the IAC, the General Medical Services Committee, extolled the virtues of what it called 'the partnership principle', that is the partnership between GPs and administrators, during what one eminent GP academic curiously called 'the happy years' of general practice.[15] This proved short-lived as in the late 1980s and early 1990s the Thatcherite new broom swept away the structures accommodating those relationships and unleashed the full force of the new NHS internal market.[16] Responding to the Griffiths report recommendation of a move 'from administration to management', the Conservative Government abandoned its reliance on professional advice and ushered in a new era in which relations between GPs and NHS managers at the local level were characterised by a sense of 'them' and 'us'.[17] The extent to which the Conservatives had departed from the principles of negotiation was demonstrated by the imposition of a new contract on a reluctant profession in 1990. Some years later, Conservative and Labour governments sought to reframe this relationship when, in England at least, they endeavoured to make GPs instruments of transforming the NHS by ceding to them unprecedented control over budgets for patient care through fundholding and then GP commissioning.[18] They hoped to capitalise on the innovative instincts of GP entrepreneurs and their deep dissatisfaction with how resources were distributed between the different parts of the NHS. The devolved governments in the rest of the UK chose not to follow this experiment. While much of the politics of general practice has continued to be determined on a UK-wide basis, that decision was symptomatic of the growing divergence in the administration of health services, and health service policy, between the constituent nations of the UK.

The government's efforts to encourage patients to see themselves as 'consumers' of healthcare led to a demand for increased scrutiny of individual GPs' performance. However, it was the trial in the early 2000s of the GP serial killer, Harold Shipman, and subsequent public inquiry which provided the greatest stimulus to what became known as clinical governance.[19] This led to a series of legislative changes which culminated in a formal process of professional reaccreditation and revalidation.[20] Having forfeited the professional monopoly of control over standards of practice, today's GPs are much less clinically autonomous than their predecessors and, since the institution of the Care Quality Commission, the British medical profession is now, arguably, among the most heavily regulated and monitored in the world. The achievements of GP commissioning, however they are assessed, may have served to distract attention from the looming crisis in general practice itself. As so many GPs directed their energies to trying to reconstruct the NHS from top to bottom, their own practices were frequently neglected. Consequently, morale plummeted, recruitment fell, overworked GPs opted for part-time working to avoid burnout, and the worsening crisis meant that the, by now hackneyed, threat of mass resignation was once again invoked.[21] Such is the magnitude of the problems facing general practice in the third decade of the twenty-first century that independent contractor status is now considered officially under threat.[22] The provisions made in the 2004 contract allowing all practices to employ salaried GPs encouraged demographic changes which have resulted in 50% of NHS GPs now being salaried.[23] However, they are not, as the profession once feared, employees of local authorities, but of practice partnerships, or, increasingly, of commercial 'corporates', some of them part of international conglomerates, which, after years of failed attempts, are now beginning to make inroads into the UK healthcare market. Meanwhile, NHS planners, together with GPs still committed to commissioning and service redesign, are, in England at least, striving to undo the last remnants of the intersectional barriers which characterised Bevan's NHS 'command and control' structure in order to create an 'integrated care system' in which GP practices are organised in 'Primary Care Networks'.[24] If the advocates of this policy are to be believed, this initiative would bring both to patients and to practitioners many of the benefits of which Addison and Dawson once dreamed. But this is a claim which has been repeated in successive NHS reorganisations and is consequently viewed with scepticism by many in the profession. The lessons of history are rarely appreciated or understood by those holding the reins of power, and it is therefore doubtful if any of those leading current NHS changes are aware of the extent to which they are retracing the steps of their many predecessors or are in any way better equipped to overcome the obstacles they encountered. A careful consideration of this pre-NHS political history of GPs and of their subsequent progress throughout the 'long' twentieth century will, hopefully, prove instructive.

Notes

1 Geoffrey Rivett, *From Cradle to Grave: Fifty Years of the NHS* (2nd ed., 1998). p. 81.
2 Anne Digby, *The Evolution of British General Practice, 1848–1948* (Oxford, 1999). p. 334.
3 Charles Webster, *The National Health Service: A Political History* (2nd ed., Oxford, 2002). p. 24.

4 Phoebe Hall, 'The Development of Health Centres,' in Phoebe Hall et al. (eds) *Change, Choice and Conflict in Social Policy* (London, 1975). pp. 277–310.

5 Rivett, *From Cradle to Grave*, p. 89. Elston Grey-Turner and Frederick M. Sutherland, *History of the British Medical Association, vol.2 1932–1981* (London, 1982). pp. 150–152.

6 Rivett, *From Cradle to Grave*, pp. 112–115. Grey-Turner and Sutherland, *History of the British Medical Association*, p. 153.

7 J.S. (Joseph Silver) Collings, 'General Practice in England Today: A Reconnaissance.' *Lancet* (25 March 1950) 255, 6604, pp. 555–585. Stephen J. Hadfield, 'A Field Survey of General Practice, 1951–52.' *BMJ* (26 September 1953) 2, pp. 683–706.

8 Rivett, *From Cradle to Grave*, pp. 169–171.

9 *Ibid.*, pp. 171–172.

10 David Wright, Sasha Mullally, and Mary C. Cordukes, '"Worse Than Being Married": The Exodus of British Doctors from the National Health Service to Canada, 1955–1975.' *Journal of the History of Medicine and Allied Sciences*, 65 (4) (2010). pp. 546–575.

11 Julian Tudor Hart, 'The Inverse Care Law.' *Lancet* (27 February 1971) 297, 7696, pp. 405–412.

12 Julian M. Simpson, Aneez Esmail, Virender S. Kalra, and Stephanie J. Snow, 'Writing Migrants Back into NHS History: Addressing a 'Collective Amnesia' and Its Policy Implications.' *Journal of the Royal Society of Medicine* 103 (10) (2010). pp. 392–396.

13 NHS (General Medical Services Contracts) Regulations 2004, part 5, clause 17.

14 John Eversley, *Continuity in a Changing World: 100 Years of GP Representative Bodies* (London, 2012). p. 37 (available at www.gpdf.org.uk).

15 BMA (General Medical Services Committee), *GMSC 75th Anniversary Booklet* (London, 1988). p. 15. David Morrell, 'Introduction and Overview,' in Irvine Loudon, John Horder, and Charles Webster (eds) *General Practice Under the NHS, 1948–1997* (Oxford, 1998). pp. 12–15.

16 Webster, *The National Health Service: A Political History*, pp. 162–207.

17 *Ibid.*, pp. 167–174.

18 National Health Service and Community Care Act 1990. Department of Health White Paper, *The New NHS: Modern, Dependable*, 1997.

19 The Shipman Inquiry Reports 1–5 (2002–2005). www.gov.uk/government/organisations/shipman-inquiry. Sir Liam Donaldson, Department of Health Chief Medical Officer, *Supporting Doctors, Protecting Patients* (London, 1999).

20 www.england.nhs.uk/professional-standards/medical-revalidation/doctors/10-steps/

21 Matthew Limb, 'GPs Threaten Mass Resignation.' *BMJ*, 352 (6 February 2016). p. i646.

22 'GPC Commits to policy that PCNs pose existential threat to independent contractor status.' www.pulsetoday.co.uk/news. 23 May 2022.

23 Eversley, *Continuity in a Changing World*, p. 13.

24 NHS Long Term Plan (2018), chapter 5. www.longtermplan.nhs.uk.

Bibliography

Primary sources

Archives

British Medical Association

Medico Political Committee minutes, agenda and documents, 1908–1938, B/231/1–26
State Sickness Insurance Committee minutes, agenda and documents, 1910–1913, B/316/1–26
Insurance Acts Committee minutes, agenda and documents, 1913–1939, B/203/1/1–31
Insurance Acts Committee minutes, agenda and documents, 1942–1948, B/203/1/34–39.
Insurance Acts Committee archives and manuscripts 1918–1939, E/144/7–9
Central Medical War Committee minutes, agenda and documents 1915–1918, B/67/1–5 and 2.
General Medical Services Scheme Committee minutes agenda, and documents, 1929–1930 B/177/1/1
General Medical Services Committee minutes, agenda and documents, 1933–1934, B/178/1
General Practice Committee minutes, agenda and documents, 1938–1948, B/182-1/1–9
Miscellaneous: Conference of Medical Organisations 1919.
Non-Panel Committee minutes, agenda and documents 1913–1914, 1917, 1923–1924, B/151/1–5
Special Committee on 'Position arising out of the Coventry case' 1918–1919, B/158/1
Special Medical Services Scheme minutes, agenda and documents 1938–1939.
County of London Panel Committee minutes, agenda and documents, 1914–1939, LMC/1–13.
Joint BMA & TUC Committee on Medical Questions, minutes, agenda and documents 1938–1939, B/431/1–13

Wellcome Institute Library

Complaints, 1917–1950, SA/BMA/D.237 Box 180
Friendly Societies and Medical Aid Institutes, 1910–1947, SA/BMA/C.102 Box 54
Medical Women's Federation, 1917–1939, SA/MWF/C.78 Box 24
Medico-Political Union, 1918–1939 SA/BMA/A.48 Box 13

National Insurance Defence Trust Minutes, 1919–1933, SA/BMA/H.10 Box 258
Partnerships and Assistants, SA/BMA/C.522 Box 139.

University of Manchester, Central University Library

Manchester Medical Associations, Newspaper Cuttings, GB133MMC7/1/3, History of Associations, GB133MMC7/2/8; Manchester Ethical Association, Tariff of Medical Fees, GB133MMC7/2/4.

Manchester Medical Guild, Rules of Members Medical Pamphlets AI.13605; Rule Books, GB133MMC7/4/1; Annual Reports, B133MMC/7/4/2; 'Reports', GB133MMC/7/4/3; Provident Dispensary Report, GB133MMC/7/4/3/1; AGM, GB133MMC/7/4/3/2; Agenda for Conference.

GB133MMC/7/4/3/3; Official Report, GB133MMC/7/4/3/4; Correspondence with BMA, GB133MMC/7/3/5.

Medical Guild Quarterly, GB133MMC/7/4/6.

NMU, Press Cuttings, GB133MMC/7/18/1; NMU Minutes 1911–1913.

BMA Lancashire & Cheshire Branch GB133MMC/7/21.

Manchester Medico Ethical Society, Guide to Fees for Insurance Committees, GB133MMC/11/1/2.

Manchester Insurance Committee, Medical Benefits Sub-Committee, GB127.M40, 1912–1948.

Report on the Manchester Medical Service, GB133MMC/11/1/2/1; Circular re Cut in Remuneration, GB133MMC/11/1/3/4, 1934; Circular re Amended Terms of Service, GB133MMC/11/1/3/5, 1934; Discontinuation of Deductions, GB133MMC/11/1/3/7, 1935.

Manchester LMPC, Formation of Committee and Scope, GB133MMC/11/2/1, 1913+.

Circular to GPs re Panel Committee, GB133MMC/11/2/1/1, 1913+; Annual Accounts of Insurance.

Doctors, GB133MMC/11/2/1/2, 1913+; LMPC Accounts, GB133MMC/11/2/1/3, 1913+; LMPC.

Circulars, GB133MMC/11/2/2/2, 1925–1936; Memorandum on Methods of Payment.

GB133MMC/11/2/2/2/1,1925; Circular on Touting for Patients, GB133MMC/11/2/2/2/14, 1920s; Circular on Joint Committee of BMA and LMPC re District Medical Services, GB133MMC/11/2/2/2/17, 1936; Handbooks for Practitioners (1, 2 and 3), GB133MMC/11/2/2/3, 1930s; Newspaper Cuttings, Opposition to the Act, GB-133MMC/11/3/2, 1912+; District Service, GB133MMC/11/3/3, 1935.

Medical Guild Quarterly, 1898–1907.

Manchester Medical Review, 1908–1909.

University of Leicester, David Wilson Library

Leicester Royal Infirmary Maternity Hospital: Essay by F.A. Alexander, E1/1/3–5, 1960; Constitution of Leicester Public Medical Service, Objects of PMS, E1/1/6, 1912+.

Union of Medical Practitioners, Working Rules, E1/1/10, Rules including Reference to Registration as Trade Union, E1/1/30, 1912, GP Membership Form, E1/1/20, 1920s;

BMA Minutes of Conference of Representatives of PMS, GP12 1941/42, E1/2/13,1942; BMJ Supplement re Trade Union Law, E1/1/20, 1948.

National Archives, Public Records Office, Kew

Ministry of Health (NHI) Records:
Registered files series 1, 1912–1968.
MH 81/26, 1929–1930, Development of NHI/Medical certification.
MH 81/28, 1929–1930, Panel Conference resolutions.
Registered files series 2, 1912–1965.
MH62/44, 1921–1922, Amendment of Regulations, Terms of service.
MH 62/107, 1919–1962, Excessive prescribing.
MH 62/109, 1926–1927, Investigation arrangements.
MH 62/116, 1918, Doctors' Terms of Service, conferences with IAC.
MH 62/117, 1919, Doctors' Terms of Service, conferences with IAC.
MH 62/118, 1919–1920 Revisions to Medical Benefit Regulations.
MH 62/119, 1919, Terms and conditions of medical service.
MH 62/ 124, 1919, Discussion papers.
MH 62/125, 1917–1919, Special grant to Panel Practitioners.
MH 62/128, 1923–1924, Summary of negotiations.
MH 62/ 175, 1931–1935, National economy, reductions in remuneration.
MH 78/96, 1919–1920, Appointment of medical referees.
MH 79/7, 1918, War Office demand for Medical Practitioners.

Kent LMC, Maidstone

Kent County Medical Committee Minutes, 1912–1913.
Kent Panel Committee and LMPC Minutes 1914– 1939 and related documents.

Lancashire and Cumbria LMCs, Preston

Lancashire LMPC Minutes, 1914–1925.
Lancashire LMPC Minutes, 1928–1931 and related documents.

North Staffordshire LMC, Stoke-on-Trent

Staffordshire LMPC Minutes, 1914–1939 and related documents.

YOR LMC (North Yorkshire), Harrogate

Group D Standing Joint Committee of LMCs and Panel Committees Minutes, 1921–1923.
Group C Standing Joint Committee of LMCs, Minutes 1923–1939.
Local Medical & Panel Committee for County of Yorkshire (North Riding) Minutes, 1932–1936.

Cheshire County Public Records Office, Chester

County Palatine of Chester LMPC Minutes, 1914–1939, NHL 7135/1–10.

Nottinghamshire County Public Records Office, Nottingham

Notts County Insurance Committee Minutes, 1912–1939, SO.NHI.1–3.
Notts County Insurance Committee Medical Benefits Sub-Committee Minutes, 1913–1926, SO.NHI/10.
Notts LMPC Correspondence 1912+, D/1440/23/20–43.
Newark LMC Minute Book, 1911–1913 DD/1440/23/1.

Government Reports

Report of the Royal Commission into the Poor Laws and Relief of Distress 1905–1909. Cmd. 4499, 1909.
Report of Sir William Plender in Respect of Medical Attendance and Remuneration in Certain Towns 1912–1913. Cmd. 6305, (the Plender Report) 1913.
Interim Report to the Minister of Health by the Consultative Council on the Future Provision of Medical and Allied Services. Cmd. 693 (the Dawson Report) 1920.
Report of the Royal Commission on National Health Insurance. Cmd. 2596, 1926.
Report of the Inter-Departmental Committee on National Expenditure. Cmd. 3920 (the May Report) 1931.
Report on Social Insurance and Allied Services. Cmd. 6404 (the Beveridge Report) 1942.
Report of the Inter-Departmental Committee on the Remuneration of General Practitioners 1945–1946, Cmd. 6810 (the Spens Report) 1946.

Other reports

Report of an Investigation into the Economic Conditions of Contract Medical Practice, British Medical Association Medico-Political Committee (BMA Contract Practice Report) 1905.
Report into the Organisation of Medical Attendance on the Provident or Insurance Basis, British Medical Association Medico-Political Committee (BMA Public Medical Services Scheme Report) 1913.
A General Medical Service for the Nation, British Medical Association Report 1930.
A General Medical Service for the Nation, British Medical Association Report (amended) 1938.
Report on the British Health Services, Political and Economic Planning (the PEP Report) 1937.

Contemporary newspapers and periodicals 1880–1948 (selective use)

British Medical Journal
Daily Chronicle
Daily Express
Daily Mail
Daily Mirror

Daily Sketch
Daily Telegraph
Fortnightly Review
Lancet
Manchester Guardian
Manchester Medical Guild Quarterly
Medical World
Nation
National Insurance Gazette
National Medical Journal
New Statesman
The Economist
The Practitioner
The Spectator
The Star
The Times
Westminster Gazette

Biography and memoirs

Addison, Christopher, Viscount, *Politics from Within, vol. 1, 1911–1918* (London, 1924).
Allen, Bernard M., *Sir Robert Morant: A Great Public Servant* (London, 1934).
Barber, Gerald, *Country Doctor* (Woodbridge, Suffolk, 1974).
Brockway, (Archibald) Fenner, *Bermondsey Story: The Life of Alfred J. Salter* (London, 1949).
Bunbury, Sir Henry (ed.), *Lloyd George's Ambulance Wagon: The Memoirs of W. J. Braithwaite* (London, 1957).
Campbell, John, *Nye Bevan: A Biography* (London, 1987).
Cox, Alfred, *Among the Doctors* (London, c. 1949).
Cronin, A.J. (Archibald Joseph), *Adventures in Two Worlds* (London, 1952), Bello Edn. 2013.
Foot, Michael, *Aneurin Bevan, 1897–1960* (abridged edn, Brivati, Brian (ed.), London, 1977).
Gosse, Phillip, *An Apple a Day* (Bristol, 1948).
Harris, Jose, *William Beveridge: A Biography* (2nd ed., Oxford, 2003).
Lane, Kenneth, *Diary of a Medical Nobody* (London, 1983).
Marks, John, *The NHS: Beginning, Middle and End? The Autobiography of John Marks* (Oxford, 2008).
Morris-Jones, Sir Henry, *Doctor in the Whipps' Room* (London, 1955).
Mullin, James, *The Story of a Toiler's Life* (London, 1921), UCD edn, 2000.
Pemberton, John, *Will Pickles of Wensleydale* (London, 1970).
Pooler, Harry W., *My Life in General Practice* (London, 1948).
Ramsay, Mabel, *The Doctor's Zig-Zag Road* (Unpublished, 1953), Royal College of Physicians, London, Archive.
Smith, Francis Maylett, *The Surgery at Aberffrwd: Some Encounters of a Colliery Doctor Seventy Years Ago* (Hythe, Kent, 1981) and *A G.P.'s Progress to the Black Country* (Hythe, Kent, 1984).

Stamp, Winifred, *Doctor Himself: An Unorthodox Biography of Harry Roberts MD, 1871–1946* (London, 1949).
Watson, Francis, *Dawson of Penn: A Biography* (London, 1951).
Wilson, McNair, *The Beloved Physician: Sir James Mackenzie* (London, 1926).

Fiction

Brett-Young, Francis, My *Brother Jonathan* (London, 1928) and *Doctor Bradley Remembers* (London, 1938).
Conan-Doyle, Sir Arthur, *The Stark Munro Letters* (London, 1898).
Cronin, A.J. (Archibald Joseph), *The Citadel* (London, 1937). Vista edn., 1996.
Layton, Frank G., *The Old Doctor* (Birmingham, 1923) and *The Little Doctor* (Edinburgh, 1933).
McLaren, Ian, *A Doctor of the Old School* (London, 1898).
Shaw, George Bernard, *The Doctor's Dilemma* (London, 1906) Penguin edn., 1946.

Other primary sources

Anon ('A Panel Doctor'), *On the Panel: General Practice as a Career* (London, 1926).
Anon ('AGP'), *This Panel Business* (London, 1933).
Ashe, Isaac, *Medical Education and Medical Interests* (Dublin, 1868).
Brackenbury, Henry Britten, *Patient and Doctor* (London, 1935).
Brend, William A., *Health and the State* (London, 1917).
Briggs, I.G., *How to Start in General Practice* (London, 1928).
Booth, Charles, *Life and Labour of the People of London* (London, 1892).
Chiozza-Money, Sir Leo, *Insurance and Poverty* (London, 1912)
Comyns-Carr, Arthur Strettel, Stuart-Garnett, William Hubert, and Taylor, James Henry, *National Insurance* (London, 1912).
Currie, John Ronald, *The Mustering of Medical Service in Scotland 1914–1919* (Edinburgh, 1922).
Gibbon, Ioan Gwilym, *Medical Benefit: A Study of the Experience of Germany and Denmark* (London, 1912).
Hardy, Horatio Nelson, *The State of the Medical Profession in Great Britain and Ireland in 1900 (Carmichael Prize Essay)* (Dublin, 1900).
Harris, R.W. (Robert William), *National Health Insurance 1911–1946* (2nd ed., London, 1946).
Harris, Robert William, and Sack, Leonard Shoeten, *Medical Insurance Practice* (London, 1924).
Herbert, S. Mervyn, *Britain's Health* (London, 1939).
Newsholme, Sir Arthur, *Medicine and the State* (London, 1932).
Orr, Douglass W. and Orr, Jean Walker, *Health Insurance with Medical Care in Great Britain* (New York, 1938).
Rowntree, Seebohm, *Poverty: A Study of Town Life* (London, 1901).
Smiles, Samuel, *Self-Help* (London, 1859) OUP edn. 2002.
Sprigge, Samuel Squire, *Medicine and the Public* (London, 1905).

Webb, Beatrice, 'Special Supplement on Professional Associations' Part II, *The New Statesman*, IX (211) (21 April 1917). pp. 1–24.

Webb, Beatrice, and Webb, Sydney, *The State and the Doctor* (London, 1910).

Woodcock, Herbert De Carle, *The Doctor and the People* (London, 1912).

Secondary sources

Abel-Smith, Brian, *The Hospitals 1800–1948: A Study in Social Administration in England and Wales* (London, 1964).

Addison, Paul, *The Road to 1945* (London, 1975).

Alborn, Timothy, 'Senses of Belonging: The Politics of Working-Class Insurance in Britain 1880–1914.' *Journal of Modern History*, 73 (2001) pp. 561–602.

Armstrong, Barbara N., *The Health Insurance Doctor: His Role in Great Britain, Denmark, and France* (Princeton, NJ, 1939).

Armstrong, David, *Political Anatomy of the Body: Medical Knowledge in Britain in the Twentieth Century* (Cambridge, 1983).

Bartrip, Paul, *Themselves Writ Large: The British Medical Association 1832–1966* (London, 1996).

Bentley, Michael, 'Boundaries in Theoretical Language About the British State,' in Green S.J., and Whiting, R.C. (eds) *The Boundaries of the State in Modern Britain* (Cambridge, 1996).

Berlant, Jeffrey, *Profession and Monopoly* (Berkley, CA, 1975).

Berridge, Virginia, 'Health and Medicine,' in Thompson, F.M.L. (ed.) *Cambridge Social History of Medicine: Britain 1750–1940* (Cambridge, 1990) pp. 171–242.

Berridge, Virginia, Harrison, Mark and Weindling, Paul, 'The Impact of War and Depression 1918–1948,' in Charles Webster (ed.) *Caring for Health: History and Diversity* (3rd ed., Buckingham, 2001) p. 141.

Blanpain, Jan, *National Health Insurance and Health Resources: The European Experience* (Harvard, MA, 1978).

Bourdieu, Pierre, *Distinction: A Social Critique of the Judgment of Taste* (London, 1984).

Bourdieu, Pierre, 'The Social Space and the Genesis of Groups.' *Theory and Society*, 14 (6) (1985) pp. 723–744.

Bourdieu, Pierre, 'The Forms of Capital,' in H. Lauder, P. Brown, J-A. Dillabough and A. H. Halsey (eds) *Education, Globalisation and Social Change* (Oxford, 2006).

Brand, Jeanne C., *Doctors and the State: The British Medical Profession and Government Action in Public Health 1870–1912* (Baltimore, MD, 1965).

Bridgen, Paul, 'Voluntary Failure: The Middle Classes and the Nationalisation of British Voluntary Hospitals, 1900–1946,' in Harris, Bernard, and Bridgen Paul (eds) *Charity and Mutual Aid in Europe and North America Since 1800* (London, 2007).

Briggs, Asa, 'The Welfare State in Historical Perspective.' Archives *Européene de Sociologie*, 2 (1961) p. 22.

Bynum, William F., *Science and the Practice of Medicine in the Nineteenth Century* (Cambridge, 1994).

Carpenter, Niles H., 'The Literature of Guild Socialism.' *The Quarterly Journal of Economics*, 34 (4) (1920) pp. 763–776.

Cherry, Steven, *Medical Services and the Hospitals in Britain, 1860–1939* (Cambridge, 1996).

Cherry, Steven, 'Change and Continuity in the Cottage Hospitals circa 1859–1948: The Experience in East Anglia.' *Medical History* 36 (1992) pp. 271–289.

Cherry, Steven, 'Before the National Health Service: Financing the Voluntary Hospitals 1900–1939', *The Economic History Review* 50 (2) (1997) pp. 305–326.

Cherry, Steven, 'Medicine and Public Health, 1900–1939,' in Wrigley, Chris (ed.) *Companion to Early Twentieth-Century Britain* (London, 2003).

Clarke, Peter, *Hope and Glory: Britain 1900–2000* (2nd ed., London, 2004).

Clegg, Hugh A., *A History of British Trade Unionism since 1889*, vol.2 1911–1933, and vol. 3 1933–1939 (Oxford, 1994).

Coburn, David, 'Medical Dominance Then and Now: Critical Reflections.' *Health Sociology Review*, 15 (5) (2006) pp. 432–443.

Cockram, Joyce, 'The Federation and the British Medical Association.' *Journal of the Medical Women's Federation,* 49 (1967) pp. 76–78.

Collin, Peter, Rudischhauser, Sabine, and Gonod, Pascale, 'Autorégulation régulée. Analyses historiques de structures de régulation hybrides = Regulierte Selbstregulierung. Historische Analysen hybrider Regelungsstrukture.' *Trivium. Revue franco-allemande de sciences humaines et sociales*, 21 (2016). Available at http//journals.openedition.org/trivium/5245

Collings, J.S. (Joseph Silver) 'General Practice in England Today: A Reconnaissance.' *Lancet* (25 March 1950) 255, 6604, pp. 555–585.

Conybeare, Sir John, 'The Crisis of 1911–1913: Lloyd George and the Doctors', *Lancet,* 15 (May 1957) pp. 1032–1035.

Cook, Chris, *The Age of Alignment: Electoral Politics in Britain 1922–1929* (London, 1975).

Cooter, Roger, 'The Rise and Decline of the Medical Member: Doctors and Parliament in Edwardian and Interwar Britain.' *The Bulletin of the Society for the Social History of Medicine,* 78 (1) (2004) pp. 59–107.

Cordery, Simon, *British Friendly Societies 1750–1914* (Basingstoke, Hants 2003).

Corfield, Penelope, *Power and the Professions in Britain 1700–1850* (London, 1995).

Corsi, Cosma, 'The Political Economy of Inclusion: The Rise and Fall of the Workhouse System.' *Journal of the History of Economic Thought,* 39 (4) (2017) pp. 453–481.

Cox, Caroline and Mead, Adrianne (eds) *A Sociology of Medical Practice* (London, 1975).

Cronin, James E., *The Politics of State Expansion: War, State and Society in Twentieth Century Britain* (London, 1991).

Crowther, Margaret Anne, *The Workhouse System, 1934-1929: The History of an English Social Institution* (London, 1981).

Daunton, Martin, 'Payment and Participation: Welfare and State Formation in Britain 1900–1951.' *Past & Present,* 150 (1996) pp. 169–216.

Daunton, Martin, *Wealth and Welfare: An Economic and Social History of Britain 1851–1951* (Oxford, 2007).

Digby, Anne, *Making a Medical Living: Doctors and Patients in the English Market for Medicine 1720–1911* (Cambridge, 1994).

Digby, Anne, 'Medicine and the English State 1901–1948,' in Green, S. J., and Whiting, R. C. (eds) *The Boundaries of the State in Modern Britain* (Cambridge, 1996).

Digby, Anne, *The Evolution of British General Practice, 1850–1948* (Oxford, 1999).

Digby, Anne, 'The Economic and Medical Significance of the British National Health Insurance Act 1911', in Gorsky, Martin, and Sheard, Sally (eds) *Financing Medicine: The British Experience since 1750* (Abingdon, Oxon, 2006), Chapter 11.

Digby, Anne, and Bosanquet, Nick, 'Doctors and Patients in an Era of National Health Insurance and Private Practice 1913–1938.' *The Economic History Review*, 41 (1) (1988) pp. 74–94.

Dixon, Michael, and Sweeney, Keiran, *The Human Effect in Medicine: Theory, Research and Practice* (London, 2000).

Domin, Jean-Paul, 'Socialisation of Healthcare Demand and Development of the French Health System (1890–1938).' *Business History*, 61 (3) (2019) pp. 498–517.

Duman, Daniel, 'The Creation and Diffusion of a Professional Ideology in Nineteenth Century England.' *Sociological Review*, 27 (1979) pp. 113–138.

Earwicker, Ray, 'A Study of the BMA/TUC Joint Committee on Medical Questions 1935–1939.' *The Journal of Social Policy*, 8 (3) (1979) pp. 335–356.

Earwicker, Ray, 'Miners' Medical Services before the First World War: the South Wales Coalfield.' *Llafur (the Journal of the Society for the* Study *of Welsh Labour History)*, III (2) (1981) pp. 39–52.

Eckstein, Harry, *The English Health Service: its Origins, Structures and Achievements* (Cambridge MA, 1958).

Eckstein, Harry, *Pressure Group Politics: The Case of the British Medical Association* (London, 1960).

Eder, Norman R., *National Health Insurance and the Medical Profession in Britain 1913–1939* (New York, 1982).

Edgerton, David, *Warfare State: Britain, 1920–1970* (Cambridge, 2006).

Eley, Geoffrey, *Modern Germany vol. 2, 'Social Imperialism'* (New York, 1988).

Elliot, Phillip, *The Sociology of the Professions* (Basingstoke, Hants, 1972).

Emrys-Roberts, Meyrick, *The Cottage Hospitals* (Motcombe, Dorset, 1991).

Eversley, John, *Continuity in a Changing World: One Hundred Years of GP Representative Bodies* (BMA, London, 2012). (available at http://www.gpdf.org.uk)

Fairfield, Letitia, 'Women Doctors in the British Forces 1914–1918.' *Journal of the Medical Women's Federation*, 49 (1967) pp. 99–102.

Finlayson, Geoffrey, 'Moving Frontier: Voluntarism and the State in British Social Welfare, 1911–1949.' *Twentieth Century British History*, 1 (2) (1990) pp. 193–206.

Foucault, Michel, *The Birth of the Clinic: An Archaeology of Medical Perception*, trans Sheridan Smith, A.M. (New York, 1975).

Foucault, Michel, 'The Subject and Power.' *Critical Inquiry*, 8 (4) (1982) pp.777–795.

Foucault, Michel, *The Foucault Effect* (Chicago, IL, 1991).

Fox, Daniel M., *Health Policies, Health Politics: The British and American Experience, 1911–1965* (Princeton, NJ, 1986).

Fraser, Derek, *The Evolution of the Welfare State* (London, 1973).

Friedson, Elliot, 'Client Control and Medical Practice.' *American Journal of Sociology*, 65 (1960) pp. 374–382.

Friedson, Elliot, *The Profession of Medicine: A Study of the Sociology of Applied Knowledge* (1st ed., New York, 1970).

Giddens, Anthony, *The Consequences of Modernity* (Cambridge, 1990).

Gilbert, Bentley B., *The Evolution of National Insurance in Great Britain: The Origins of the Welfare State* (London, 1966).

Gilbert, Bentley B., *British Social Policy 1914–1939* (London, 1970).

Godber, Sir Charles, 'The Domesday Book of British Hospitals.' *Bulletin of the Society for the Social History of Medicine*, 32 (1983) pp. 4–12.

Gorsky, Martin, 'Friendly Society Health Insurance in Nineteenth Century England,' in Gorsky Martin, and Sheard, Sally (eds) *Financing Medicine: The British Experience since 1750* (Abingdon, Oxon, 2006a) Chapter 9.

Gorsky, Martin, 'The Gloucestershire Extension of Medical Services Scheme: An Experiment in the Integration of Health Services in Britain before the NHS.' *Medical History* 1 (2006b) pp. 499–512.

Gorsky, Martin, 'The British National Health Service 1948–2018: A Review of the Historiography.' *Social History of Medicine,* 21 (3) (2008) pp. 437–460.

Gorsky, Martin. 'The Political Economy of Health Care in the Nineteenth and Twentieth Centuries,' in Jackson, Mark (ed.) *The Oxford Handbook of the History of Medicine* (Oxford, 2011a).

Gorsky, Martin, 'Local Government Health Services in Interwar England: Problems of Quantification and Interpretation.' *Bulletin of History of Medicine*, 85 (2011b) pp. 384–412.

Gorsky, Martin, 'Local Government Health Services in Interwar England: Problems of Quantification and Interpretation.' *Bulletin of Medical History*, 85 (2011c) pp. 384–412.

Gorsky, Martin, 'Voluntarism in English Health and Welfare: Visions of History,' in Lucey, Donnacha Sean, and Crossman, Virginia (eds) *Healthcare in Ireland and Britain from 1850: Voluntary, Regional and Comparative Perspectives* (London, 2014).

Gorsky, Martin, Mohan, John, and Willis, Tim, 'Hospital Contributory Schemes and the NHS Debates 1937–1946: The Rejection of Social Insurance in the British Welfare State?' *Twentieth Century British History,* 16 (2) (2005) pp. 170–192.

Gosling, George Campbell, *Payment and Philanthropy in British Healthcare, 1918–1948* (Manchester, 2017).

Granshaw, Lindsay, "Fame and Fortune by Means of Bricks and Mortar': The Medical Profession and Specialist Hospitals in Britain 1800–1948,' in Granshaw, Lindsay and Porter, Roy (eds) *The Hospital in History* (London, 1989).

Green, David B., *Working-Class Patients and the Medical Establishment: Self-help in Britain from the Mid-Nineteenth Century to 1948* (Aldershot, Hants, 1985).

Green, David B., 'Medical Care in Britain Before the Welfare State.' *Critical Review,* 7 (4) (1993) pp. 479–495.

Grenfell, Michael (ed.), *Pierre Bourdieu: Key Concepts* (2nd ed., Abingdon, Oxon, 2012).

Grey-Turner, Elston, *History of the British Medical Association 1932–1972* (London, 1982).

Grigg, John, *Lloyd George: The People's Champion 1902–1911* (London, 1978).

Grigg, John, *Lloyd George: From Peace to War 1912–1916* (London, 1985).

Gunn, Simon, 'Translating Bourdieu: Cultural Capital and the English Middle Class in Historical Perspective.' *British Journal of Sociology*, 56 (2005) pp. 49–64.

Hadfield, Stephen J., 'A Field Survey of General Practice, 1951–52.' *BMJ*, vol.2 (26 September 1953). pp. 683–706.

Halevy, Elie, *History of the English People in the 19th Century. Vol.5, 'Imperialism and the Rise of Labour'* (London, 1961).

Hall, Phoebe, 'The Development of Health Centres,' in Hall, Phoebe, Land, Hilary, Parker, Roy and Webb, Adrian (eds) *Change, Choice and Conflict in Social Policy* (London, 1975).

Harris, Bernard, *Origins of the Welfare State* (Basingstoke, Hants, 2004).

Harris, Bernard, 'Social Policy by Other Means? Mutual Aid and the Origins of the Welfare State in Britain during the Nineteenth and Twentieth Centuries.' *Journal of Policy History*, 30 (2) (2018) pp. 202–235.

Harris, Bernard, Gorsky, Martin, Guntupalli, Aravinda Meera, and Hinde, Andrew, 'Long-Term Changes in Sickness and Health: Further Evidence from the Hampshire Friendly Society.' *Economic History Review*, 65 (2) (2012) pp. 719–745.

Harris, Jose, *Unemployment and Politics 1886–1914* (Oxford, 1972).

Harris, Jose, 'Political Thought and the Welfare State 1870–1940: An Intellectual Framework for British Social Policy.' *Past & Present*, 135 (1992) pp. 116–141.

Harris, Jose, *Private Lives, Public Spirit: Britain 1870–1914* (2nd ed., London, 1994).

Hart, Julian Tudor, 'The Inverse Care Law.' *Lancet* (27 February 1971), 297, pp. 405–412.

Hart, Julian Tudor, 'Going to the Doctor,' in Cooter, Roger, and Pickstone, John (eds) *Companion to Medicine in the Twentieth Century* (London, 2000).

Hart, Julian Tudor, 'Storming the Citadel: From Romantic Fiction to Effective Reality,' in Michael, Pamela, and Webster, Charles (eds) *Health and Society in Twentieth Century Wales* (Cardiff, 2006) pp. 208–215.

Hay, James R., *The Origins of the Liberal Government Reforms 1906–1914* (London, 1983).

Hayward, Rhodri, *The Transformation of the Psyche in British Primary Care* 1870–1970 (London, 2014).

Hennock, E.P. (Ernest Peter) 'Poverty and Social Theory in England: The Experience of the Eighteen Eighties.' *Social History* 1 (1) (1976) pp. 67–91.

Herzlich, Claudine, 'The Evolution of Relations between French Physicians and the State between 1880 and 1980.' *Sociology of Health and Illness* 4 (4) (1982) pp. 241–253.

Hill, Bradford Austin, 'The Doctor's Day and Pay.' *Journal of the Royal Statistical Society*, 114 (1) (1951) Series A (General) pp. 1–34.

Himmelfarb, Gertrude, *Poverty and Compassion: The Moral Imagination of the Late Victorians* (New York, 1992).

Holloway, S.W.F., 'Medical Education in England 1830–1858: A Sociological Analysis.' *History*, 49 (167) (1964).

Honigsbaum, Frank, *The Struggle for the Ministry of Health, 1914–1919* (London, 1970).

Honigsbaum, Frank, *The Division in British Medicine: A History of the Separation of General Practice from Hospital Care 1911–1968* (London, 1979).

Honigsbaum, Frank, 'The BMA/TUC Alliance and the Beveridge Report.' *Bulletin of the Society for the Social History of Medicine*, 32 (1983) pp. 18–19.

Honigsbaum, Frank, *Health, Happiness and Security: The Creation of the National Health Service* (London, 1989).

Honigsbaum, Frank, 'Christopher Addison: a Realist in Pursuit of Dreams,' in Porter, Dorothy and Roy (eds) *Doctors, Politics and Society: Historical Essays* (Amsterdam, 1993).

Horrobin, Gordon, 'Professional Mystery: The Maintenance of Charisma in General Medical Practice,' in Dingwall, Robert and Lewis, Paul (eds) *The Sociology of the Professions* (London, 1983).

Huerkamp, Claudia, 'The Making of the Modern Medical Profession 1800–1914: Prussian Doctors in the Nineteenth Century,' in Cocks, Geoffrey and Jarausch, Konrad H. (eds) *German Professions 1800–1950* (Oxford, 1990).

Inkster, Ian, 'Marginal Men: Aspects of the Social Role of the Medical Community in Sheffield 1790–1850,' in Woodward J. and Richards D. (eds) *Healthcare in Popular Medicine in Nineteenth century England: Essays in the Social History of Medicine* (London, 1977).

Jackson, Ben, *Equality and the British Left: A Study in Progressive Political Thought 1900–1964* (Manchester, 2007).

Jefferys, Kevin, 'British Politics and Social Policy During the Second World War.' *The Historical Journal* 30 (1) (1987) pp. 123–144.

Jenkinson, Jacqueline, *Scotland's Health, 1919–1948* (Bern, 2002).

Jenkinson, Jacqueline, 'A 'Crutch to Assist in Gaining an Honest Living': Dispensary Shopkeeping by Scottish General Practitioners and the Responses of the Medical Elite 1852–1911.' *The Bulletin of the Society for the Social History of Medicine*, 86 (1) (2012) pp. 1–36.

Jenkinson, Jacqueline, 'More 'Marginal Men': A Prosopography of Scottish Shopkeeping Doctors in the Late Nineteenth and Early Twentieth Centuries.' *Social History of Medicine*, 29 (1) (2016) pp. 89–111.

Jewson, Nicholas, 'Medical Knowledge and the Patronage System in Eighteenth-Century England.' *Sociology*, 8 (1974) pp. 369–385.

Johnson, Terence J., *The Professions and Power* (London, 1972).

Jones, Esyllt, 'Nothing Too Good for the People: Local Labour and London's Interwar Health Centre Movement.' *Social History of Medicine*, 25 (1) (2011) pp. 84–102.

Jones, Helen, *Health and Society in Twentieth Century Britain* (London, 1994).

Joyce, Patrick, *The State of Freedom: A Social History of the British State since 1800* (Cambridge, 2013).

Kent Local Medical Committee, *The History of Kent Local Medical Committee 1912–2012* (2nd ed., Harrietsham, Kent, 2012).

Kidd, Alan J., 'Historians or Polemicists? How the Webbs Wrote Their History of the English Poor Laws.' *Economic History Review*, 40 (3) (1987) pp. 400–417.

Kidd, Alan J., *State, Society and the Poor in Nineteenth Century England* (Basingstoke, Hants, 1999).

Kidd, Alan J., The 'Liberal State': Civil Society and Social Welfare in Nineteenth Century England.' *The Journal of Historical Sociology*, 15 (1) (2002) pp. 114–119.

King, Steven, 'Poverty, Medicine and the Workhouse,' in Reinarz, Jonathan, and Schwarz, Leonard (eds) *Medicine and the Workhouse* (Rochester, NJ, 2013).

Koven, Seth, and Michel, Sonya, 'Womanly Duties: Maternalist Policies and the Origins of the Welfare State in France, Germany, Great Britain and the United States, 1880–1920.' *American Historical Review*, 95 (4) (1990) pp. 1076–1108.

Lane, Joan, *A Social History of Medicine* (London, 2001).

Larkin, Gerald, *Occupational Monopoly and Modern Medicine* (London, 1983).

Lawrence, Christopher, *Medicine and the Making of Modern Britain, 1700–1920* (London, 1994).

Levene, Alysa, 'Between Less Eligibility and the NHS: The Changing Place of Poor Law Hospitals in England and Wales, 1929–39.' *Twentieth-Century British History*, 20 (3) (2009) pp. 322–345.

Levene, Alysa, Powell, Martin, and Stewart, John 'Patterns of Municipal Health Expenditure in Interwar England and Wales.' *Bulletin of the History of Medicine,* 78 (3) (2004) pp. 635–669.

Levene, Alysa, Powell, Martin, and Stewart, John, 'The Development of Municipal General Hospitals in English County Boroughs in the 1930s.' *Medical History,* 50 (2006) pp. 3–38.

Levy, Hermann, *National Health Insurance: A Critical Study* (Cambridge, 1944).

Lewis, Jane, *The Politics of Motherhood: Child and Maternal Welfare in England 1900–1939* (London, 1980).

Lewis, Jane, 'Providers, Consumers, the State and the Delivery of Healthcare Services in Twentieth Century Britain,' in Wear, A. (ed.) *Medicine and Society: Historical Essays* (Cambridge, 1993) pp. 317–345.

Lewis, Jane, and Brookes, Barbara, 'The Peckham Health Centre, 'PEP', and the concept of General Practice during the 1930s and 1940s.' *Medical History,* 27 (1983) pp. 307–350; 'A Reassessment of the Work of the Peckham Health Centre 1926–1951.' *Health and Society,* 61 (2) (1983) pp. 307–350.

Little, Ernest Muirhead, *History of the British Medical Association 1832–1932* (London, c. 1933).

Loudon, Irvine, *'The Concept of the Family Doctor.' Bulletin of the History of Medicine,* 58 (3) (1984) pp. 347–352.

Loudon, Irvine, *Medical Care and the General Practitioner, 1750 to 1850* (Oxford, 1986a).

Loudon, Irvine, 'Death in Childbed from the Eighteenth Century to 1935.' *Medical History,* 30 (1986b) pp. 1–41.

Loudon, Irvine, 'Midwives and the Control of Maternal Care,' in Marland, Hilary and Rafferty, Anne Marie (eds) *Midwives, Society and Childbirth: Debates and Controversies in the Modern Period* (London, 1997).

Loudon, Irvine, Horder, John, and Webster, Charles (eds), *General Practice Under the NHS, 1948–1997* (Oxford, 1998).

Lowe, Rodney, *The Welfare State in Britain Since 1945* (3rd ed., Basingstoke, 2005).

MacLaren, Atholl, 'Fifty Years On: How a Fledgling Health Service Proved Its Worth,' in Locke, Chris (ed.) *General Practitioners in Nottinghamshire, 1948–1998: A Health Service Record* (Nottingham, 1999).

Macleod, Roy M., 'The Frustration of State Medicine 1880–1899.' *Medical History,* 11 (1) (1967a) pp. 15–40.

MacLeod, Roy M., 'Law, Medicine and Public Opinion: The Resistance to Compulsory Health Legislation, 1870–1907', *Public Law* Summer (1967b) p. 211.

MacNicol, John, *Politics of Retirement in Britain 1878–1948* (Cambridge, 1998).

Maehle, Andreas-Holger, 'Beyond Professional Self-interest: Medical Ethics and the Disciplinary Function of the General Medical Council of the United Kingdom, 1858–1914.' *Social History of Medicine,* 33 (1) (2020) pp. 41–56.

Mann, Michael, *The Sources of Social Power (vol 2): The Rise of Classes and Nation States, 1790–1914* (2nd ed., Cambridge, 2012).

Marks, Lara, *Metropolitan Maternity: Maternal and Infant Welfare Services in Early Twentieth Century London* (Amsterdam, 1996).

Marland, Hilary, *Medicine and Society in Wakefield and Huddersfield, 1780–1870* (Cambridge, 1987).

Marland, Hilary, 'A Pioneer in Infant Welfare: The Huddersfield Scheme, 1903–1920.' *Social History of Medicine*, 6 (1) (1993) pp. 25–50.

Marland, Hilary and Rafferty, Anne Marie (eds) *Midwives, Society and Childbirth: Debates and Controversies in the Modern Period* (London, 1997).

Marshall, T.H. (Thomas Humphrey), 'The Recent History of Professionalism and Social Policy.' *Canadian Journal of Economics and Political Science*, 5 (3) (1939) reprinted in Marshall T.H., *Sociology at the Crossroads* (1963) pp. 150–170.

McDonald, Andrew, 'The Geddes Committee and the Formulation of Public Expenditure Policy, 1921–1922.' *The Historical Journal*, 32 (1989) pp. 643–674.

McKibbin, Ross, *The Ideologies of Class: Social Relations in Britain 1880–1950* (Oxford, 1990).

McKibbin, Ross, 'Politics and the Medical Hero: A.J. Cronin's 'The Citadel'.' *English Historical Review*, 123 (502) (2008) pp. 651–678.

McLarren-Caldwell, Janis, *Literature and Medicine in Nineteenth Century Britain* (Cambridge, 2004).

Morgan, Jane and Kenneth, *Portrait of a Progressive: The Political career of Christopher Viscount Addison* (Oxford, 1980).

Morgan, Kenneth O., *Consensus and Disunity: the Lloyd George Coalition Government, 1918–1922* (Oxford, 1978).

Morgan, Kenneth O., *Labour in Power, 1945–1951* (2nd ed., Oxford, 1987).

Morrell, David, 'Introduction and Overview,' in Loudon, Irvine, Horder, John and Webster, Charles (eds) *General Practice Under the NHS, 1948–1997* (Oxford, 1998).

Morrice, Andrew, "Strong Combination': The Edwardian BMA and Contract Practice,' in Gorsky, Martin, and Sheard, Sally (eds) *Financing Medicine: The British Experience since 1750* (Abingdon, Oxon, 2006) ch. 10.

Morris, A.D., 'Two Colliery Doctors; the Brothers Armstrong of Treorchy,' in Cule, John (ed.) *Wales and Medicine: An Historical Survey* (Llandysul, Ceredigion, 1975).

Mottram, John, 'State Control in Local Context: Public Health and Midwife Regulation in Manchester, 1900–1914,' in Marland, Hilary and Rafferty, Anne Marie (eds) *Midwives, Society and Childbirth: Debates and Controversies in the Modern Period* (London, 1997) pp. 136–139.

Negrine, Angela, 'Practitioners and Paupers: Medicine at the Leicester Union Workhouse, 1867–1905,' in Reinarz, Jonathan, and Schwarz, Leonard (eds) *Medicine and the Workhouse* (Rochester, NJ, 2013).

Neville, Julia, 'Explaining Local Authority Choices in Public Hospital Provision in the 1930s: A Public Policy Hypothesis.' *Medical History* 1, vi (2012) pp. 48–72.

O'Hara, Glenn, and Gosling, George Campbell, 'Healthcare as Nation-Building in the 20th Century: The case of the British National Health Service,' in Weindling, Paul (ed.) *Healthcare in Private and Public from the Early Modern Period to 2000* (Oxford, 2015).

Park, Robert E., 'Human Migration and the Marginal Man.' *American Journal of Sociology*, 33 (1927–1928) pp. 881–893.

Parry, Noel and Jose, *The Rise of the Medical Profession: A Study of Collective Social Mobility* (London, 1976).

Pater, John E., *The Making of the National Health Service* (London, 1981).

Pearson, Robert, and Williams, Geraint, *Political Thought and Public Policy in the Nineteenth Century: An Introduction* (London, 1984).

Pelling, H.M. (Henry Mathison), *Population, Politics and Society in Late Victorian Britain* (London, 1969).

Perkin, Harold, *The Rise of Professional Society: England since 1880* (2nd ed., Abingdon, 2002).

Peterson, M. Jeanne, *The Medical Profession in Mid-Victorian London* (London, 1978).

Peterson, M. Jeanne, 'Gentlemen and Medical Men: The Problem of Professional Recruitment.' *Bulletin of the Society for the Social History of Medicine*, 58 (4) (1984) pp. 457–473.

Pickstone, John, 'Production, Community and Consumption: The Political Economy of Twentieth Century Medicine,' in Cooter, Roger, and Pickstone, John (eds) *Companion to Medicine in the Twentieth Century* (London, 2000).

Pierson, Christopher, *Beyond the Welfare State? The New Political Economy of Welfare* (Cambridge, 1991).

Poovey, Mary, *Making a Social Body: British Cultural Formation 1830–1864* (Chicago, IL, 1995).

Porter, Dorothy and Porter, Roy, 'The Politics of Prevention: Anti-Vaccinationism and Public Health in Nineteenth Century England.' *Medical History*, 32 (1988) p. 231.

Porter, Roy, 'Lay Medical Knowledge in the Eighteenth Century: The Evidence of the Gentleman's Magazine.' *Medical History*, 29 (1985a) pp. 138–168.

Porter, Roy, 'The Patient's View: Doing History from Below.' *Theory and Society*, 14 (2) (1985b) pp. 175–198.

Powell, Martin, 'An Expanding Service: Municipal Acute Medicine in the 1930s.' *Twentieth-Century British History*, 8 (3) (1997) pp. 334–347.

Powell, Martin, 'Coasts and Coalfields: The Geographical Distribution of Doctors in England and Wales in the 1930s.' *Social History of Medicine*, 18 (2) (2005) pp. 245–263.

Poynter, F.N.L. (Frederick Noel Lawrence) (ed.), *Medicine and Science in the 1860s* (London, 1968).

Renwick, Chris, *Bread for All: The Origins of The Welfare State* (2nd ed., London, 2018).

Rew, Mabel, 'Looking Back', *Journal of the Medical Women's Federation*, 49 (1967) pp. 84–86.

Riley, James C., *Sick Not Dead: The Health of British Working Men During the Mortality Decline* (London, 1997).

Rimlinger, Gaston V., 'Welfare Policy and Economic Development: A Comparative Historical Perspective.' *Journal of Economic History*, 26 (1966) p. 566.

Rivett, Geoffrey, *From Cradle to Grave: Fifty Years of the NHS* (London, 1997).

Robinson, Paul (ed.), *The Foucault Reader; an Introduction to Foucault's Thought* (London, 1984).

Rose, Nikolas, 'Government, Authority and Expertise in Advanced Liberalism.' *Economy and Society*, 22 (3) (1993) p. 292.

Rose, Nikolas, and Miller, Peter, 'Power Beyond the State: Problematics of Government.' *The British Journal of Sociology*, 43 (2) (1992) pp. 173–205.

Routh, Guy, *Occupation and Pay in Great Britain* 1906–1979 (2nd ed., London, 1980).

Rubinstein, William D., 'Britain's Elites in the Interwar Period 1918–1939,' in Kidd, Alan, and Nichols, David (eds) *The Making of the British Middle Class? Studies of Regional and Cultural Diversity since the Eighteenth Century* (Stroud, Glos, 1998).

Rueschemeyer, Dietrich, 'Political Autonomy and the Social Control of Expertise' in Dingwall, Robert and Lewis, Paul (eds) *The Sociology of the Professions* (London, 1983).

Searle, Geoffrey R., *The Quest for National Efficiency: A Study in British Politics and National Thought 1899–1914* (Oxford, 1971).

Searle, Geoffrey R., *A New England? Peace and War 1886–1918* (Oxford, 2004).

Seaton, Andrew, 'Against the "Sacred Cow": NHS Opposition and the Fellowship for Freedom in Medicine, 1948–72.' *Twentieth Century British History*, 26 (3) (2015) pp. 424–449.

Sheard, Sally, 'The Roots of Regionalism: Municipal Medicine from the Local Government Board to the Dawson Report,' in Lucey, Donnacha Sean, and Crossman, Virginia (eds) *Healthcare in Ireland and Britain from 1850: Voluntary, Regional and Comparative Perspectives* (London, 2014).

Simpson, Julian M., Esmail, Aneez, Kalra, Virender S. and Snow, Stephanie J., 'Writing Migrants Back into NHS History: Addressing a 'Collective Amnesia' and Its Policy Implications.' *Journal of the Royal Society of Medicine*, 103 (10) (2010) pp. 392–396.

Smith, F. B. (Francis Barrymore), *The People's Health, 1830–1910* (Canberra, 1979).

Stacey, Margaret, *The Sociology of Health and Healing* (London, 1988).

Starr, Paul, *The Social Transformation of American Medicine: The Rise of a Sovereign Profession and a Vast Industry* (New York, 1982).

Stears, Marc, *Progressives, Pluralists and the Problems of the State: Ideologies of Reform in the United States and Britain 1909–1926* (Oxford, 2002).

Stears, Marc, 'Guild Socialism,' in Bevir, Mark (ed.) *Modern Pluralism: Anglo-American Debates since 1880* (Cambridge, 2012).

Stevens, Rosemary, *Medical Practice in Modern England: the Impact of Specialization and State Medicine* (New Haven, CT, 1935).

Stewart, A.B. (Alexander Bernard), 'Health Centres of Today.' *Lancet*, 16 March 1946, pp. 392–393.

Stewart, Clara, 'History of the Federation.' *Journal of the Medical Women's Federation*, 49 (1967) 70.

Stewart, John, 'Socialist Proposals for Health Reform in Interwar Britain: The Case of Somerville Hastings.' *Medical History*, 39 (1995) pp. 338–357.

Stewart, John, '"For a Healthy London": The Socialist Medical Association and the London County Council in the 1930s.' *Medical History*, 42 (1997) pp. 417–436.

Stewart, John, *The Battle for Health: A Political History of the Socialist Medical Association 1930–1951* (Abingdon, Oxon, 1999).

Swift, Paul, *Presidents of the Nottingham Medico Chirugical Society* (Grantham, Lincs, 2001).

Taylor, Arthur J., *Laissez-faire and State Intervention in 19th Century Britain* (London, 1972).

Taylor, Becky, Powell, Martin and Stewart, John, 'Central and Local Government and the Provision of Municipal Medicine, 1919–1939.' *English Historical Review*, 122 (2007) pp. 397–426.

Taylor, Stephen, *Good General Practice* (Oxford, 1954).

Thane, Pat, *Foundations of the Welfare State* (London, 1982).

Thompson, Steven, 'A Proletarian Public Sphere: Working-Class Provision of Medical Services in South Wales, 1900–1948,' in Borsay, Anne (ed) *Medicine in Wales, 1800–2000: Public Service or Private Commodity?* (Cardiff, 2003).

Thompson, Steven, 'Unemployment, Poverty and Women's Health in Interwar South Wales,' in Michael, Pamela, and Webster, Charles (eds) *Health and Society in Twentieth Century Wales* (Cardiff, 2006).

Thompson, Steven, 'The Mixed Economy of Care in the South Wales Coalfield, c.1850–1950,' in Lucey, Donnacha Sean, and Crossman, Virginia (eds) *Healthcare in Ireland and Britain from 1850: Voluntary, Regional and Comparative Perspectives* (London, 2014).

Titmuss, Richard M., *Essays on the Welfare State* (Boston, MA, 1969).

Trainor, Richard, 'Neither Metropolitan Nor Provincial: The Interwar Middle Class,' in Kidd, Alan, and Nichols, David (eds) *The Making of the British Middle Class? Studies of Regional and Cultural Diversity since the Eighteenth Century* (Stroud, Glos, 1998).

Turner, E.S. (Ernest Sackville), *Call the Doctor: A Social History of Medical Men* (London, 1958).

Turner, John, "Experts' and Interests: David Lloyd George and the Dilemmas of the Expanding State 1906–1919,' in MacLeod, Roy (ed.) *Government and Expertise: Specialists, Administrators and Professionals 1860–1919* (Cambridge, 1988).

Vaughan, Paul, *Doctors' Commons: A Short History of the British Medical Association* (London, 1959).

Vernon, James, *Modern Britain: 1750 to the Present* (Cambridge, 2017).

Waddington, Ivan, 'General Practitioners and Consultants in Early Nineteenth Century England,' in Woodward, J. and Richards, D. (eds) *Healthcare in Popular Medicine in Nineteenth century England: Essays in the Social History of Medicine* (London, 1977).

Waddington, Ivan, *The Medical Profession in the Industrial Revolution* (Dublin, 1984).

Waddington, Ivan, 'The Movement towards the Professionalisation of Medicine.' *British Medical Journal*, 301 (6754) (1990) pp. 688–690.

Waddington, Keir, 'Unsuitable Patients: The Debate Over Outpatient Admissions, the Medical Profession and the Late Victorian Hospitals.' *Medical History*, 42 (1998) pp. 26–46.

Watkins, Steve, *Medicine and Labour: The Politics of a Profession* (London, 1987).

Webster, Charles, 'Healthy or Hungry Thirties?' *History Workshop Journal,* 13 (1982) pp. 110–129.

Webster, Charles, 'General Practice under the Panel: The Last Phase.' *Bulletin of the Society for the Social History of Medicine*, 32 (1983) pp. 20–23.

Webster, Charles, *The Health Services Since the War, Volume 1, Problems of Healthcare: The National Health Service Before 1957* (London, 1988).

Webster, Charles, 'Conflict and Consensus: Explaining the British Health Service.' *Twentieth Century British History*, 1 (2) (1990a) pp. 115–151.

Webster, Charles, 'Doctors, Public Service and Profit: General Practitioners and the National Health Service.' *Transactions of the Royal Historical Society*, 40 (1990b) pp. 197–216.

Webster, Charles, 'The Metamorphosis of Dawson of Penn,' in Porter, Dorothy and Roy (eds) *Doctors, Politics and Society: Historical Essays* (Amsterdam, 1993).

Webster, Charles, 'The Politics of General Practice,' in Loudon, Irvine, Horder, John, and Webster, Charles (eds) *General Practice and the National Health Service 1948–1997* (Oxford, 1998).

Webster, Charles, 'Medicine and the Welfare State, 1930–1970,' in Cooter, Roger, and Pickstone, John (eds) *Companion to Medicine in the Twentieth Century* (London, 2000).

Webster, Charles, *The National Health Service: A Political History* (2nd ed., Oxford, 2002).

Webster, Charles, 'Devolution and the Health Service in Wales, 1919–1969,' in Michael, Pamela, and Webster, Charles (eds) *Health and Society in Twentieth Century Wales* (Cardiff, 2006).

Weindling, Paul, 'Health and Medicine in Interwar Europe,' in Cooter, Roger, and Pickstone, John (eds) *Companion to Medicine in the Twentieth Century* (London, 2000).

Welshman, John, 'The Medical Officer of Health: Watchdog or Lapdog?' *Journal of Public Health Medicine*, 19 (1997) pp. 443–450.

Welshman, John, *Municipal Medicine: Public Health in Twentieth Century Britain* (Oxford, 2000).

West, Michael, 'One Hundred Years of an Association of Physicians.' *Quarterly Journal of Medicine*, 100 (2007) pp. 151–183.

Whiteside, Noel, 'Central Control and the Approved Societies: Access to Social Support under the Interwar Health Insurance Scheme.' *Bulletin of the Society for the Social History of Medicine*, 32 (1983) pp. 16–19.

Whiteside, Noel, 'Counting the Cost: Sickness and Disability among Working People in an Era of Industrial Recession 1920–1939.' *The Economic History Review*, 40 (1987) pp. 228–246.

Whiteside, Noelle, 'Private Agencies for Public Purposes.' *Journal of Social History*, 12 (2) (1983) pp. 165–193.

Widgery, David, *Health in Danger: The Crisis in the National Health Service* (London, 1979).

Willis, Tim, 'The Bradford Municipal Hospital Experiment of 1920: The Emergence of the Mixed Economy in Hospital Provision in Interwar Britain,' in Gorsky, Martin and Sheard, Sally (eds) *Financing Medicine: The British Experience since 1750* (Abingdon, Oxon, 2006) pp. 130–144.

Winter, Jay M., *The Great War and the British People* (2nd ed., Basingstoke, Hants, 2003).

Wright, David, Mullally, Sacha and Cordukes, Mary C., '"Worse Than Being Married": The Exodus of British Doctors from the National Health Service to Canada, 1955–1975.' *Journal of the History of Medicine and Allied Sciences*, 65 (4) (2010) pp. 546–575.

Young, Linda, *Middle-Class Culture in the Nineteenth Century: America, Australia and Britain* (Basingstoke, Hants, 2003).

Youngson, A.J. (Alexander John), 'Medical Education in the Later Nineteenth Century: The Science Take-Over.' *Medical Education*, 23 (1989) pp. 480–491.

Unpublished documents

John H. Marks, *The History and Development of Local Medical Committees, Their Conference and Its Executive* (Edinburgh University MD Thesis 1974).

Websites

www.gmc-uk.org
www.gov.uk
www.gpdf.org.uk
www.hansard.parliament.uk
www.historymatters.group.shef.ac.uk
www.england.nhs.uk
www.longtermplan.nhs.uk
www.themdu.com
www.nhs.history.net
www.pulsetoday.co.uk
www.rcgp.org.uk

Index

For Product Safety Concerns and Information please contact our EU
representative GPSR@taylorandfrancis.com
Taylor & Francis Verlag GmbH, Kaufingerstraße 24, 80331 München, Germany